CLINICAL JUDGMENT

CLINICAL

JUDGMENT

ALVAN R. FEINSTEIN, M.D.

PROFESSOR OF MEDICINE AND EPIDEMIOLOGY,
YALE UNIVERSITY SCHOOL OF MEDICINE;

CHIEF, DIVISION OF CLINICAL BIOSTATISTICS,
WEST HAVEN VETERANS ADMINISTRATION HOSPITAL

ROBERT E. KRIEGER PUBLISHING COMPANY
HUNTINGTON, NEW YORK

ORIGINAL EDITION 1967
Reprint 1968, 69, 73, 74, 76

Printed and Published by
ROBERT E. KRIEGER PUBLISHING CO., INC.
BOX 542, HUNTINGTON, NEW YORK, 11743

©Copyright 1967 by
THE WILLIAMS & WILKINS COMPANY
Reprinted by arrangement

Library of Congress Catalog Card Number 67-19517
ISBN 0-88275-141-7

Printed in the United States of America

In memory of my father

In memory of my father

Contents

Contents

PROLOGUE: By Way of Background

Many people who have read this manuscript in its current or ancestral forms have suggested that I introduce the book by describing how some of its concepts came into being. The introduction would be optional—unnecessary for readers who regard any kind of preface as a nuisance, but available for those who may want to know more about a book's background either before or after they read it. Therefore, this prologue.

Medawar[1] has complained that scientific writing is often intellectually "fraudulent" because the careful organization given to the published material does not reflect the way things happened. Since few human ideas are truly original, a scientist's creative thoughts generally represent the conquest of his own ignorance. To get his mind through to a "liberating concept" that is often obvious to an untutored observer, the scientist may have to overcome many intellectual restrictions— the boundaries of his specialized focus, the incrustations of his previous training, and the fashions of his current pre-occupations.

After conquering his ignorance, the scientist presenting the "new" ideas in print may be reluctant to discuss how much ignorance he had to overcome. He may describe, in a pattern of gradual deduction, thoughts that came to him as sudden revelation or unexpected insight. He may omit many of the things he did initially, include others he did not do until much later, or sometimes put first what he thought of last. To provide orderly logic for his written exposition, he may thus shuffle and revise almost every item in his own mental sequence of "discovery". I have committed many such shufflings and revisions for this

1

book, and my effort in this prologue, for the sake of the record, is to recall the way things happened.

Some years ago, I became responsible for directing the clinical activities of an epidemiologic investigation comparing the effectiveness of new anti-streptococcal agents in preventing recurrent attacks of acute rheumatic fever.[2] The project's statistical procedures and laboratory methods had been excellently designed for the primary research goals of identifying streptococcal infections and evaluating prophylaxis. My job, in the clinical part of the project, was mainly to supervise the care of the patients and the collection of clinical data ancillary to the prophylaxis research.

It was a job for which I had had no special educational background beyond the advantages of undergraduate and graduate medical training at several excellent institutions. Not having had any intensive exposure in the laboratory technology of rheumatic fever, I concentrated on studying the patients of our clinic and in the associated hospital-convalescent home.

Soon after I began this new work, while making ward rounds one day, I heard a faint but unequivocal diastolic murmur along the left sternal border of a patient in whom no murmurs had been noted either by the resident physician of our hospital or by the physicians who had just referred the patient to us. After I demonstrated the murmur to our resident physician, he agreed that it was there and that he had failed to recognize it.

The correction of the resident's error was a simple event—part of the ordinary daily routine of clinical activities and training. Yet, as I later thought about the event, it assumed greater significance. Since the resident physician and I might have been the only two doctors who were going to listen to this patient's heart at our institution, the murmur would have been undetected had I not found it. The patient would have been discharged with the same diagnosis of "no heart disease" with which she had arrived. If the murmur persisted, it would probably be found at some later date by another auscultator. Since the murmur would never have been cited previously, however, the new auscultator might falsely conclude that it was new, and might then falsely conclude further that the murmur had arisen from insidious scarring of an aortic valve whose damage had previously been clinically imperceptible.

The insidious development of scarring in valves that initially seemed undamaged has long been regarded as a major pathogenetic mechanism in rheumatic heart disease. I began to wonder how many patients might have developed such "scarring" as a fallacy of clinical ausculta-tion. *De novo* rheumatic heart disease—absent on initial examination of a rheumatic patient and found in another examination some time later—might certainly occur by insidious scarring of a valve, but could also be "created" by two iatrogenic mechanisms: the abnormal mur-mur might have been present on both auscultatory examinations al-though undetected initially; or it might have been absent on both ex-aminations, but erroneously diagnosed as present on the second. The whole concept of insidious *de novo* rheumatic scarring seemed to de-pend on clinical auscultation of the heart, and yet auscultators could sometimes be wrong.[3, 4]

Moreover, I had no way of knowing how often *I* might be wrong. I could constantly check the resident staff, but no one was checking me. My auscultatory decisions could seldom be confirmed by direct anatomic inspection during necropsy or surgery, because very few of our patients died or needed operations. Moreover, the indirect evi-dence of angiocardiography and cardiac catheterization was seldom available, because most of our patients were not sick enough to justify these special diagnostic tests. My only way of routinely confirming my own conclusions, therefore, was the auscultatory opinion of consult-ant colleagues whose reliability I could not ascertain and had to ac-cept on faith. I could not even determine whether I was consistent in my own day-to-day auscultatory decisions, and whether I might be a "misser" or "maker" of significant murmurs.

For my own curiosity, I began to insist that auscultation on ward rounds and in our research clinic be performed before the examiner re-ceived any other information about the patient. Until completing auscultation, an examiner was not to know the results that others had found or that he himself might have noted in patients he had examined before. If the examiner disagreed with his colleagues or with himself, the discovery of his own discrepancies, or of theirs, would be enlighten-ing to all of us. Since cardiac size in rheumatic patients was another crucial diagnostic decision made by human observation and interpre-tation, we also began to examine X-ray films with this same type of initial objectivity. In developing these techniques, we had no conscious motives of innovation or of science; we just wanted to become more skillful in our clinical work. Any scientific advances emerging from our research project were presumably to come mainly from the laboratory part of the investigation.

In one sense, however, the clinical motivation was distinctly scientific. The basic decision for each patient in our investigation was the diagnosis of an attack of acute rheumatic fever. A patient had to have this diagnosis before we could admit him to the project, and a subsequent recurrent attack was the "endpoint" by which we measured the failure or success of prophylaxis. Although we could rely on laboratory tests for detecting streptococcal infections, we could not make the diagnosis of rheumatic fever from any single laboratory test or other objective procedure. To receive the rheumatic diagnosis, a patient must fulfill specific clinical criteria,[5] which demand that he have either arthritis, chorea, carditis, erythema marginatum, or subcutaneous nodules appearing in appropriate circumstances and combinations. The identification of each clinical entity that is a constituent of these criteria depends on a physician's subjective interpretation of visible, audible, or palpable clinical evidence. Our attempt to improve the examination procedures was therefore a scientific necessity for the main diagnostic decisions of our research.

In using the new "objective" techniques of examination, my colleagues and I soon began to discover many disagreements and inconsistencies. This discovery was not surprising, since all clinicians realize that human observers vary greatly in the way they perform and interpret their examinations. What was surprising and somewhat disturbing, however, was that we had been taught nothing in medical school or in subsequent training to prepare us for the existence of these variations, for dealing with them, or for anticipating the consequences they might have in clinical science. Throughout centuries of medical education, students have almost unquestioningly accepted the word of their teacher or "chief" as definitive, and neither he nor his students ever seemed to discuss the possibility that his latest word might not agree with his previous one, or with the word of "chiefs" elsewhere.

Although interpretations made by human observers are the main source of the basic data used in pathology, radiology, and clinical activities, the "science" transmitted in medical training usually omitted the problem of testing reliability and standardizing performance of the human examining "apparatus". Only in the past decade have medical investigators begun seriously to contemplate issues in "observer variability".[6] When our own work began, we had no idea that the concept had the name of "observer variability" and we were unaware of the few studies already performed elsewhere of variability in other aspects of clinical examination.

Our main concern, in fact, was not to investigate observer variability but to remove it as much as possible in the members of our staff. The approach was based on a systematic exploration of reasons for disagreements in the results of our examinations. Each examiner had to identify the specific features that made him reach such diagnostic conclusions as *normal, abnormal, enlarged,* or *mitral regurgitation.* We rejected such diagnostic explanations as "it just sounds (or looks) that way", and we insisted that the examiner specify all the acoustic or visual characteristics he had noted in making his decision.

As we "dissected" our interpretations in this manner, it soon became apparent that the main problems of observer variability were in neither the eyes nor the ears of the observers. We all saw and heard essentially the same things, but each observer used different ingredients in his criteria for description and interpretation of the observations. Some examiners had only a few ingredients in their criteria, while other examiners had many. For example, the loudness, transmission, pitch, and quality of an apical systolic murmur might be noted by both of two examiners, but one examiner might note nothing else about the murmur, while the other examiner might record such additional properties as the duration, site of maximal loudness, and variations in loudness with respiration and thoracic position.

The identification of observational elements in our criteria thus enabled us to recognize the many distinctive properties of cardiac noise that had to be specifically cited during auscultation. After we disciplined ourselves to cite all those properties, we discovered that everyone not only heard the same thing, but also usually described the same thing. With the additional descriptive observations available, we could then establish specific criteria for diagnostic interpretation, making provision for each of the different types of acoustic property we were observing. As we began to use the new criteria, many of our previous disagreements and inconsistencies in diagnosis became infrequent or vanished. Similar improvements occurred when analogous procedures were used for the interpretation of roentgenograms.

Concomitant with these techniques, we began to apply the "team" concept so prevalent in modern research. When a rheumatic patient is examined at monthly intervals by different individual examiners, his auscultatory diagnosis may change back and forth from "no heart disease" to various types of heart disease, according to the diagnostic criteria of each new examiner. To avoid such bizarre oscillations, we

insisted that a diagnosis not be changed until auscultation was performed objectively by a "team" of examiners whose consensus would
eliminate a single member's idiosyncrasies.

As a result of these procedures,[7, 8] our group became more reliable
in making the diagnosis of "carditis" and of other clinical features in
rheumatic fever. We still did not think of these activities as being particularly scientific. We did them because our job was to make diagnostic decisions, and it was easier to settle arguments with data and
specific criteria than with dogma and authoritarian decree.

As the improved diagnostic data became available, we then began
to use the clinical distinctions for other types of correlation. In those
correlations, the patients were classified into subgroups with either
"no carditis", "mild carditis", or "severe carditis". Each subgroup
also did or did not have the various non-cardiac manifestations of
rheumatic fever. When the prognosis, therapeutic results, and other
features of rheumatic fever were correlated for each of these clinical
subgroups, many previously confusing aspects of the disease became
clarified.

For each of the different subgroups, we became able to predict,
with considerable accuracy, the duration of the rheumatic attack,[9] the
likelihood of post-therapeutic "rebounds",[10] the persistence or disappearance of residual heart disease,[7, 11] the likelihood of rheumatic recurrences,[12] the cardiac effects of rheumatic recurrences,[12, 13] and the
reasons for many existing controversies in the evaluation of therapeutic
agents.[14] With this information, we could develop effective therapeutic
maneuvers for preventing "rebounds",[15] for removing the somatic and
psychologic debilitation of unnecessarily long bed rest, and for encouraging normal physical activities for patients without significant
cardiac impairment.[16] These decisions were beneficial to the patients,
and were based not on the intuitions of "clinical experience", but on
the analysis of quantified evidence. The results observed in the different clinical subgroups gave us numerical data to support the validity
of our choices in treatment.

We also found that at least three traditional concepts about pathogenetic mechanisms in rheumatic fever were probably incorrect:

1) Contrary to long-standing beliefs, patients *without* initial clinical evidence of carditis seldom developed "insidious valvular scarring" [11] and seldom developed valvular damage in rheumatic recurrences.[13] Some of the contrary evidence for the conventional beliefs
had probably come from auscultatory inconsistencies.

2) Patients treated "early" for rheumatic fever often had no residual heart disease, but the cardiac triumph was usually due neither to prompt treatment nor to the effectiveness of anti-inflammatory agents. In its pattern of clinical behavior, rheumatic fever tended to "lick at the joints and bite at the heart" and, conversely, to lick at or spare the heart when it bit the joints.[17] Because of this inverse clinical pattern, many patients with severe arthritis had no carditis, but sought treatment promptly after onset of the joint pain; patients with carditis but no joint pains seldom had symptoms severe enough to evoke early medical attention.[18]

3) The rebound phenomenon after discontinuation of steroid therapy was not caused by either prolonged or inadequately treated rheumatic activity. The rebounds, in all likelihood, represented the clinical appearance of the "accumulated" inflammatory stimulus whose overt expression had been previously suppressed by the anti-inflammatory treatment.[19]

Almost all the contrary beliefs and previous difficulties in analyzing many of these problems seemed to arise from the variability of clinical observation and from failure to classify the constituent patients in the spectrum of rheumatic fever. If these different subgroups of patients were all lumped together with a common diagnosis of "rheumatic fever", carditis might be abundant in the rheumatic patients of one medical center and infrequent in the patients of another. The manifestations, prognoses, and therapeutic outcomes of the rheumatic fever populations at these two centers would be quite different, but the reason for the difference might be unrecognized because all the distinctive subgroups had been combined as "rheumatic fever". Moreover, even if the two medical centers tried to divide their patients into distinct clinical subgroups, the results might still not agree because the basic observations were made with subtle but important discrepancies in the techniques of examination.

The improvement of clinical methods—in observation, in criteria, and in subgroup classification—had thus enabled us to clarify several problems that had bothered clinicians for many years. Among the contributions made by these different methods, the role of classification had been particularly important. Separating the diverse clinical spectrum of rheumatic fever into subgroups of patients with common properties had been a tactic of fundamental importance in our work. To illustrate the distinctions in classification, I began to draw some special diagrams. I used a circle to represent patients who all had a single common property (such as arthritis) and another, overlapping circle to represent patients with another property (such as carditis). The overlap of the circles would denote patients with both properties; the non-overlapping sectors would denote patients who had one property or the other but not both.

I began using such multi-circle diagrams in illustrations presented both in print[17, 20] and in lectures. Many physicians are accustomed to seeing drawings in which a single circle is "sliced", like a pie, into radial segments that show the proportional distribution or percentages of some total entity. The circles I drew were used in a quite different way: they contained no quantitative distinctions and the "partitions" were performed not by the radial lines of a "pie", but by the overlap of several other circles. Although the new circular diagrams were initially unfamiliar and looked peculiar, the concepts usually became clear after a few words of explanation and a few moments of thought. A colleague once asked me why I persisted in using circles for the diagrams. Why not triangles, hexagons, or some other shape? I replied at the time that I did not know why: the circles just appealed to me esthetically.

One day I had the thought that what we had done in improving our techniques of clinical observation and analysis might even be called *science*. We had made our basic observational data more reliable than before; by classifying the data appropriately, we had identified and enumerated situations that previously were unquantified; consequently, we had rectified several traditional conceptual errors and we had, in particular, increased the precision of our clinical predictions in prognosis and therapy. To be able to discern natural phenomena with predictable precision was surely one of the hallmarks of science, even though the work was purely clinical.

I then began to suspect that analogous improvements in clinical observation and classification might be equally illuminating for such non-rheumatic chronic disorders as coronary artery disease, diabetes mellitus, hypertension, and cancer. These diseases also have a diverse spectrum of clinical manifestations, and are also enmeshed in many controversies about natural history, prognosis, and therapy. Perhaps some of the many intellectual dissensions about these diseases were also attributable to observer variability, and to the lumping together of different subgroups of patients who, although joined by the same diagnostic name, should have been separated according to clinical distinctions that might have major biologic importance.

With these suspicions, I began to wonder about the identification of clinical subgroups in diseases other than rheumatic fever. There seemed to be certain clinical properties that could be noted in all patients with a particular disease, and that could be used to classify them regardless of what that disease was. After my adventures with rheumatic fever, I believed that one such clinical distinction was the mode of detection of a disease: whether it was found by "accident" or whether the patient had come to a doctor complaining of symptoms caused by that disease. Another distinction in classification might be the pattern of clinical features: the particular combination of signs and symptoms present in an individual patient. I wrote an editorial[21] to state these beliefs, and then began to give serious thought to developing a specific system for classifying clinical distinctions in human illness.

I soon stopped. The procedure was too complex and confusing. Too many different properties and variables were present simultaneously in too many different combinations. I could find no way to classify all the concomitant distinctions that had to be managed. Every time I thought I had a workable system, it always omitted a feature of major importance. I gave up the idea of a specific classification procedure, and resumed work on other things.

One evening, after showing some of my circular diagrams during a lecture on rheumatic fever, I was approached from the audience by a man* I had not seen for 15 years. We had been students together in several courses taken during graduate training that had given us both Master's degrees: his in physics, mine in mathematics. Neither of us knew that the other had later abandoned the physical sciences to enter medicine; he was now a radiologist and I an internist. After we exchanged greetings and reminiscences, he said, "I see that you're using Boolean algebra." For a moment, I did not know what he meant— and then the recognition came. Those overlapping circles: they were not just a fanciful whim in illustration. They were the type of Venn diagram devised to illustrate the "sets" studied in symbolic logic and in Boolean algebra. I had spent many hours with those mathematical topics during my graduate work before entering medical school, but, after years of thinking medical thoughts, I had completely forgotten about Venn's symbolism. When I started to draw clinical concepts, insisting on circles rather than other shapes, I had no conscious recollection of Venn diagrams, or of any other inherently mathematical relationships. I was illustrating clinical medicine, not mathematics.

* Dr. Harold Lehrer.

After savoring the surprise revelation that Venn diagrams had waited all those years to be evoked from my subconscious memory, I paid no further attention to them. I had just moved to a new academic job, conducive to studying spectral patterns in diseases other than rheumatic fever, and I was pre-occupied with trying to design ways of evaluating those patterns. Once again I began to think about the general theme of clinical classification. It was the unsolved crucial problem, the lock whose key I kept looking for and could not find.

On a pleasant spring night at about 1 A.M., I was ready to go to sleep after an evening of unsuccessful struggle with systems of classification. None of my approaches had worked. The problem was that every system of classification I had ever known in biology or in physical science was designed for mutually exclusive categories. A particular chemical element was sodium, potassium, or strontium, but not two of those, or all three. An animal might be either fish or fowl, not both. But a patient might have many different clinical properties simultaneously. I wanted to find mutually exclusive clinical categories for classifying patients, but I could not get the different categories separated. They all seemed to overlap, and I could find no consistent way to separate the overlap.

Just as I was about to fall asleep, I remembered the conversation a few months earlier about Boolean algebra and Venn diagrams. I suddenly saw a solution for the problem: I did not have to remove the overlap; I could preserve and classify it. Boolean algebra and Venn diagrams were a perfect intellectual mechanism for classifying overlap; they were an ideal way to distinguish multiple properties that could be present or absent, alone or in combination.

I returned to my desk, and, in less than half an hour, I completed construction of the classification system that had been so evasive. In broad outline, the system was applicable to any human disease, yet it made provision for the many clinical specificities distinctive to each individual disease. My old sense of mathematical esthetics was gratified, since the system represented the induction from particular observation to general formulation. More importantly, the system seemed clinically pertinent and valid.

To contemplate its clinical validity, I spent the next four hours wandering the streets of New Haven, thinking about every type of disease I could possibly recall, and checking that the clinical details of those diseases did indeed fit the classification system. During that review of diseases, I had the hunch that the new system ought to be particularly valuable for clarifying certain aspects of cancer, and I planned the design of research to test that hunch. I could find no important exceptions to the general validity of the system, and I had decided on the main course of my research for the next few years; I returned home exhausted, and fell asleep.

After some long and particularly difficult writing, I completed an account of the new taxonomic system for classifying the different clinical subgroups that constitute the diverse spectrum of a human disease. Without those classifications, clinicians had often analyzed each disease as though it were a single homogeneous fruit salad, rather than a mixture of heterogeneous fruits. Many of our misunderstandings and confusion about the biology of disease had arisen because different clinicians, seeing different mixtures of patients with the same disease, had been neglecting the clinical distinctions of the patients and referring only to the morphologic and other non-clinical characteristics of the disease. By distinguishing and analyzing the clinical components separately, we should be able to clarify many aspects of biologic behavior in human disease; we should be able to prognosticate more accurately and to evaluate therapy more effectively.

I wrote the paper with a delightful feeling of serendipity. During my days in graduate school as a mathematician, my wildest imagery had not conceived of the possibility that the abstract mathematics I was studying would ever have any kind of practical application. Now the abstract mathematics had an immediate clinical value; it could help bring science to many aspects of what had hitherto been regarded as medical artistry. I sent the finished paper for pre-publicational review to several friends who were also clinical investigators, and I awaited their enthusiastic response.

The paper (in that version) was never published. To my dismay, my academic colleagues showed little or no enthusiasm, although some other friends who were not clinical investigators—a medical statistician and several practicing clinicians—responded with enthusiasm and excitement. My main concern, however, was to rouse the clinical investigators who I thought would find the work particularly useful, but they seemed to have missed the point.

Where had I failed? The paper wasn't that badly written; I had even received some compliments on its lucidity. The mathematics wasn't that difficult to grasp; it had been understood by several readers with much less mathematical training than the investigators. And surely the clinical principles seemed clear enough. Yet my fellow clinical investigators, whose intellects and clinical judgment I greatly respected, had not perceived what I was saying. Why?

I struggled with that question for several weeks, trying to decide whether the problem was mine, theirs, or ours. I then realized that there were probably two reasons for the difficulty. The first was that my academic colleagues, although excellent clinicians, seldom made specific use of clinical data in their research analyses. Their investigations dealt mainly with mechanisms of disease, rather than with management of patients, and most of their research data came either from animals or from the results of patients' laboratory tests. Without the need to classify clinical symptoms and signs for specific analysis, these colleagues had seldom encountered such classifications as a challenge in research. Accordingly, they were not likely either to view the problem as important or to be stimulated by a proposed solution.

Another probable reason for the difficulty was that these particular colleagues, when working in bedside activities away from their laboratories, were superb clinicians with excellent clinical judgment. Performing the non-research service functions of clinical teaching and care, they already had their own good systems of clinical classification. Although each colleague might have used a different system that was non-reproducible or even undescribable, he had been using the system for years and had found that it worked reasonably well for his clinical judgments. A new system that required formal specification and organized categories for clinical distinctions might seem unnecessary and disconcerting.

This latter perception about my colleagues' clinical judgment gave me my first conscious "insight" into what the classification system really did. All good clinicians use a distinctly clinical type of reasoning, called *clinical judgment,* for making decisions about prognosis and therapy of patients. We often refer to a clinician's judgment as being good or bad according to the wisdom with which he makes those decisions. The reasoning in this type of clinical thinking is quite different from the deductive logic employed to establish diagnosis, etiology, or pathogenesis of a patient's disease. Clinical judgment depends not on a knowledge of causes, mechanisms, or names for disease, but on a knowledge of patients. The background of clinical judgment is clinical experience: the things clinicians have learned at the bedside in the care of sick people. In acquiring this experience, every clinician has to use some sort of intellectual mechanism for organizing and remembering his observations. I had inadvertently worked out a rational description for at least a part of this intellectual mechanism. The system of clinical classification was a coherent, logical technique for cataloging the information used as a basis for clinical judgment. With that realization, I then re-wrote and simplified my original paper on classification, emphasizing the value of Boolean algebra and clinical taxonomy in the clinical judgment with which doctors plan and appraise treatment. This new version of the work was the form in which it was first published.[22]

While all this was going on, I was intensively surveying the medical records of large numbers of patients with carcinoma of the lung, to test my earlier hunch about the value of the new classification system in cancer. My hunch was based on Ian MacDonald's hypothesis of "biologic predeterminism" [23] for cancer. He had suggested that many cancers detected in a state suitable for cure by surgical resection had been found "early" not because of prompt diagnosis but because the tumors grew slowly. The hypothesis was consistent with many clinical caprices of neoplasia, but had been difficult to prove because there was no good way of classifying the biologic behavior and rate of growth of a cancer in its human host. If MacDonald was right, the symptoms produced by a tumor should be an index of its behavior and rate of growth—and the new system of classification offered a way to categorize symptoms. Besides, we had already noted an analogous phenomenon in rheumatic fever:[18] the patients treated "early" had shown good results not because of the treatment but because the relatively "benign" cases were the ones detected most promptly.

Cancers could produce essentially three main types of symptoms: primary, systemic, and metastatic. In the course of nature and of clinical activities, patients with cancer would be impelled to seek medical attention for diverse reasons, and would be detected with various combinations of some, all, or none of these symptoms. As we classified the different "symptomatic stages", we could predict that the favorable slow-growing tumors (and the best survival rates) were most likely to occur in two specific symptomatic subgroups: the patients detected by accident while asymptomatic; and those who had a *long* duration of primary symptoms, without developing any systemic or metastatic symptoms.

This prediction was fulfilled by the results obtained in our study of lung cancer;[24] a subsequent study showed analogous data for cancer of the rectum.[25] MacDonald's hypothesis was correct, and we had found a way to prove it. The results completed a classical scientific cycle: the experiences with one disease, rheumatic fever, had led to the formulation of a general system of clinical classification. The general had then led back to the particular, with the system applied successfully in an entirely different disease—cancer. In cancer, as in rheumatic fever, the use of clinical taxonomy had clarified the biologic behavior of disease, and had improved the evaluation of prognosis and therapy.

Shortly thereafter, I had the last of the "insights" to be recorded here: a clinician performs an experiment every time he treats a patient. The experiment has purposes different from those of laboratory work, but the sequence and intellectual construction are the same: a plan, an execution, and an appraisal. Yet we had never been taught to give our ordinary clinical treatment the scientific "respect" accorded to a laboratory experiment. Treatment was supposed to be an "art", a humanistic application of established modes of therapy.

But what mode of therapy was "established"? The patient had to have confidence in his doctor's choices—but what choices would doctors really be confident about? Honest, dedicated clinicians today disagree on the treatment for almost every disease from the common cold to the metastatic cancer. Our experiments in treatment were acceptable by the standards of the community, but were not reproducible by the standards of science.

Clinical judgment was our method for designing and evaluating those experiments, but the method was unreproducible because we had been taught to call it "art", and to consign its intellectual aspects to some mystic realm of intuition that was "unworthy"of scientific attention because it was used for the practical everyday work of clinical care. Not recognizing ordinary treatment as an experiment, our medical teachers had taught us an experimental science of the laboratory—a science whose methods could not be satisfactory for studying the live human beings who were the "material" of our work at the bedside.

I began to contemplate the way we used scientific principles in the experiments performed during our daily clinical activities. Many defects were already apparent; others became evident with further thought. Methods of improving the defects also became apparent; I had even begun to use some of the improvements before recognizing that the procedure was a necessity of experimental science. The product of all that thinking was then organized into a logical arrangement, presented as a series of four articles, entitled "Scientific Methodology in Clinical Medicine". The series was published by the *Annals of Internal Medicine,* in four consecutive installments during September–December, 1964.[26] The gratifying response to those articles—in favorable comments from colleagues in all branches and specialties of clinical medicine—led to the plan for this book.

At first I thought the book would be easy to prepare. After the large amounts of time and effort spent in writing those four articles, I assumed that only minor editorial alterations would be necessary for aptly combining the articles into a collected unit of publication. When I began to write this book, however, I discovered with chagrin (and pleasure) that I had many new items to add. I wanted to include a few minor "new" ideas; to discuss many historical aspects of diagnostic classification that had not been covered in the previous work; to add some comments about computers, which I had begun to use in my own research;[27] and to revise some of the original writing in the hope of clarifying certain concepts that had been difficult for previous readers. Thus, Chapters 1, 5, 6, 7, 10, and 20 of this book contain entirely new material; Chapters 2, 4, 8, 9, 12, 14, 15, 16, and 21 have been expanded much beyond their analogous earlier contents; and many parts of other chapters have been augmented or revised.

The concepts discussed here may sometimes seem "philosophic", but every topic, term, and example is derived from practical clinical activities, and many of the illustrations come from problems I have studied myself. I have not attempted to survey every aspect of the selected issues, or to include the encyclopedic details of a traditional textbook; and I fear I may have omitted reference to many people with whose work I should be familiar but am not. Instead, as a clinician writing primarily for other clinicians and for medical students, I have tried to provide a background for further thought, and to establish a basis for restoring clinicians' self-respect and scientific pride in their own work. I trust that my fellow clinicians—sharing my sentiments and motives—will recognize that the adverse criticism of many traditional clinical procedures is accompanied by constructive suggestions of improvements. In those criticisms, I have tried, with undiminished respect for the past, to separate archaisms, sustained only by the hoary custom of intellectual inertia, from the old cherished clinical activities that are still valuable and as modern as tomorrow.

Each chapter in the book has been written as an essay that can stand alone, but the essays are interconnected and follow a definite order that is "rational" rather than "chronologic". Chronologically, in clinical work at the bedside, we first observe and then reason with the data. In the discussion here, I have reversed that order because I believe clinicians will not be motivated to improve the basic clinical observations until we first establish scientific procedures and purposes for what we do in reasoning with those observations.

Although much of the descriptive material in these essays can be read quickly, all of it follows a patterned argument of logic, and some of it contains new forms of mathematics. I make no apologies for having tried to simplify the "new" mathematics. It is merely an adjunct to clinical work, a means of illustrating the principal regions and landmarks of clinical topography. The mathematics has only the secondary role of providing lines and colors for the map; the main goal is the identification of different clinical terrains. Mathematics has no value in helping us understand nature unless we begin by understanding nature. To start with mathematical formulations and to alter nature so that it fits the assumptions is a procrustean *non sequitur* unfortunately all too prevalent in contemporary "science". What emerges is tenable and sometimes even elegant as mathematics, but is too distorted by its initial assumptions to be a valid representation of what goes on in nature. I therefore prefer to work from the inside out, rather than from outside in: as a clinician trying to find whatever mathematics fits clinical medicine, rather than as a mathematician pouring clinical phenomena into a preconceived mathematical mold.

I have tried to make the discussions of logic and mathematics as clear as I know how—but they are still logic and mathematics, and they cannot be read with the same rapid facility used for conventional descriptive articles in medicine or biology. Some of my friends have noted that an occasional difficulty in understanding the text disappeared once they began reading instead of racing, and that other problems in comprehension were clarified by re-reading an earlier chapter after a subsequent chapter had been completed.

I have already acknowledged[28] my gratitude to the many people whose encouragement and suggestions contributed to the original four articles from which this book evolves. I should now like to thank many institutions and people for various forms of help directly associated with this book.

Much of the data and many of the concepts presented here were developed during research activities supported at various times by Irvington House, by the West Haven Veterans Administration Hospital, and by specific project grants from the Division of Chronic Diseases of the United States Public Health Service, the National Heart Institute, the National Cancer Institute, the Connecticut Division of the American Cancer Society, and Fluid Research Funds of the Yale University School of Medicine. The editors of the *Annals of Internal Medicine* (Dr. J. Russell Elkinton), of the *New England Journal of Medicine* (Dr. Joseph Garland), and of *Nature* (Dr. John Maddox) have kindly permitted me to repeat portions of material that originally appeared in their journals.

Parts of the manuscript specifically prepared for this book have been improved by suggestions from many friends, some of whom also aided in the earlier articles. Although these friends should not be held responsible for either content or presentation, their help is gratefully acknowledged here: Drs. Paul B. Beeson, Harold O. Conn, Nelson A. Gelfman, Saul Jarcho, Mary F. Keohane, Lester S. King, Harold Lamport, Robert J. Levine, Stephen E. Malawista, Jennifer R. Niebyl, Jack L. Paradise, Robert G. Petersdorf, Jacques M. Quen, Walter H. Sheldon, Helen L. Smits, Lloyd G. Stevenson, and William A. Tisdale.

I should like to thank the colleagues who, as research associates or students, have contributed their talents to some of the recent investigation cited here: Helen L. Bidwell, Linda A. George, H. Teresa Hatch, Joyce A. Pritchett, and Carol R. Schimpff; and Drs. Edgar A. Hull, Neal Koss, and Harlan Spitz. The staff of the Historical Library of the Yale University School of Medicine, particularly Madeline E. Stanton and Elizabeth H. Thomson, have graciously and patiently guided me to the treasures of medical thought that unite us today with our predecessors of the world of the past. The staff of the Yale University Computer Center, particularly Professor Robert F. Rosin, have, with equal grace and patience, introduced me to thoughts for the world of the future. My free-hand drawings have been capably converted into illustrations by Mrs. Virginia Simon, and my long-hand into typescript by Mrs. Lorraine MacI. Phillips, Mrs. Evelyn R. Fogarasi, and Miss Elizabeth Tartagni. Several critical problems in esthetics were solved with the perceptive help of Sam Feinstein and Thorpe Feidt.

Finally, anyone who tries to retreat into thinking with dispassionate intellect must be sustained by human warmth. I know no words to express adequate thanks to the family, friends, and colleagues whose affection provides that sustenance.

PART I

The Clinician's Challenge in Experimental Science

1. Clinical Judgment and the Experiments of Clinical Therapy

Despite many revolutionary changes in the technology, concepts, and practice of medicine during the past half century, there remains a single common title to distinguish a doctor who treats sick people: he is a clinician. The clinician may be a family physician or a consultant, a general practitioner or a specialist. His professional work may be only with patients, or he may also devote time to teaching, research, or other medical activities. Regardless of whatever else a doctor is or does, he acts as a clinician when he performs the traditional medical function of treating a patient.

A clinician need not be the only doctor who contributes to a patient's welfare. Biochemists, microbiologists, radiologists, and pathologists may help in diagnosis. Pharmacologists, epidemiologists, and geneticists may give background information about new drugs, vaccines, or familial diseases. But the clinician provides treatment. The word *clinician* comes from the Greek κλινικος, which means *bed;* and the word *patient* comes from the Latin *pati*, which means *to suffer*. The clinician is the doctor at the sufferer's bedside, the doctor who accepts responsibility for the life entrusted to him by the patient, the doctor who plans the strategy and executes the tactics of therapeutic care.

In caring for patients, clinicians constantly perform experiments. During a single week of active practice, a busy clinician conducts more experiments than most of his laboratory colleagues do in a year. Although clinicians do not usually regard ordinary patient care as a type

21

of experiment, every aspect of clinical management can be designed, executed, and appraised with intellectual procedures identical to those used in any experimental situation. The experiments of bedside and laboratory differ fundamentally not in their basic intellectual construction, but in their materials and modes of inception.

In laboratory work, the experimental material is an intact animal, a part of a person or of an animal, or an inanimate system; in clinical treatment, the material is an intact human being. In laboratory work, the investigator initiates the experiment at a time of his own convenience, and chooses his material without regard to its desire or consent for participation. In clinical treatment, the material initiates the experiment, which begins when a patient decides to seek medical aid, thereby volunteering as a subject for therapy and choosing the time, place, and clinician who will serve as investigator.

The patient's goal in seeking medical attention creates two other major differences—in motives and premises—between laboratory and clinical experiments. In laboratory work, the usual motive is inquiring: to gain a new understanding of some mechanism of nature. In clinical treatment, the main motives are remedial or prophylactic: to change what nature has done or to prevent what it may do. In laboratory work, the premise is innovative: the goal is to test a new hypothesis or a new procedure. In ordinary clinical treatment, the premise is repetitive: the goal is to reproduce (or surpass) the best results of experiments conducted before in similar circumstances. A clinician chooses treatment in a new situation by reviewing what was done and what happened in previous situations that resembled the one at hand; he then selects whatever mode of treatment had the most successful outcome in the past.

The concept that a clinician performs experiments in his routine therapeutic activities is entirely consistent with the definition offered by Claude Bernard,[29] who is often regarded as a founder of experimental discipline in medicine. Said Bernard, "We give the name experimenter to the man who applies methods of investigation, whether simple or complex, so as to make natural phenomena vary, or so as to alter them with some purpose or other. . . ." In establishing this definition, Bernard was interested mainly in the physiologist's search for understanding mechanisms of disease, but the definition clearly fits the clinician's work in therapeutic management.

Not all experiments performed on patients have the remedial motives and repetitive premises of ordinary therapy. To learn new facts about human illness, or to test new therapeutic agents, clinicians may perform other types of experiments with people who are sick or healthy. If the experiment is planned to learn new facts about physiology, biochemistry, pathogenesis, symptoms, signs, or human behavior, the motives are inquiring rather than remedial or prophylactic. If a new therapeutic procedure is untried or untested, the clinician has no previous experiences from which to make a repetitive experimental hypothesis. Without any past results, he must develop new premises based on the immediate rather than previous circumstances.

These inquiring, innovating investigations are the activities customarily regarded as clinical experiments. The ethics of such experiments have become an active concern not only of clinicians, but also of philosophers, lawyers, and other students of human morality.[30-32] In the experiments of ordinary clinical treatment, however, the purpose is not to gain new knowledge but to repeat a success of the past. The morality of these conventional experiments is seldom questioned, either because they are not regarded as "experiments", or because their procedures are accepted as well-established and repeatable. Although man is used as an object of experiment in both innovative and conventional therapy, the modern clinician's virtue is generally prodded only to justify the new, not to validate the old.

Yet many aspects of conventional contemporary therapy are neither repeatable, validated, nor universally regarded as well-established.[33] Radical surgery and irradiation therapy in cancer, for example, have both been available for more than 60 years, but their therapeutic contributions in many neoplasms remain obscure and controversial.[34] Although anticoagulants, antibiotics, hypotensive agents, insulin, and steroids have been available for 15 to 40 years, many of their true effects on patients and diseases are unknown or equivocal. Clinicians are still uncertain about the best means of treatment for even such routine problems as a common cold, a sprained back, a fractured hip, a peptic ulcer, a stroke, a myocardial infarction, an obstetrical delivery, or an acute psychiatric depression.

For all of these, and for many other standard problems of ordinary clinical treatment, contemporary clinicians constantly perform experiments that lack the scientific qualities of valid evidence, logical analyses, and demonstrable proofs. In an era of calculators and computers, many prognoses are made as vague statistical generalities that are often individually inapplicable and erroneous. At a time of potent drugs and formidable surgery, the exact effects of many therapeutic procedures are dubious and shrouded in dissension—often documented either by the unquantified data of "experience" or by grandiose statistics whose mathematical formulations are so clinically naive that any significance is purely numerical rather than biologic. In the words of Norbert Wiener,[35]

> The average paper which appears in our medical journals is characterized by a childishness in statistical techniques which is simply ridiculous and inexcusable. A new disease is first recognized in those cases in which it is fatal or at least seriously disabling. It is thus given a high rate of mortality. Later on, improved techniques of diagnosis identify the same pathologic process at a much earlier stage. It is found that most of these newly identified cases are relatively mild and the mortality rate drops sharply. "Aha," says the author of a paper, "see how effective my therapeutic measures have been!"

This lamentable state of science in clinical therapy is generally accepted impassively by both the lay and the medical public. The layman—impressed by the magnificent equipment, expensive research, and well-publicized activities of modern medical centers—believes that therapeutic science must be making major "breakthroughs" in its intellectual problems. The medical public—more cognizant of the clinician's unsolved basic problems in therapy—often assumes that the problems are either too complex for scientific solution or unworthy of scientific investigation. These assumptions about the scientific complexity and value of clinical therapy have become fundamental issues in modern medicine.

THE COMPLEXITY OF HUMAN DATA AND REASONING

For each patient who undergoes treatment, a clinician observes at least three different types of data. The first type of data describes a *disease* in morphologic, chemical, microbiologic, physiologic, or other impersonal terms. The second type of data describes the *host* in whom the disease occurs. This description of the host's environmental background includes both the personal properties of the host before the disease began (such as age, race, sex, and education) and also the properties of the host's external surroundings (such as geographic location, occupation, and financial and social status). The third type of data describes the *illness* that occurs in the interaction between the disease and its environmental host. The illness consists of clinical phenomena: the host's subjective sensations, which are called "symptoms", and certain findings, called "signs", which are discerned objectively during the physical examination of the diseased host. When the diseased host seeks medical attention, he becomes a patient, and the clinician's work begins.

The clinician uses these three types of data to make decisions about the present, past, and future of the patient. The decisions consist of determining a present diagnosis (which gives the disease a name and tells what is wrong), a past etiology and pathogenesis (or how it got that way), and a future prognosis and therapy (or what to do about it). Of these various decisions, only the choice of prognosis and therapy is distinctively clinical. Diagnosis, etiology, and pathogenesis of disease can often be discerned effectively by non-clinical doctors, remote from the bedside. The clinician, however, must examine the patient to make effective decisions about treatment.

The data that describe the disease can often be obtained by examining the patient's fluids, cells, tissues, excreta, roentgenograms, graphic tracings, and other derivative substances. The patient's personal environmental data can often be elicited by nurses, secretaries, social workers, or other interviewers with little or no clinical training. The clinical symptoms and signs of the patient's illness, however, are determined only by a doctor skilled in the clinical procedures of history-taking and physical examination.

In using all these data for planning treatment, the clinician's reasoning can broadly be divided into two categories: therapeutic and environmental. The therapeutic decision deals with the mode of treatment: a choice of diet, drugs, surgery, radiotherapy, physiotherapy, psychotherapy, combinations of these and other agents, or no specific agent of treatment. The environmental decision deals with the management of the host: a choice of methods of communication, accommodation, and human interchange that will best enable the sick host to bear the burdens of both ailment and treatment. The therapeutic decision answers the question, "What is the best treatment for this particular ailment?" The environmental decision answers the question, "How should that treatment be managed or modified for this particular person?" In the reasoning of therapeutic decision, the patient is a case—a representative instance of disease and illness—for which treatment is chosen after comparison with results obtained in similar previous cases. In the reasoning of environmental decision, the patient is a unique person for whom each aspect of management must be individualized.

For example, after getting a biopsy report that the lump in a patient's breast is a cancer, the clinician's therapeutic decision is whether to remove the lump alone; the breast alone; the breast and part of the chest wall; or the breast, chest wall, and various chains of lymph nodes; and whether to give radiotherapy or chemotherapy (or both) before the operation, after the operation, or instead. After choosing treatment for this particular instance of breast cancer, the clinician's environmental decision then determines the way he explains the diagnosis and therapeutic plans to the patient, and the way he helps her adapt to the subsequent personal, social, psychic, and other consequences.

A clinician's privilege and power in clinical therapy is his ability to make both the therapeutic and the environmental decisions concomitantly. The clinician combines treatment for the patient, as a personal case of disease, with concern for the patient, as a personal instance of mankind, into the unified mixture that is clinical care. The process of observation and reasoning used for these decisions is as diverse as the intricacies of human thought, and is performed differently by each clinician. Because so many different types of data are involved, because so many elements of the data are difficult to specify, and because clinicians and patients are so diverse, the process is usually regarded as an art-like, sometimes mystical, often intuitive procedure, which seldom merits and seldom fulfills the intellectual demands of scientific thought.

When a laboratory investigator makes decisions in conducting an experiment, we require that the ingredients of his reasoning be explicitly defined. We insist that he be able to specify his methods, his data, and his interpretations of the data, and that the specifications be precise and reproducible. When a clinician makes decisions in the experiments of therapy, we generally assume that the procedure is too complex for scientific documentation. The clinician is usually permitted to justify his work on the basis of "hunch", intuition, or a nebulously defined previous "clinical experience". His decisions are allowed a rationale that need not be overtly rational, and reasons that need not be particularly reasonable. If the clinician seems knowledgeable and authoritative, and if his reputation and results seem good, he can be condoned the most flagrant imprecisions, vagueness, and inconsistency in his conduct of therapy. The clinician does not even use a scientific name for his method of designing, executing, and appraising therapeutic experiments. He calls it *clinical judgment.*

THE INTELLECTUAL WORTHINESS OF CLINICAL THERAPY

Among the many ideas subjected to scientific investigation, the *idea* of clinical treatment may not appeal to a scientist concerned mainly with discovering new basic truths about nature. Even if he acknowledges conventional treatment as an experiment, the "basic scientist" may not deem it a worthy scientific challenge because the experiments of routine therapy seldom have innovating premises and purely inquiring motives.

To a clinician, however, the idea of treatment is not merely important; it is paramount. The care of a patient is the ultimate, specific act that characterizes a clinician. It differentiates him from all other medical doctors, biologists, and students of human illness. Its obligation is transmitted as the heritage of his profession. Its performance is his unique contribution to the multifarious services exchanged by mankind to sustain human civilization and life. If treatment is an unimportant experiment, a clinician has no useful purpose for his medical existence.

Nevertheless, the basic intellectual problems of treatment receive comparatively little attention in contemporary clinical research. The clinicians of modern academic medical centers have become increasingly concerned with laboratory investigation of pathogenesis of disease or mechanisms of cellular biology. The problems of clinical therapy are often dismissed as a mere application of the "basic science" studied in the clinical investigator's laboratory. Behind this dismissal is the traditional belief that the therapeutic aspects of medicine can never be a "science" and that clinical judgment can never be "scientific".

*   *   *

The purpose of these essays is to revise that traditional belief. There is surely no inherent sanctity or immunity in clinical judgment to spare it from receiving the critical examination of basic principles that has been given to all other aspects of clinical medicine during the past few decades. With the development of new technologic advances, clinicians have re-evaluated and altered their methods of gathering many types of data, making diagnoses, and delivering treatment. The alterations have created or improved the medical science produced in such places as the laboratory, the X-ray suite, the pharmacy, and the operating room. These technologic advances have changed the mechanical equipment and inanimate methods a doctor uses for doing things, but not the cerebral equipment and rational methods he uses for thinking about what he does.

The intellectual technology of clinical judgment—the methods of acquiring evidence and organizing clinical thought—has not received the same attention that contemporary clinical scientists have given to chemical, mechanical, electronic, and other new inanimate methods for observing and assessing tangible materials. Yet clinical judgment has a distinctive methodology for dealing with the tangible data of human illness; and clinical judgment now—uniquely in medical history —has both the obligation and the opportunity to be accomplished with scientific taste, discretion, and quality. Never before have clinicians had to make decisions about therapeutic agents capable of such spectacular benefits and such devastating harm. Never before have clinicians had available the intellectual assistance of new mathematical and computational systems to help manage the complex data assessed in the therapeutic decisions.

One of the main causes of the traditional belief that clinical judgment is beyond the reach of science is the failure of clinicians to distinguish the different types of observations and reasoning that are the components of clinical judgment. By dividing the observational data into descriptions of disease, illness, and host, and by analyzing the therapeutic and the environmental decisions separately, clinicians can discern the ingredients of clinical judgment. After those ingredients are discerned, their defects and possible improvements can be contemplated. If all three types of data and both types of decision are considered only as a single entity, scientific principles cannot be conveniently applied to the mixture. The multiple human personal attributes considered in the environmental decisions are often too complex to be cataloged, analyzed, and rationally dissected by any conventional contemporary logic. The clinician's approach to evaluating the patient exclusively as a person is still an artful aspect of care that depends on human perception and understanding. These components of clinical care are properties of heart and spirit, of instinct and psyche, and cannot be easily identified, assessed, or quantified by ordinary methods of reasoning.

The environmental decisions of clinical care, however, constitute only one part of the observations and reasoning of clinical judgment. The other main part is the selection and appraisal of therapeutic agents. This aspect of clinical judgment is a product of the clinician's mind, of his cultivated intellect and knowledge. The therapeutic decisions of clinical judgment require valid evidence, logical analyses, and demonstrable proofs. Their scientific quality can be discerned, assessed, and improved by the same rational procedures used for any other act of experimental science.

These therapeutic decisions are often regarded as scientifically unapproachable because they depend on clinical and personal data obtained and analyzed by human beings observing other human beings. Although a disease can often be appraised by inanimate scientific methods, the sick person must be studied by the specifically human techniques of clinical observation and clinical reasoning. The procedures used to obtain the data must provide for all the complexities of people, and must be motivated and performed with human perception. Nevertheless, both the acquisition and the evaluation of the data can be done with scientific reasoning. Clinicians have complacently accepted the traditional but unproved doctrine that their clinical activities are too human and too complex for science.

If the clinical judgment used in therapeutic experimentation is so scientifically defective today, it is not because the clinician's human capacities impede science, but because he has failed to use his human capacities in a scientific manner. He applies scientific methods to analyze the patient as a case of disease, but not as a case of human illness; to edify the agents of treatment but not the choice of appropriate agents; to improve the procedures of the laboratory but not the procedures of the bedside. The clinician tries to be scientific in the use of inanimate objects, but not in the use of his own sensory organs and brain. He often believes his own human equipment is a hindrance, not an advantage, and an apology, rather than an incentive, for science in his clinical work.

The argument of these essays is that clinicians can bring science to clinical judgment by better exercise of the very human capacities that appear to impair it, and by giving increased attention not to laboratory substances and inanimate technology, but to sick people and the human methods of evaluating sick people. The personal environmental management of a patient is a challenge to the clinician's judgment as a humanistic healer. The treatment of the patient is a challenge to the clinician's judgment as an experimental scientist. It is this latter aspect of clinical judgment—the performance and appraisal of therapeutic decisions—with which these essays are primarily concerned.

2. The Evolution of Clinical Investigation

Until the past few decades, the research of clinicians and non-clinicians at academic medical centers could be sharply distinguished. Today, however, because of major changes in the orientation of clinical investigation, the research of clinical academicians frequently resembles the work of their non-clinical colleagues. Both types of investigation often have the same sites, materials, methods, and objectives.

The site of most clinical investigation has been moved from bedside to laboratory. The material formerly was patients; it now often consists of animals, substances derived from patients or animals, or inanimate systems. The old bedside methods of clinical investigation enabled academicians to care for patients and to do research as a unified intellectual process, using the same techniques for both activities. Today a clinical investigator must often develop two different sets of methods for his academic work: one set for his clinical service in teaching and treating at the bedside, and the other for his research in the laboratory. The clinical academician's old objectives in research were directly concerned with better ways of managing illness in sick people; he now often approaches that objective more remotely, by studying basic mechanisms of disease and of biology. Thus, contemporary clinical investigation is still *clinical* in name because it is done by members of academic clinical departments, but the research is often not *clinical* in function.

For example, during the period from 1953 to 1965, in research descriptions submitted as "abstracts" for the annual meetings of the

31

American Society for Clinical Investigation and of the American Federation for Clinical Research, the percentage of projects containing human material progressively declined from 88% to 62%; the percentage of disease-oriented projects fell from 79% to 58%, of patient-centered projects from 40% to 15%, and of specifically therapeutic projects from 8% to 2%. During this same interval, the percentage of research activities that had neither human material nor a disease orientation rose from 6% to 26%.*

The new direction in the investigative activities of clinicians has evolved from the desire, first advanced more than a century ago mainly by Claude Bernard, to bring the discipline of active experimental research into clinical medicine. The need for experimentation in medicine was later emphasized in the United States by the establishment of two new stimulating forces that included the word *experimental* in their titles: the *Journal of Experimental Medicine,* founded in 1896, and the *Society for Experimental Biology and Medicine,* in 1903. The influence of these two respected organizations helped to direct clinical investigators away from the passive observations and imprecise descriptions then prevalent in bedside research. Instead, clinicians began to seek the active experiments and numerical precision of the laboratory.

The laboratory, at that time, was the only place where a clinical investigator could hope to perform scientific experiments. Even if Claude Bernard and other experimenters of that era had recognized the active experimental character of clinical therapy, they could not have expected to achieve scientific quality in the routine treatment of patients. Diagnosis was too imprecise and fallible: the X-ray was non-existent or primitive; chemical and hematologic methods were just beginning to supplement the developing bacteriologic aid of the laboratory; and the regular use of biopsy and endoscopy was not to appear for decades. Consequently, diagnosis could seldom be objectively confirmed during the life of the treated patient, and the human diseases treated in therapeutic experiments could seldom be reproducibly identified.

Moreover, even when diagnosis was accurate, the agents of therapy were generally nondescript and ineffective. Surgery was confined mainly to the amputation of appendages and to a limited number of intra-abdominal procedures; thoracic, neurologic, cardiovascular,

* These figures are taken from an analysis[36] of the "abstracts" submitted to the annual meetings of these two organizations. Each percentage here represents the mean of two values, one from each organization, for the cited categories of research.

plastic, prosthetic, and transplantational operations were yet to come. With uncommon exception, drugs were botanical extracts and mixtures whose active principles had not yet been isolated. There were no readily available antibiotics; diuretics; antimetabolites; anticoagulants; coagulants; blood transfusions; glandular arrays of insulin, thyroid, estrogens, adrenocortical steroids, pituitary derivatives, and other hormones; infusions of electrolytes; vitamins; or many other agents of modern therapy. Consequently, the clinician of that era could seldom decide when to attribute his meager therapeutic successes to nature or to therapy, and he could seldom ascertain which aspect of a successful therapeutic regimen was responsible for the success. In those diagnostic and therapeutic circumstances, a clinician seeking active scientific experiments had to look for something other than the treatment of sick people.

If he still wanted to study people, however, there was little he could do that was actively experimental. Human morality generally forbade experiments that were innovative or potentially harmful to his human subjects. With living people as his experimental material, he could not test new drugs or operations directly; he could not isolate organs or tissues from the rest of the body; he could not use noxious substances to induce the diseases whose causes and mechanisms he wanted to study. To do active scientific experiments in that era, therefore, the clinician had to reject people as the objects of research. The experiments of conventional human therapy were scientifically unattractive, and other experiments that were scientifically attractive were unfeasible in human beings. Instead, the clinical investigator turned to animals and to the laboratory to study "models" of human disease.

By exchanging the bedside for the laboratory, the investigator found a constantly available supply of experimental material that he could control, manipulate, dissect, and, if necessary, destroy. He also found many other advantages and luxuries of science. In the laboratory, he could make his experimental procedures specific and reproducible; he could use reagents, equipment, and techniques that had been developed, standardized, and calibrated in the flourishing growth of chemistry and physics; he could replace the anecdotal terminology of human observation by the numerical data of dimensional measurement.

For many decades, the academic clinician preserved his clinical orientation, and did research directly applicable to human disease. By laboratory studies of substances derived from sick people, he discerned, defined, and correlated elements of disease that were previously unknown and undetectable at bedside examination. By inducing analogs of human disease in animals, he investigated etiology and pathogenesis not with the undocumented conjectures of the past, but with precise numerical data. By testing new drugs and operations on animal disease models, he developed pharmaceutical and surgical procedures of unprecedented therapeutic specificity and power.

As time progressed, however, many clinical investigators began to find that a clinical orientation was often an impediment to laboratory science. The laboratory investigation of a patient's products could provide diagnostic correlations and identifications of disease, but not "active" experiments with the disease in its host. The models of disease induced in animals did not evolve in the same natural patterns as human illness, and could not really supplant sick people for accurate studies of human prognosis and therapy. And even for studies of etiology and pathogenesis, the induction of disease in animals was often unsatisfactory: many human diseases could not be induced in animals; many animal replicas were too disparate from the original human model to be adequately comparable; and satisfactory models, when produced in living animals, still contained many variables that could not be sufficiently isolated.

A strict orientation to disease, moreover, prevented clinical investigators from attaining what Bernard had called the object of the experimental method—"finding the relations which connect any phenomenon with its immediate cause"—and from pursuing this object by the principles of reductionist biology that Bernard had suggested: "We must reduce the phenomena to experimental conditions as definite and simple as possible . . . , reducing all the vital manifestations of a complex organism to the play of certain organs, and the action of these organs to the properties of well-defined tissues or organic units." [37] In contrast to the original intact unit studied by bedside clinicians and other organismal biologists, the unit of investigation in reductionist biology was to be a part of the original organism, or an intact but simpler organism.

Accordingly, many academic clinicians reduced the magnitude of phylum, organism, or part in the material used for research. Having started with man or other mammals, the investigators went phylogenetically downward to fowl, fish, invertebrates, or unicellular organisms. Having begun with intact organisms, the investigators began to work with smaller and smaller parts of organisms, progressively descending to organs, tissues, cells, cellular constituents, molecules, and electrons.

Since clinical training did not provide the sophistication needed for this type of laboratory research, the educational preparation of a clinician for an investigative career was modified. Additional postgraduate clinical training was often replaced or supplemented by "residencies" in laboratory work. The methods of such domains as microbiology and chemistry became regarded as "basic sciences" that would enable clinicians to do research using precise technology, and choosing problems from all of biology and nature. Although the problems approachable by these scientific methods often had few or no immediately evident clinical relationships, the academic clinician had good justification for his new activities: the scientific search for basic truths of nature should not be constrained by any limited objectives; the clarification of normal biologic and molecular function would eventually lead to better understanding of the deranged functions encountered in human disease.

This intellectual transition in the objectives of clinical research was aided by a simultaneous transition in its financing. Until the past two decades, only a few medical institutions in the United States could provide support for the necessary laboratories and clinical investigators. Now, with the availability of ample funds from federal and other sources, the clinical departments of almost every American medical school have become centers of "basic clinical research". The facilities, salaries, and numbers of clinical investigators have increased markedly, so that the investigators form a large cadre of clinical faculty, devoting full time to their academic work as investigators, teachers, and clinicians. The clinicians of the community, as part-time faculty members, were formerly responsible for most of the teaching and patient care at medical schools; this responsibility is now increasingly assigned mainly to the full-time clinical investigators, who divide their efforts between "basic science" in the laboratory and clinical service at the bedside. The division of time between the two sites often favors the laboratory for reasons other than pure science: prestige and advancement in the academic clinical hierarchy are more frequently a reward for laboratory accomplishment than for clinical skill.

These intellectual and other incentives to "basic research" have produced a revolutionary change in the focus of clinical investigation. Clinicians had originally entered the laboratory to do active scientific experiments concerned with human disease. To exploit the scientific opportunities of the laboratory, however, clinicians began to divert their investigative attention from both man and disease. The transition took clinical investigators from the traditional clinical problems of prognosis and therapy to the traditional medical problems of etiology and pathogenesis; from organismal whole to reductionist part; and from living patient to biologic molecule.

This change in the orientation of clinical investigation has had many repercussions in the clinical and pedagogical world outside the investigator's laboratory. Some of the major effects are evident in the way that contemporary academic clinicians allocate resources, provide care, teach students, and relate to other clinicians in the community.

In the allocation of medical resources, clinical research that is not specifically related to human disease tends to be wasteful both of the clinician's distinctive talents and of the unique material available to him for investigation in the wards and clinics of the medical center. A clinician's singular talents for examining, appraising, and managing sick people at the bedside are left unused when he does laboratory work, but are not possessed by many of the colleagues whose technologic skills he emulates in the laboratory. Moreover, the specific clinical problems of human prognosis and therapy can be adequately investigated only in patients. Thus, by electing to do his research in the laboratory, the clinician believes he can be more scientific than at the bedside, but he discards his clinical skills to compete as a scientist with non-clinicians who are often better prepared than he for laboratory work, and he leaves unexplored at the bedside the basic clinical problems that only he can solve.

In the care of patients, the application of research science formerly depended on the patients as direct sources of data; the symptoms, signs, and personal properties discerned from examination of patients at the bedside were the main observations used for analysis. Today, the major scientific variables used in clinical strategy often come from patients only indirectly; patients provide the substances that yield the data discerned from examinations in the laboratory. The scientific aspects of modern clinical care are therefore often focused more on the patient's laboratory identification as a diseased organism than on his bedside identity as a sick person.

In the teaching of medical students, the clinical investigator's primary scientific interest in laboratory procedures is often reflected in the topics he discusses at or near the bedside.[38] In many of his non-pedagogic activities, the investigator is intellectually concerned not with the care of patients but with the care of animals and of laboratory equipment. His research interests and devotion to scientific data obtained away from the bedside have inevitably reduced both the time he spends in communication with sick people and the attention he gives to information received directly from them. Consequently, his clinical discussion of a diseased patient may often dwell more on the elements of the disease revealed in the laboratory than on the features of the patient observed at the bedside. The student may learn about the clinical application of science in laboratory problems but not in patient care.

In the relationship between academic clinicians and the practitioners of the community, a new and insidious schism has developed. The old antagonism between town and gown was based on a competition for patients. The full-time members of the old academic clinical faculty often practiced as clinical rivals of community practitioners who held only part-time or no appointments at the medical school. As the full-time positions in the clinical faculty have become increasingly occupied by clinicians whose principal interest is laboratory investigation, the old discord between town and gown has developed into a new conflict that is more subtle and sometimes intramural. The new schism is intellectual, rather than financial, and based on focus, rather than locus. It depends not on the site of a clinician's practice, but on his research activities.

Behind the new schism is the belief that a clinician performs acts of science when he works in the laboratory but not when he takes care of patients. When he studies the problems of deranged human biology at the bedside, he is a mere clinician; when he does research in the laboratory, he is a scientist. The schism tends to divide clinical medicine into "two cultures", one containing the artful practicing clinicians of the community, and the other, the scientific investigating clinicians of the medical school. The separation is between service and science, between the practitioner of the bedside and the professor of the laboratory. The hiatus between these two cultures has steadily increased at most medical centers despite attempts to "educate" the practicing clinician with special lectures and courses in "basic science". The schism has even been openly acknowledged at some medical schools where the clinical faculty is divided into two platoons—the part-time practitioners who fulfill many of the academic clinical responsibilities for teaching and patient care, and the full-time clinical investigators who do the laboratory research.

The antagonisms produced by the new schism are humanistic and intellectual. From the bedside, the practicing clinician often condemns the clinical investigator for a lack of concern with the problems of sick people. From the laboratory, the clinical investigator often disdains the absence of science in the clinician's bedside art.

*　　　*　　　*

Despite these associated difficulties and disadvantages, the value of laboratory research by clinicians is indisputable. The laboratory work of clinical investigators has brought so many scientific improvements to clinical medicine that no single list of accomplishments can do justice to the total achievement. By applying a clinical orientation to work done with the methods of physical and non-clinical biologic science, clinical investigators have successfully introduced to bedside medicine most of the chemical, radiologic, electronic, and other advances of modern technology. Our contemporary clinical enlightenment in understanding causes of disease, in clarifications of pathogenesis, in the accuracy and precision of diagnosis, and in the availability of potent, specific therapeutic agents is all directly attributable to the clinical investigators who bridged the gap between the science of the laboratory and the service of the bedside. These clinical applications of "basic science" required that laboratory research be done by clinicians familiar with clinical problems, able to deal with the patients who were often observed during the research, and ready to transfer and communicate the new knowledge for clinical use. Even some of the contemporary investigative activities that seem so remote from clinical medicine may eventually bring many practical clinical advances.

There can be no legitimate quarrel with the necessity and desirability for continued laboratory research by clinicians. Many of the existing problems of clinical medicine and many of the new problems uncovered by future research at the bedside (or in the laboratory) can be solved only by further experimental investigation in the laboratory. These essays are intended to propose clinical studies not as a preferable alternative to laboratory research, but rather as an additional and equally valid opportunity for scientific clinical investigation.

The opportunity for contemporary clinicians to regard clinical work as an additional challenge in experimental science is actually attributable, paradoxically, to the laboratory research that has brought so many improvements to modern diagnostic procedures and therapeutic agents. With radiography, biopsy, endoscopy, and contemporary laboratory tests, diseases can be diagnosed during life, accurately and early. With modern pharmacology and surgery, treatment has become potent and specific. These improvements have removed two insurmountable handicaps that prevented Claude Bernard and older generations of clinical investigators from seeking science in the active experiments of therapy. A patient's disease can now be reproducibly identified; the agents of therapy can now be isolated and effective. Consequently, in every act of contemporary prognosis and therapy, clinicians can perform active scientific experiments as deliberate and distinct as any work done in the laboratory.

The chaotic state of contemporary prognosis and therapy reflects the failure of academic and non-academic clinicians to exploit their opportunities for achieving scientific performance in the routine experiments of the bedside. Surrounded by a scientific revolution that has identified molecules, enzymes, and genes, and possessing the most powerful therapeutic armamentarium in medical history, clinicians remain deplorably uncertain of when and how to use the magnificent agents at their disposal. A century ago, Claude Bernard referred to clinical therapy as "fanciful medicine which may involve the greatest dangers, by surrendering the health and life of the sick to the whims of an inspired ignoramus." [39] The modern era of "clinical science" that followed Bernard has already produced such unnecessary, hazardous, or tragic therapeutic procedures as hysterectomy for non-specific backache, gastropexy and nephropexy for "visceroptosis", total extraction of teeth for rheumatoid arthritis, and the iatrogenic catastrophes of mismatched blood transfusions, skin cancer due to irradiation for acne, retrolental fibroplasia due to oxygen for prematurity, and, most recently, the phocomelia induced by thalidomide. All of these unfortunate therapeutic procedures were carried out by well-intentioned, honest, dedicated, apparently enlightened clinicians working with the scientific diagnostic methods and therapeutic agents of modern medicine.

The scientific deficiencies of contemporary clinical therapy are often ascribed to clinicians, either for failing to solve the economic problems that keep new modes of treatment from being available ubiquitously, or for failing to understand the advances of laboratory research. The deficiencies *are* attributable to clinicians, but not for those reasons.

The economic arrangements for delivering treatment are basic problems in the logistics of medical care, not in the science of therapy. The scientific problem is which agents to deliver, and to whom. Should open-heart surgery, even if available everywhere, be done for all patients with rheumatic or congenital heart disease? If long-term anticoagulant therapy could be made convenient and inexpensive, would it still be worth its hazards in coronary and cerebrovascular disease? When hyperbaric oxygen chambers exist in every community, will they do more good than harm in the treatment of acute myocardial infarction and other disorders? If every cancer could be detected before or shortly after the onset of symptoms, would we really cure a higher percentage of the victims? If we can make radical surgery, irradiation, or chemotherapy available for everyone with cancer, can we effectively separate the cases in which these agents may be beneficial from those in which the treatment may only add agony to mortality? Do all peripheral arterial aneurysms need replacement by prostheses? Does a patient paralyzed by a stroke benefit as much from complex physical maneuvers and drugs as he does from the attention itself and the efforts to help him adjust to a new life? Are a drastic diet and intensive insulin regulation really necessary in all diabetic patients for preventing vascular deterioration? Should digitalis be maintained for the lifetime of every patient whose heart has ever decompensated? Should *all* hypertensive patients receive a pharmacologic reduction of blood pressure in the hope of preventing strokes, arteriosclerosis, and renal failure?

The answers to these and scores of other therapeutic questions are still unknown or highly controversial today, although the questions have existed ever since the accurate diagnostic methods and potent therapeutic agents became available years ago. The answers remain unknown and controversial, despite many attempts to answer them in the existing plethora of "retrospective surveys" and "prospective trials". These surveys and trials are often unproductive of answers because, with all their elaborate statistics, they usually are not scientifically reproducible investigations. The individual reports are often limited to collections, by unreproducible methods, of the data derived from individual acts of treatment assessed by equally unreproducible methods. The contentions and dissensions of the published reports then cannot be properly confirmed or refuted because the original work can seldom be meaningfully appraised or repeated. Errors and misconceptions can become established, accepted, and diffused because they cannot be suitably tested and rectified. Unless the scientific methods of both innovative and conventional clinical therapy are made more sensible and reproducible, the widespread distribution of modern therapeutic agents may provoke iatrogenic tragedies worse, individually and collectively, than any already known in medical history.

A better economic system for delivering the available agents of treatment is clearly not the answer to fundamental scientific questions in clinical therapy. Nor can the answers come only from understanding the knowledge gained in laboratory research. Even if clinicians understood and applied every new advance of laboratory science, they still could not improve the critical scientific defects of modern therapy. The clinician's experimental material in therapy is distinctly different from the cadavers, human parts and substances, animals, and inanimate systems of the laboratory; the clinician's material is an alive, whole, sick person. One of the oldest principles of science, dating back to the writings of Aristotle,[40] is that the methods of an experiment must be adapted to the material. The methods of laboratory research provide neither the technology nor the judgment for the *clinical* study of people.

For the experiments of ordinary clinical therapy, the clinician must be able to identify the similar situations he has seen in the past and to evaluate successful results. His methods of identification and evaluation must, in the treatment of sick people, account for many properties that are uniquely human, and that are neither encountered nor managed in the material studied by laboratory methods. The human symptoms, signs, and personal properties that distinguish patients occur only at the bedside and are discernible only by clinical methods of examination. As scientific necessities for reproducibly identifying illness and host in therapeutic experiments, the bedside data must be acquired, interpreted, and organized by methods specifically designed for the various human beings who are the observers and the observed.

To the clinician who abandoned the bedside for the laboratory years ago in search of active scientific experiments, an opportunity for experimental research now occurs every time a patient is treated. The clinician seeking scientific investigation can now find it in the same clinical activities that motivated him to become a *medical* doctor and that gave him his primary training and skills. If he wants to do experimental research in clinical science, he can find basic challenges in the many types of investigation needed to convert the artful experiments of clinical therapy into acts of science. Not just with laboratory methods, but with clinical skills, clinical settings, and the sick people who constitute clinical material, clinicians can develop a scientific methodology of their own.

3. Scientific Method in Clinical and Laboratory Experiments

No one would want to use an electron microscope for studying a baseball pitcher's ability to throw a curve ball, and few people would look with naked eye for the actomyosin bands in the fibrils of a muscle. If we wanted to measure the circumference of a biceps, we would not employ an electromyograph, nor would we expect a measuring tape to demonstrate the electrical discharge that accompanies the contraction of muscle fibers. Although a particular muscle may have each of these four properties—gross size, microscopic bands, electrical discharge, and curve-ball throwing—they represent different structures and functions, and must be observed by different techniques. If the investigated muscle unit and its possessor are intact, the muscle has a measurable circumference and can participate in throwing a curve ball. If the muscle is observed as isolated fibers, it has bands and electrical potential. The isolated fibers cannot throw a curve ball; the intact muscle has no grossly visible bands.

Throughout all of biology and nature, the form (or structure) and the function of an observed entity always change as the entity changes. As organism is reduced to organ, organ to tissue, tissue to cell, cell to molecule, and molecule to sub-atomic particle—every time the unit of observation is changed, the forms and functions of the new unit are different from those present before. If an investigator wants to study the forms and functions of that new unit, he must correspondingly change his techniques of observation. For a muscle fiber, he may need an electron microscope and an electromyograph. For an intact gross muscle, he may need a tape measure and his naked eye. These techno-logic distinctions were summarized by Aristotle in his comment that the methods of an experiment must be adapted to its material. Different material, different forms and functions; different forms and functions, different methods of observation.

This basic principle of science is constantly overlooked, ignored, or avoided in contemporary "basic clinical science". Clinicians use excellent techniques for observing and analyzing animals or the parts of a person as the entities of the laboratory, but inadequate techniques for studying a whole person as the human entity of the bedside. The general hope seems to be either that the defects of bedside techniques will somehow vanish after further advances in laboratory research, or that human problems can be circumvented through the study of sub-human material. A perceptive clinical investigator who recognizes that bedside defects will not be corrected by laboratory techniques, and that the avoidance of clinical problems will not eliminate the problems, often feels inextricably trapped. He wants to work as a scientist, but he believes that clinical techniques contain so many inevitable, unredeemable human flaws that the principles of "the scientific method" cannot be applied at the bedside. The rest of this chapter is intended to demonstrate the fallacy of this belief, and to propose an emergence from the apparent trap.

"The scientific method" is an intellectual concept. It refers to the quality with which an experiment is designed, executed, and appraised. Almost anyone can make some plans, carry them out, and see what happens. The scientific quality of the activity depends on the methods used for making and consummating the plans, and for observing and interpreting what happens.

In *every* aspect of experimental construction by the scientific method, the performance of clinical therapy is identical to a laboratory investigation. The differences between clinical treatment and laboratory work are not in the rational aspects of scientific method, but in the procedures—in the *methodology*—used for design, execution, and appraisal of the experiments. These procedures include the techniques used for *preparation* of material, selection of *maneuver,* and observation of *response.*

1) In *preparation,* a material is selected and arranged—by identifying, classifying, and perhaps altering it—for the maneuver that follows. A laboratory investigator, for example, designs the preparation of an experiment by removing the adrenals from a group of healthy rats and

by performing a sham operation on another group, to be used as controls. In ordinary clinical therapy, the clinician designs the preparation of the experiment by examining a patient, arriving at a diagnostic classification, estimating a prognosis, and choosing a mode of treatment.

2) The experimental *maneuver* is imposed by nature or by man; it may be merely a natural course of events, or it may include various manipulations of the material beyond the alterations performed in the initial preparation. In the cited laboratory experiment, the maneuver may consist of injecting adrenocorticotropin (ACTH) into both groups of rats. In clinical therapy, the maneuver is the administration of treatment, or the clinician may elect to give no specific treatment, allowing nature to take its course.

3) The *response* is observed as and after the prepared material undergoes the maneuver. In the laboratory experiment, the observed response may be the urinary excretion of 17-ketosteroids (17-KS). In clinical treatment, the patient's subsequent reactions constitute the response.

In the intellectual usage of "scientific method", the *design* of an experiment is the plan for arranging the *preparation,* performing the *maneuver,* and observing the *response;* the *appraisal* of the experiment is the plan for evaluating the results by means of correlations, analyses, and conclusions. In *correlations,* one type of data is compared (or associated) with another. The data can come from any of the observations made during the preparation, maneuver, and response, but the most common experimental correlations are between something observed in the initial preparation and something in the subsequent response. In *analyses,* the significance and meaning of the correlations are determined. In *conclusions,* the analyses are interpreted, if possible, to answer the original questions of the experiment, and to establish knowledge that may clarify the past, illuminate the present, and anticipate the future.

For example, in the cited laboratory experiment, the investigator makes correlations that compare the range and mean values for 17-KS in adrenalectomized rats with those of the controls. After analyzing the correlations, he draws conclusions about the role of adrenal glands and ACTH in the production of 17-KS. In ordinary clinical treatment, the clinician correlates the post-therapeutic events with the patient's previous state and with what was predictable had the patient been left untreated. The clinician then analyzes these correlations and draws conclusions about the effectiveness of the treatment in that patient. By combining data from a series of such experiments in the same patient or in many patients, the clinician can perform additional correlations and analyses for evaluating the general effectiveness of the treatment.

Clinicians can thus apply, at the bedside, exactly the same principles of scientific method that are used for any other experiment. Because the unit material of clinical therapy is a person, however, the procedures used to design and appraise experiments scientifically at the bedside must be drastically different from the technology of laboratory work. Some of the common principles of these scientific procedures, and some of the problems in applying them in the laboratory and at the bedside, are discussed in the sections that follow.

DESIGN OF EXPERIMENTS

A scientific investigation must fulfill at least three principles *before it begins:*

1) The material prepared for the experiment must be identified, and its characteristics, or mode of preparation, must be clearly stipulated.

2) The apparatus for observing critical variables must be standardized for consistency and accuracy.

3) The experimental material must be divided identically, one part to be used for experimental maneuver and the other for "control" comparison.

These three principles—stipulation, standardization, identical division—are essential for scientific work. The first two make the prepared material and the observed data reproducible; the third enables valid assessment of experimental effects. An investigation that does not fulfill these three principles is defective at its core, and cannot be rectified by *any* subsequent analysis or contrivance of the results.

STIPULATION OF PREPARED MATERIAL

In the laboratory, the investigator usually obtains his material originally from some standard source of supply and then prepares it for the experiment by certain procedures or manipulations, using purified reagents and standardized equipment. His material is essentially "healthy", and he creates its "disease". He can readily define, describe, and repeat what he prepared, since he arranged its "history".

At the bedside, the investigator receives his patients in a state of disease already prepared in an experiment begun by nature. Before the investigator can begin his intended experiment in therapy, he must first engage in the separate investigation of diagnosis, trying to identify what nature has done. Since he did not prepare his received material, he tries to learn its mode of development and to classify its present state. To learn its development, the investigator relies on the ability of the diseased human preparation, unique among investigative materials, to talk and to describe a history the investigator could not arrange. To classify its state, the investigator establishes a diagnosis, based on the information obtained by history, augmented by physical examination, and confirmed (whenever possible) by laboratory tests.

STANDARDIZATION OF APPARATUS

The data of the laboratory are usually observed by measurement with precise apparatus, calibrated and standardized for accuracy both inherently and in operation by technicians. Moreover, the apparatus and techniques used to prepare the material for the experiment often differ from those used to observe the variables of experimental response. (For example, a chemical extract of mitochondria is prepared by one set of procedures; its uptake of radioactive substances is measured in an altogether different way.)

The data of the bedside are human symptoms, signs, and personal properties, assessed by a human apparatus—the clinician. Both the apparatus and the data it collects are fraught with human imprecision, yet seldom does the apparatus get standardized or the data validated. Moreover, the symptoms and signs that indicate the developmental preparation of a patient's clinical state are observed by the same human apparatus that is later used to assess the subsequent symptoms and signs of therapeutic response. Thus, when the apparatus functions improperly, its errors are doubled and compounded.

IDENTICAL DIVISION

In the laboratory, inanimate material is easily divided into identical parts by simple physical separation. Living organisms cannot be divided into identical parts and hence must be arranged into identical groups. Since the laboratory investigator gets pristine material and prepares it by defined techniques, he can easily repeat his preparation of an experimental unit as often as necessary to get the desired number of similar units for his identical groups.

At the bedside, diseased patients give the investigator no such option. He must take them as he finds them, and identify them as best he can. In the clinical experiments of prognosis, therapy, and other types of correlation, he must attempt to divide his clinical material for the comparison of similar groups. The comparison of similar groups, as subjects and "controls" in experiments or for other purposes, is essential for scientific procedures and requires not merely that such groups be formed, but that their contents be as alike as possible.

APPRAISAL OF EXPERIMENTAL RESPONSE

For its reasoning and conclusions to be valid, an investigation must fulfill the following principles *after* it begins:

1) The observation period must be long enough for pertinent events to be noted.

2) The data on both sides of a correlation must be appropriate and clearly specified.

3) Important correlations must be analyzed to determine to what extent their numerical distinctions are significant or possibly attributable to chance.

4) The features or events held responsible for significant relationships must be evaluated as direct or indirect, causal or co-existent.

5) The experimental results must be established as having come from a valid sampling of the "universe" they supposedly represent or to which their conclusions will be extrapolated.

These principles—adequate duration, specificity of correlation, statistical significance, identification of cause, and valid extrapolation—are basic to scientific reasoning.

ADEQUATE DURATION

Most experiments in the laboratory take relatively little time. They are sometimes completed in a day and rarely take longer than a year. The investigator usually designs them for results that quickly answer a question. Having complete control of his enclosed or caged material, he need seldom consider whether his preservation of the material will be affected by the world outside his laboratory. Since he has few moral responsibilities to the material beyond humane care, he can conclude the experiment whenever he wishes, discarding what he observed, of "sacrificing" it to perform post-mortem examination.

Clinical investigations do not allow such freedom. The human diseases presented to the investigator are natural experiments he could not begin and often cannot change; they may last for decades before their conclusion by death. To see the total spectrum and duration of disease as well as the isolated portions that appear in admissions to the hospital, the investigator must arrange for further observations under everyday conditions. His data may thus come from such diverse sites as other hospitals, private medical offices, out-patient clinics, schoolrooms, prisons, military installations, epidemiologic and public health field stations, and factories. In addition to needing the appropriate facilities, the personnel who make the observations may need to cope not only with the disease, but with multiple external factors that affect the diseased patient's willingness or ability to permit himself to be observed. In undertaking such studies, an investigator must be ready to accept the responsibilities of caring for people, to wait for answers to his questions, to sustain his curiosity for long periods of time, to work in situations that may not always provide pathologic data, to accept many frustrations when he is denied opportunity for critical examinations, and to recognize that all his efforts may sometimes be unproductive. For such investigations, the clinician must often have personal qualities and temperament different from those needed in laboratory work.

SPECIFICITY OF CORRELATION

In the laboratory, the investigator prepares his material, creates the experimental sequence of events, and obtains precise experimental results. These circumstances help clarify his choice of features to be correlated, and give him appropriate, accurate data for the correlations.

Because human illness has so many intricate and sometimes obscure variables, the clinical investigator often has difficulty in deciding which variables to correlate. The sequence he assigns the variables may come from conjecture rather than observation, and the data that describe the variables may have dubious accuracy. He can get impressive-looking results by analyzing the correlations with the same statistical and computational devices used for laboratory data, but these devices cannot correct inaccuracy, supply omissions, eliminate erroneous assumptions, or rectify correlations of variables that were improperly chosen or inadequately described.

STATISTICAL SIGNIFICANCE

To workers in animal and human biology, the application of analytic statistical techniques has provided an intellectual liberation comparable to that given physicists years ago by quantum mechanics and the Heisenberg uncertainty principle.[41] Heisenberg's demonstration that essential, irremovable uncertainties occur during observation of the physical behavior of particulate matter is also applicable to the complex, frequently random variations in the biologic phenomena of living organisms. For assessing the variations in these phenomena, statistical analysis helps biologists to distinguish random chance from likely trend, and likely trend from general rule.

Statistical analysis has been used often and effectively as a powerful tool for these biologic refinements, but, like many other powerful tools, it has also been used inappropriately and erroneously. The statistical analysis of biologic data has little value, and may actually impair progress, if the statistician is pre-occupied with numerical distinctions and ignores the biologic sources and meaning of the numbers, or if the biologist is pre-occupied with causal speculations, and ignores or distorts the numerical distinctions. In medicine, a single well-studied case may seem statistically meaningless, but it can sometimes establish or refute an important clinical concept. A single case report was all that was necessary, for example, to demonstrate that insulin could save the life of a patient in diabetic coma, to show that antibiotic treatment could cure subacute bacterial endocarditis, or to prove that certain patients may have long survival despite untreated breast cancer.

Conversely, the numerical distinctions found in large amounts of medical data may sometimes be statistically significant, but clinically or therapeutically meaningless. Suppose a population of private patients is treated for meningitis by drug A, and a population of skid-row derelicts by drug B. The numerical data may show significantly better therapeutic results for A than B, yet the differences may have nothing to do with the therapy. Because derelicts with meningitis are often comatose or stuporous before treatment begins, their results will be much worse than those of the private patients who come to treatment in a milder stage of the disease. This type of biologic-sociologic distinction may be neglected, however, when the "statistically significant" differences in therapeutic results are attributed to the two different agents used to treat the "same" disease at a municipal hospital and at a private referral clinic.

Laboratory workers and clinicians often forget that statistical analysis, despite its power, has many limitations. It may demonstrate the precison of data, but cannot verify their basic accuracy; it may indicate the variations in a sampling, but cannot denote how appropriately the sampling represents the total "universe"; it may signify that a certain relationship is likely to have a specific cause, but it does not specify the cause, or confirm the choice of whatever is deemed to be the cause.

For biologic use of statistical analysis, the amount of data must be large enough for application of the appropriate formulas. To obtain large amounts of data, the laboratory investigator can repeat his experiment exactly, as many times as he must. Since his experimental material is defined reproducibly and his observational apparatus is calibrated, he can decide that significant statistical relationships are due to the effects of the experimental maneuver, rather than to variations in the original material or in the observational apparatus.

For the amount of clinical data to be large enough for analysis, the bedside investigator must often combine the results from many patients. The combination may frequently include patients studied at different times, in different places, and by different examiners. Statistically significant relationships found in therapeutic surveys and trials may thus often be due not to therapy, but to unrecognized variations in clinical material or in clinical examiners.

IDENTIFICATION OF CAUSE

After determining that a result of an experimental maneuver is significant and not due to variations in the original material or in the observational apparatus, investigators try to determine how or why the maneuver caused the result. If the material is inanimate, it cannot change itself or its reactions, so the investigator need consider only the experimental maneuver as a cause of any subsequent change. Living material, however, has inherent biologic capacities to grow, heal, or otherwise change itself. Living human material, moreover, has psychic properties, not present or noteworthy in the study of lower animals, that can affect many reactions and sensations in the state of human illness. Hence a patient's improvement after treatment may often be due not to the therapeutic agent, but to his natural powers of recuperation or to diverse psychic effects.

Unless an investigator recognizes that these biologic and psychic causes can change the course of a human illness, he may fall into the frequent, widespread, and traditional clinical fallacy of *post hoc ergo propter hoc* reasoning: the clinician gives a therapeutic agent, the patient gets better, and the clinician concludes that the agent must have been responsible. In the specious self-deception of *post hoc* clinical reasoning, many a drug, diet, or device of ancient and modern medicine has been given false credit for improvements that really were due to nature or to man himself.

In contemplating the general problem of *cause* in experimental work, moreover, clinical investigators have an additional, separate issue not present in laboratory research. In the laboratory, the investigator "caused" the preparation of his material, so his search for cause can be confined only to analyzing how the experimental maneuver produced the subsequent results. The clinical investigator, however, did not create the disease in his material, and must try to decide what caused the disease as well as what caused the experimental therapeutic responses of the diseased patient.

VALID EXTRAPOLATION

Having observed and correlated the results, determined the statistical significance of the correlations, and evaluated their cause, the investigator would then like to extrapolate his findings to allow more general application. To do this, he must be sure that the general material or population to which he extrapolates was validly represented by the selected portion used in his experiment.

Laboratory material, which is obtained, prepared, and manipulated precisely, can usually be made a truly random sampling of other material just like it. At the bedside, however, no two instances of a human disease are exactly alike. The content of two collections of patients with the same disease can differ considerably, making extrapolation of the results difficult, hazardous, or false.

*   *   *

Although these scientific principles of experimental design and appraisal are commonly violated in clinical work, clinicians need not feel uniquely culpable. The violations have been, and still are, present in the activities of every form of experimental investigation, with every type of material. A recitation of the errors produced by the violations can readily be obtained from review of the history of *any* scientific domain, and from comparison of concepts that were once fashionable with those that have survived.

The use of intact human beings as the material of clinical therapeutic experiments does not preclude scientific principles of design and appraisal. The principles are much more difficult to attain at the bedside than in the laboratory, however, because of the overt and subtle complexities that distinguish sick people from animals, from inanimate substances, and from each other. Since clinical methodology must cope with these complexities, its major problems are in the precision and reproducibility with which clinicians identify the condition and responses of sick human beings. The identifications must account for *all* of the pertinent, distinctive manifestations of human ailments.

Although certain aspects of methodology in therapeutic experiments have been helped by the contemporary use of statistical techniques, placebo comparisons, and double-blind procedures for execution of certain experiments, these improvements are merely peripheral. They are devices imposed for the analysis of results, but they fail to deal with more basic aspects of the results. The fundamental techniques of clinical methodology remain egregiously defective for acquiring and classifying the elemental data of the bedside: symptoms, signs, and other personal features of sick people.

These clinical and personal data are the responsibility of the clinician. He is the principal apparatus that observes and interprets the data as variables of human illness. The scientific function of this human apparatus is gravely impaired when the clinician's observations are imprecise and unstandardized, and when his interpretations are made without appropriate criteria and without vigorous attempts to achieve uniformity and consistency. Clinicians usually accept these methodologic defects complacently, attributing them to the frailty of human capacities, and concluding that, since the flaws are traditional, they must also be inevitable. Yet his human sensory organs give a clinician the power to make many observations of which no inanimate instrument is capable, and his human mind enables him to make constant scientific improvements in the way he performs his observations and interpretations. The clinician cannot begin to improve these functions, however, until he recognizes himself as a unique and powerful piece of scientific equipment. He can then contemplate and, if necessary, revise the fundamental aspects of what he does and how he thinks when he collects the human data for which he is the main, and often the only, perceptual apparatus.

4. Conceptual Barriers
to Clinical Science

A clinician who wants to contemplate the scientific performance of his bedside procedures soon finds his paths of thought blocked by a series of obstacles. The obstacles are deeply imbedded in the basic matrix of his clinical thinking, put there by most of the teaching he received in medical school and perpetuated by his subsequent training, reading, and experience. The obstacles are a group of hallowed beliefs, transmitted as intellectual legacies by teacher to student, and from one medical generation to the next. Each of these beliefs is like an axiom—an established principle, which, though not a necessary truth, is universally accepted.

There are at least five such axioms—in clinical ideas about scientific motivation, reasoning, observation, correlation, and classification—that are major conceptual barriers to clinical science:

1) In motivation, the clinician believes that the main incentive for scientific research is to discover the *cause* of natural phenomena and that phenomena whose causes are unknown cannot be properly managed.

2) In reasoning, the clinician believes that his intellectual organization of clinical observations is rationally amorphous—that his thinking has too many intricate and unquantified elements to be expressed in the mathematical structures used for other types of scientific analysis.

3) In observation, the clinician believes that his descriptions of symptoms and signs cannot be scientifically precise because they often

54

contain nouns, adjectives, verbs, and adverbs rather than the numerical dimensions of measurement.

4) In correlation, the clinician believes he finds a constant association between the abnormal structures and abnormal functions that occur in human illness.

5) In classification, the clinician believes that he adequately identifies human illness by categorizing sick people with diagnostic names that represent the morphologic and laboratory abnormalities of disease.

Each of these beliefs is widely disseminated, long established, and seldom questioned; each has achieved the secure status of tradition; and each is either inappropriate, obsolete, or mistaken.

MOTIVATION, AND THE GOALS OF SCIENTIFIC RESEARCH

Anyone who explores nature always wonders about the *why* of the *what* he observes. Yet he seldom can find out *why,* and when he does, each answer raises a new series of questions. Because the sequence of questions is endless, scientists cannot find ultimate answers for the *why* of nature's manifestations. After a certain stage in the questioning, the matter reverts to philosophers or theologians, who seldom provide unanimous replies.

Claude Bernard, who so keenly looked for causes of natural phenomena, was willing to settle for a satisfactory *how.* He regarded his scientific objective as "defining the conditions necessary to the appearance of the phenomenon". Said Bernard,[42]

> The nature of our mind leads us to seek the essence or the *why* of of things . . . (but) experience soon teaches us that we cannot get beyond the *how.* . . . We know how water can be made; but why does the combination of one volume of oxygen with two volumes of hydrogen produce water? We have no idea. In medicine it is equally absurd to concern one's self with the question 'why'. . . . [To know] the inmost nature, or the absolute, in the simplest phenomenon, would demand knowledge of the whole universe. . . . Man behaves as if he were destined to reach this absolute knowledge; and the incessant *why* which he puts to nature proves it. . . . If our feeling constantly puts the question *why,* our reason shows us that only the question *how* is within our range. . . . This is true of all experimental sciences in which we reach only relative or partial truths, . . . but this knowledge is

enough to broaden our power over nature. Though we do not know the essence of phenomena, we can produce or prevent their appearance.

In seeking the *why* rather than the *how* of natural phenomena in human illness, clinicians may forget the many medical triumphs achieved in the past without knowledge of "cause" or even of diagnosis of a disease. For example, sanitation of water supply and pasteurization of milk have prevented many diseases whose identities and "causal" agents were still unknown when these public health procedures were first introduced. Lind's oranges and lemons had begun to eliminate scurvy from the British Navy before anyone suspected the existence of vitamins; Jenner's vaccination was preventing smallpox long before the causal virus was discovered. Generations of patients with acute gouty arthritis have been helped by colchicine, although its mechanism of action is just now becoming clarified via studies in frog skin,[43] and although we still do not know the cause of gout. Surgeons have presumably cured many breast cancers by operative excision, although the cause of breast cancer is no better known today than it was in the time of Halsted.

Moreover, in seeking knowledge of "cause", clinicians may forget that the etiologic information does not always provide prompt help in treatment. For example, we have known for many decades that one type of familial hemolytic jaundice is "caused" by spherical red blood cells, and, for more than a decade, that another type, with sickle-shaped cells, is due to specific abnormalities in the hemoglobin molecule. Yet the treatment for both these diseases is essentially the same now as it was before the new knowledge of pathogenesis was acquired. A specialist in physical rehabilitation may know with certainty that his patient's paraplegia was caused by an automobile accident, a bullet wound, or a local reaction to spinal anesthesia. This knowledge of cause, however, plays little role in the physiatrist's choice of braces, wheelchairs, and other mechanical therapeutic devices; the cause has come and gone, but the illness still needs treatment.

Clinicians have known, for almost a century, that Koch's bacillus "causes" tuberculosis, but our knowledge of *how* and *why* remains incomplete. We still do not know why or even how the bacillus does its work, why it is sensitive to certain drugs but resistant to others, and why only certain human hosts are clinically susceptible to the disease. We have learned the general sequence of pathogenesis in tuberculosis, but we do not know the exact reactions responsible for the tissue changes, or the exact chemical mechanisms of those reactions. After we learn the chemical mechanisms, we shall want to know the molecular mechanisms. And after we learn the molecular mechanisms, we shall want to know the electronic mechanisms. And after that, . . .

The search for causes of phenomena is incessant, always important, and always attractive. Of course clinicians will want to know all they can about each *how*, and each subsequent *how* thereafter. And of course clinicians, like all other scientists, will continue to ask *why*. When a scientist stops wondering *why*, his ideas have ended. But if he is willing to recognize that his *why* is composed of a sequence of *how*'s, he can then decide what kind of question to ask of the phenomenon he observes. "How does it occur?" is one question. "How do I keep it from occurring?" and "How do I change it?" are two others.

All three of these *how*'s are legitimate, respectable, and fundamental scientific questions, but the first deals with the cause and mechanism of disease, and the next two, with prevention and management. In contemporary clinical investigation, a predominant emphasis has been given to finding the *how*'s of cause and mechanism. These are always worthy scientific goals. An improved knowledge of etiology and pathogenesis, although desirable for its own sake, may contribute much more to clinical medicine than just the possibility of practical aid in treatment: many diseases may be eliminated once their causes and mechanisms are known. Etiology and pathogenesis of disease, however, are not the only worthy goals in clinical science. As long as any human illness exists, clinicians will continue to be confronted with problems in therapy, and will have to continue seeking basic answers to the equally worthy *how*'s of prevention and management.

These therapeutic *how*'s can be asked and sometimes answered without a knowledge of cause and mechanism. When they are, the process is often described by the scientifically "dirty" word, *empiric*. This word comes from the Greek εν πειρα, *in experiment,* and its older meaning was "founded on experiment". Only in modern times has the word come to refer to quackery, or to an almost disreputable "reliance on practical experience alone".[44]

Was William Withering a quack? His work was purely *empiric*. He observed a phenomenon of nature that was called "dropsy". He learned to modify the outcome of that phenomenon, predictably and consistently, by treating it with preparations of foxglove leaf.[45] He learned, predictably and consistently, how much of the preparation to give for successful results, and when to stop. He knew little or nothing about myocardial metabolism, end-diastolic ventricular pressure, and glomerular filtration rate, and he was probably wrong in many of his anatomic cardiac diagnoses. Today, we know many things of which Withering was ignorant; we have changed the name of the phenomenon from "dropsy" to "congestive heart failure"; and we have purified and standardized his foxglove extract into various preparations of digitalis. Yet we still encounter the same condition he described, and we still treat it—getting successes not too much better than his—with the same drug he tested, and with the same therapeutic directions he gave. His *empiric* ability to predict, to reproduce, and to modify phenomena of nature was an act of science when he did it, and its scientific validity has been proved by time.

The search for etiology and, particularly, for pathogenesis of disease is not a clinician's only important outlet in scientific research, and is not readily available to him as a *clinical* activity. He cannot manipulate his bedside material for the types of experiments needed to answer basic scientific questions about *how* a disease develops. The clinician does, however, constantly perform other types of experiments, in treating his bedside material, that are fundamentally important and desperately in need of science. His therapeutic experiments have a purpose different from the investigation of pathogenesis; they use different methods, and ask a different *how.*

A clinician's experimental goals in treating sick people are just as intellectually challenging as those of his laboratory colleagues who explore etiology and pathogenesis of disease. Moreover, the clinical goals are often more attainable than those of laboratory experiments, for the clinician's *care* can always give comfort to his patients even when his scientific *treatment* fails. The therapeutic motive of changing nature, instead of just understanding it, does not bar a clinician from science. He has only to ask the right questions.

REASONING, AND THE MATHEMATICAL ORGANIZATION OF DATA

In its broadest sense, mathematical symbolism is a method of describing the relationships of things that people think about. Each symbol represents a thing or a property called a *variable,* and the arrangement of symbols shows how those variables are related to one another. The arrangement also indicates the places where numbers are to be inserted for identifications of magnitude and for interpretive or statistical analysis. In biology, mathematics provides three main types of organizational arrangement for different variables.

ORDERING TWO COMPARABLE DIMENSIONS

This type of common, simple mathematical arrangement requires no more than a knowledge of greater or less, before or after. For example, we know almost without thinking that an event that occurred 3 seconds after zero time precedes an event that occurs at 4 seconds, or that a dimension of 180 cm. is longer than one of 170 cm. This kind of mathematical ordering is so obvious that it is done almost subconsciously. Its "equations" are depicted by the familiar symbols: $>$, $=$, and $<$.

DEPENDENCY OF TWO OR MORE CONTINUOUS VARIABLES

This type of mathematical procedure is also familiar to biologists. It provides the equations of straight lines or curves that represent the dependent relationship between one continuous variable and another. The variables are "continuous" because they can extend through an indefinite range of numerical values; the relationship is "dependent" because each value of one of the variables corresponds to at least one value of the other as changes occur.

The equations for such relationships can be simple or complicated, and are provided by the binomial and polynomial structures of algebra, analytic geometry, and the calculus. For example, two variables that relate to each other linearly (as a straight line) are expressed in the form $y = mx + b$. If a variable decreases in time proportionately to the amount present at each moment, the equation is $y = -k'(dy/dt)$. This differential equation, which may be integrated and written as $\log_e y = C - kt$ or $y = y_0 e^{-kt}$, is a standard representation of chronologic decay of radioactivity.

CLASSIFICATION OF MULTIPLE, DISCRETE, INDEPENDENT VARIABLES

This type of mathematics is relatively new (little more than a century old) and is unfamiliar to most biologists. It is concerned with variables that are attributes (or properties) characterizing an object or group of objects at a specific time, rather than with the changes of one variable in relation to changes in another variable. The "new" mathematics describes the relationships of classes or sets of objects having many different attributes, rather than the way one particular attribute may be affected by changes in another. As mathematical variables, these attributes are "multiple", because a single object can possess many distinct properties; "discrete" (or "noncontinuous"), because each attribute can be characterized with only a finite number of descriptive categories; and "independent", because the presence or absence of one attribute often has no bearing on whether some other attribute is present or absent in the same object.

For example, a person may possess such properties as number of fingers, hair color, pregnancy, and serum sodium. The properties are obviously "multiple", and they are also "independent", since changes in hair color may not affect the number of fingers, and so forth. As variables, the number of fingers, hair color, and pregnancy are "discrete". A particular person can have only 0 to 10 fingers (perhaps a few more for people with supernumerary digits); the color of human hair is described with only a limited collection of adjectives (brown, black, blond, etc.), and the person is either pregnant or non-pregnant. Serum sodium, on the other hand, is a "continuous" variable. Although its human range may be limited to the zone from 85 to 170 meq. per 100 ml., a particular value can be 135, 135.1, 135.14, or 135.139, etc., according to the precision with which it is measured.

In using traditional mathematics, we seek equations to express a person's growth or gain in weight as a "function" of time, or the changes in his serum sodium in relation to changes in blood glucose. In the new form of mathematics, we use symbols to indicate that the person (at a fixed time) is short or tall, fat or thin, eunatremic or hyponatremic, hypoglycemic or hyperglycemic. We do this not to show that his blood sugar depends on his weight or that his serum sodium is related to his height, but to characterize him as having or not having each of the cited attributes. With this characterization, we can distinguish him from some other person whose attributes are different.

The new mathematical techniques used for such characterizations are provided by set theory, symbolic logic, and Boolean algebra. Despite their novelty, these new mathematical concepts are relatively simple and easy to learn. (They will be described in greater detail in Chapter 10.) The type of thinking used in the "new" mathematics is entirely different from that of the "old" mathematics, but its principles can be grasped well enough for practical usage by any intelligent adult willing to give the subject one or two hours of concentrated attention. The concepts require no previous familiarity or skill with the "old" mathematics, and are readily comprehended by the grade-school children to whom the "new" mathematics is now being taught.

These new forms of mathematics make profound and perhaps revolutionary contributions to the reasoning of clinical medicine. The properties used in the new mathematical characterizations can be qualitative or anecdotal descriptions, and need not be numerical dimensions. The new symbolism permits a codification for all the different properties, however multiple, that an object may possess. Consequently, the new mathematical techniques can be employed to indicate the many qualitative features that distinguish people as units of illness, and to demarcate the different properties that are present or absent—alone or in overlapping combinations—in the clinical subgroups of complex populations of human disease.

With these new techniques, a formal mathematical structure can be established for the clinical reasoning applied in the deductive logic of diagnosis, in the inductive predictions of prognosis, and in the quantitative assessment of therapy.

OBSERVATION, AND THE USE OF NUMBERS

Ever since Kelvin[46] stated the doctrine that measurement was a prerequisite to science, biologists have been trying to measure, and clinicians have felt lost. A clinician could measure height, blood pressure, urinary volume, and cardiac output, but how could he measure headache, angina pectoris, dysuria, or anxiety? What could a clinician possibly do to measure *all* of the subjective sensations, qualitative signs, and personal reactions that were inevitable parts of the data noted in clinical observation? Quite clearly, if science depended on dimensional measurement, a clinician could never attain science; he could never escape his inability to find dimensional expressions for many phenomena of the bedside.

For the past half century, the clinician's usual way out of this scientific dilemma has been to escape the phenomena of the bedside. In order to measure, he has measured what he could measure: not the variables he observed clinically, but the entities he observed in the laboratory. By using laboratory technology, clinicians have improved precision in previous measurements of disease entities, and have learned to measure many entities that were previously either unrecognized or assessed only qualitatively. Consequently, modern clinicians have become adept at getting measurements for everything in medicine except the unique clinical evidence observed at the bedside. For clinical science, Kelvin's doctrine has had the same practical implication that Frank Knight[47] noted for it in social science: "If you cannot measure, measure anyhow."

These para-clinical activities in measurement depend on the beliefs that number is the "language" of science, and that statistical analysis is an important part of the "grammar". The beliefs are correct, but the current concept of measurement is not. The contemporary biologic ideas of measurement are often restricted only to *mensuration:* the use of a scale or some other type of "yardstick" to determine a dimension that represents the amount of some substance. Many clinical investigators today believe that this kind of dimensional mensuration is the only form of measurement.

There is another type of measurement, however, that also produces numbers: counting. In this alternative form of measurement, the number represents the *enumeration* of a group of entities that have been categorized as similar units; the counted number is the sum of the units present in a particular situation. A counted number is just as *numerical* as a dimensional number. A quantity of particles, events, or people is just as much of a measurement as the quantity of a chemical substance present in blood—but one type of number is measured by enumeration and the other by mensuration. A counted number is a sum of individual units; a dimensional number is a proportional amount of some unit (such as grams, ounces, or minutes) demarcated on a scale. A counted number is an integer; a dimensional number can be an integer or a fraction. A counted number answers the question, "How many?"; a dimensional number answers the question, "How much?".

Although both types of measurement produce a number, the scientific reliability of the number depends on the fundamental observational procedures of *identification* and *comparison*. In dimensional measurement, the entity to be assessed is a particular attribute or substance contained within an observed collection or mixture of substances. The entity is first identified by extracting or in some way isolating it from the mixture in which it is contained; the isolated entity is then given dimension by comparing its magnitude on a previously calibrated scale. In enumerational measurement, the entity to be assessed is already a unit, and the measurement consists of finding a particular category in which the unit is to be counted. The entity is first identified by observing its many different attributes; the identified entity is then classified as a member of some particular subgroup after its attributes are compared with those of other units in the subgroup.

Thus, for example, we determine the amount of uric acid in blood by applying chemical methods to isolate uric acid, and scalar methods to assess its magnitude. We decide to count a patient as having or not having tophaceous gout by observing his various attributes (including his joints, subcutaneous tissues, and uric acid value), and by comparing his attributes with those of other patients who have tophaceous gout.

The critical features of mensuration are thus *isolation* of the entity and *calibration* of the scale. The critical features of enumeration are *observation* of the attributes and *criteria* for their classification. If the methods for chemical isolation and scalar assessment are reliable, the uric acid will be measured correctly. If the methods of clinical observation and criteria for classification are reliable, the patient will be counted correctly as having tophaceous gout.

The search for "measurement" should not obscure the realization that precise identifications and comparisons are the basis of "measurement" and that scientific *precision* requires precision in what a number represents, and not merely a number alone. Clinical phenomena can constantly be evaluated to yield numerical data, but the numbers will often arise from counting units whose basic identifications are verbal rather than dimensional. Many of the attributes, events, or patients counted as clinical units are often identified by dimensional measurement, but many others require verbal description. (Thus, a patient's height, weight, and temperature are dimensionally measured; his race, sex, and symptoms are verbally described.) Almost all the important observations of pathology and most of the symptoms and signs observed clinically depend on verbal description—on the use of words rather than numbers.

There is no ordinary method, for example, of dimensionally measuring the difference in physical appearance between a man and a woman. Yet a child can give a precise description of most of the distinctions. There is no ordinary method of dimensionally measuring the firmness of a carcinoma, the fluctuation of an abscess, the croak of a rhonchus, or the rasp of a murmur. Yet each of these distinctions can be described precisely. There is no ordinary method of dimensionally measuring the locations, qualities, and other characteristics of the different types of pain produced by toothache, migraine, pleurisy, abdominal cramps, or angina pectoris. Yet each pain can be differentiated distinctly and precisely by verbal description. A dimensional measurement of duration can be made for a pain that begins acutely at a specific moment, but not for a pain that starts insidiously. The dimensional duration of the two pains may not be needed, however, to determine their origin and significance. The descriptive properties of acute onset or of insidious onset are *precise* features of the two types of pain and can often be used to distinguish between them with scientific exactness.

These distinctions between dimensional numbers and counted numbers are also reflected in the way the numbers are statistically analyzed. Before the analysis begins, the numbers must first receive an arrangement that correlates or associates the variables they represent. If the variables are few, dependent, and dimensional, their relationship can usually be portrayed by drawing a curve on a graph, and by "fitting" that curve with a binomial, polynomial, or differential equation from ordinary algebra and the calculus. In the statistical analysis of such curvilinear relationships, we determine the coefficients used for writing the equation that best approximates the curve (or line), and we obtain an indication of how well the equation fits the data. If the variables, however, describe the multiple, independent, discrete attributes of different patients, the relationships between variables and counted numbers cannot be drawn as a curve on an ordinary graph, and cannot be expressed in the conventional "old" mathematical systems just cited.

To correlate the variables used for characterizing and counting different patients, we often use *tables* rather than *graphs*. A "point" on a graph represents the *dimensional* "intersection" of an abscissa and ordinate that are the measured quantities of independent and dependent variables. A "cell" in a table corresponds to a "point" on a graph, and represents the *logical* "intersection" (defined later in Chapter 10) of two variables that may be discrete, independent, and verbally described rather than continuous, dependent, and dimensionally measured.

In planning the arrangement of variables to indicate these logical "intersections" in a table, we can use the mathematics of set theory and Boolean algebra. In giving the "tables" a visual portrayal analogous to "graphs", we can use the Venn diagrams discussed later in Chapter 10. These techniques identify and compare the patients enumerated for such tabular statistical data as percentages, and for such analytic statistical tests as χ^2.

The differences in the "units" of material observed clinically and those observed in the laboratory thus require methodologic distinctions so drastic that even the systems of mathematical analysis, as well as the techniques for getting numbers, must be different. Laboratory workers often measure dimensions, and equate. Clinicians often classify cases, and count. These differences in mathematical management of numerical data are so basic that two different systems have been necessary for the computer devices now popular in scientific research. The difference between the devices (expressed in over-simplified form) is that the analog computer measures dimensions, and its circuits use the differential and integral equations of continuous variables; the digital computer counts units, and its circuits use the Boolean algebra of discrete variables.

With modern mathematical systems of data management, and with appropriate attention to acquisition of the data, clinical studies of bedside therapy can now achieve the main principle of Kelvin's demand for scientific measurement. The individual attributes of patients may still be described verbally, but the data will be expressed in numerical form as the sums of counted patients or of counted attributes.

These scientific quantifications cannot be achieved, however, until clinicians give as much attention to precision in verbal description as they now give to precision in measured dimension. Attention to precise verbal description is not unusual in biologic science. Some of the greatest achievements of modern biology and medicine—including the work of Mendel, Virchow, Darwin, Pavlov, and all the contemporary research in electron microscopy and chromosomal characteristics—have been based not on dimension alone, but on precise observation and verbal description.

Instead of zealously seeking dimensional measurement for symptoms, signs, and other human properties that cannot be dimensionally measured with precision or convenience, clinicians must seek ways of improving the value of their own verbal clinical descriptions of these entities. The clinical examination of patients is frequently dismissed as unreliable because the data are not always reproducible. Yet the unreliability is often attributable to the examiner, not the patient. Patients may describe symptoms imprecisely or inconsistently because of defects not in the history, but in the history-taker. Physical signs may change from one examination to another only because the examiner has changed.

The subsequent chapters of this book will demonstrate some of the ways in which clinical data are used as necessary constituents of scientific analyses in prognosis and therapy. For symptoms and signs to attain their full scientific potential, however, they must be reliable as basic observational data, and the observations must be performed not by laboratory techniques or by measuring devices incapable of the performance, but by an irreplaceable human medical apparatus—the clinician.

CORRELATIONS, AND BIOLOGIC "DISSOCIATION" OF FORM AND FUNCTION

A primary concept of biology is that form and function are constantly associated. Birds, having wings, fly; fish, having fins, swim; men, having legs, walk. The human eye sees, the ear hears, the brain thinks, the heart beats, the stomach absorbs, and the uterus incubates. In all these aspects of biology, so beautifully analyzed by Darwin,[48] D'Arcy Thompson,[49] and others, the general form of an organism or organ, and its function, are directly correlated. The principle is so basic and so well-established, when appropriate, that we almost never stop to realize all the violations we constantly see around us.

In normal human biology, for example, we can find two baseball players whose biceps' circumferences, actomyosin bands, and electromyograms are identical. Yet one player throws an effective curve ball and the other does not. Two human stomachs may appear identical in their shape, size, mucosa, and exposure to food; yet one stomach may consistently secrete more acid each day than the other. Provoked by the same cutaneous pain stimulus, one healthy person may be tormented; another may remain stoic. We can regularly find two people with identical anatomic structures in brain, and identical scores on some quantified test of intelligence. Yet one person may be an imaginative but careless worker; the other may be careful but unimaginative.

As Szent-Györgi[50] has said, "There is no real difference between structure and function; they are two sides of the same coin. If structure does not tell us anything about function, it means we have not looked at it correctly." In contemporary biology, there are still many entities awaiting correct observation. Hundreds of distinctions in uniquely human functions cannot now be explained by the known structural characteristics of the people, organs, tissues, or cells that perform the functions. A day may come when *all* of these normal functional distinctions in structures, ranging from cells to people, will be explainable by differences found in their molecular or inframolecular components and configurations. But that day is long distant, and only the most hypermetropic of visionaries can foresee it on any current horizon. Until that day comes, we shall have to assess and describe curve-ball throwing, acid secretion, reactions to cutaneous pain, and human imagination with methods and vocabularies disparate from those used to characterize the corresponding structure of muscle, stomach, skin, or brain.

In human disease, the frequency of dissociation between abnormal structure and abnormal function has established our contemporary diagnostic practices in clinical medicine. The reason clinicians do a complete physical examination "routinely", instead of examining just the regions suggested by a patient's symptoms, is to find structural abnormalities that have produced no symptoms. The reason we order many "routine" roentgenograms and laboratory tests, instead of confining our tests to those indicated by the overt clinical abnormalities, is to find diseases that have produced neither symptoms nor signs. In an *asymptomatic* patient we do the complete physical examinations and tests to find an unsuspected heart murmur, retinal exudate, or prostatic nodule; we order the diagnostic adjuncts that will detect clinically inapparent lung cancer or tuberculosis by chest roentgenogram, rectal cancer by sigmoidoscopy, chronic leukemia by white blood cell morphology, or atrio-ventricular block by electrocardiogram. Whenever we get a positive result in one of these examinations of an asymptomatic patient, we have found another instance in which gross structure and clinical function were dissociated in human disease.

This frequent dissociation of diseased form and function is also the reason for ordering so many diagnostic tests in patients who *do* have overt symptoms and signs. Years ago, for example, we thought that almost all patients with hemoptysis, fever, weight loss, and pulmonary râles had tuberculosis. Today we know that many such patients may have carcinoma, viral pneumonia, bronchiectasis, or many other diseases—so we order roentgenograms, bacterial cultures, Papanicolaou smears, and biopsies to help us distinguish the different anatomic lesions that can produce identical abnormalities in clinical function.

Not only do the structural lesions of a disease often fail to correlate with *clinical* dysfunctions, but the lesions also often fail to correlate with the dysfunctions discernible in *laboratory* tests. For example, the histologic character of the nephritis detected in a biopsy of renal tissue often has no relationship to the amount of azotemia; the atrial septal defect demonstrated by angiocardiography does not indicate whether or not the atria are fibrillating in the electrocardiogram. So clinicians order the biopsy *and* the measurement of blood urea nitrogen, the angiocardiogram *and* the electrocardiogram.

There are many human diseases, of course, in which form and function, or clinical manifestation and laboratory manifestation, are well correlated. A clinician's ability to diagnose disease purely from its clinical manifestations depends on the frequency of these correlations. We know that angina pectoris, a function, regularly correlates with coronary arteriosclerosis, a form. We know that yellow-colored skin, a clinical manifestation, regularly correlates with hyperbilirubinemia, a laboratory test; that the clinical manifestation of cyanosis regularly correlates with the laboratory manifestation of hypoxemia; or that the clinical finding of "lid-lag" is regularly associated with the high serum protein-bound iodine of hyperthyroidism.

Nevertheless, even these entities may occasionally be dissociated. Anginal pain may arise from pulmonary hypertension, not coronary disease; coronary disease may produce no angina. Skin may look yellow because of hypercarotenemia; a serum bilirubin value may be elevated without evident clinical jaundice. Cyanosis may be due to methemoglobinemia; a hypoxemic patient may be too anemic to look cyanotic. Lid-lag may sometimes occur in healthy people or in euthyroid patients with pulmonary disease; the exophthalmos associated with the lid-lag and hyperthyroidism may persist long after treatment has made the patient euthyroid or even hypothyroid; hyperthyroidism may produce no lid-lag; and an elevation of protein-bound iodine, associated with neither lid-lag nor hyperthyroidism, may be due to residual deposits of iodine dye used in a previous gall bladder X-ray examination.

The very profusion of adjunctive diagnostic tests in clinical medicine today is a direct result of the frequent dissociation between the forms and functions of diseased human biology. Clinicians order these tests in order to bring the specificity of science to the separate identification of both form and function. After achieving this specificity, however, clinicians generally obscure it in the language used for diagnostic and therapeutic identifications of sick people. A patient's clinical state is often identified by a phrase describing an abnormal structure *or* an abnormal function but not both.

If abnormal structure and abnormal function could always be correlated, so that one constantly implied the other and vice versa, the brevity of many incomplete diagnostic phrases would be justified. In clinical medicine, however, form-function dissociations occur so frequently that profound errors in communication and reasoning are produced by abbreviated diagnostic statements. The abbreviations may permit a particular diagnosis of morbid anatomy to imply the existence of an abnormal function that is not always present. The term *myocardial infarction,* for example, usually conveys the clinical idea of chest pain, yet many patients with myocardial infarction have no chest pain. The term *cancer* or *carcinoma* conveys the idea of a disseminating lethal malignancy, yet basal cell carcinoma of the skin seldom disseminates beyond its local region, and some patients with other carcinomas (in such locations as breast) have refused treatment and have died of other causes. *Schizophrenia* often suggests a huddled body in the back wards of a state mental hospital, but many schizophrenic patients walk the streets, function well at work, and sometimes even achieve high public office. *Duodenal ulcer* suggests abdominal distress, but many ulcer patients are pain-free. *Endometriosis,* which suggests abnormal gynecologic bleeding or cramps, may be an unexpected discovery to a gynecologist operating to remove an asymptomatic mass that he initially thought was a fibroid.

In the examples just cited and in many others, the diagnostic name of a disease is inadequate to distinguish the diverse functional effects that can occur in different patients who have the same pathologic lesion. To identify a patient, rather than a disease, the name of an abnormal structure is not enough. Yet clinicians, when communicating in speech or in writing, persist in identifying sick people by means of incomplete diagnostic phrases that obscure both the patient's initial clinical situation and the results of the therapy. In the clinical literature, for example, the results of treatment for "duodenal ulcer" are often reported without indicating whether the ulcer was bleeding or not, or painful or not. The report of treatment for "bleeding peptic ulcer" may specify neither the presence or absence of previous pain, nor the anatomic location of the ulcer in stomach or duodenum. Many other distinctions of illness are constantly omitted from the reported analyses of treatment for "peptic ulcer"—and then internists and surgeons wonder why so many disagreements exist about the many different medical and surgical modes of treatment that are available for the ulcers.

We see the chaos of contemporary literature in the anticoagulant treatment of "myocardial infarction", where the reported results are seldom separated and correlated for clinical subgroups that did or did not have chest pain, shock, congestive heart failure, or cardiac arrythmias. In the treatment of diabetes mellitus, we read of strict diet versus no diet, rigid regulation of blood sugar or regulation of only urinary acetone—in reports that make no distinction between a diabetic patient who is fat or thin, and "brittle" or "non-brittle" in the ability to remain normoglycemic without frequently developing insulin shock. In these and in many other chronic diseases, the clinical features of the treated patients are regularly omitted in the analysis of therapeutic results.

After scrupulously obtaining the diverse data that precisely distinguish the clinical, laboratory, and morphologic dissociations of form and function in human disease, the clinician then often proceeds to obliterate his patient's distinctions by consolidating them into a short identifying phrase that is called a "diagnosis".

CLASSIFICATION, AND SYSTEMS OF TAXONOMY

The word taxonomy stems from the Greek τάξις, *arrangement* or *order*, and νομος, *law*. Although *taxonomy,* as a word, refers to "classification" or to "systems of categorization", the term *taxonomy* has for several centuries connoted the branch of biology which deals with the "classification of animals and plants according to their natural relationships".[44] As a term of designation, *taxonomy* is obviously applicable to many other systems of classification. There is a taxonomy of library books (one such taxonomy is called the Dewey Decimal System), of chemical elements (called the Periodic Table), of words (published in a thesaurus or dictionary), of occupations, of colors, of postage stamps, and of almost any collection of entities that have enough in common to warrant a classified distinction of their differences. As a name, *taxonomy* is preferable to *system of classification* because it is shorter and because a single taxonomy may include several different systems or aspects of classification.

In contemporary science, taxonomy has become an important creative intellectual discipline. Modern technology is constantly providing many new types of data that need classification, and modern systems of data management require discrete, specific arrangement of the information into numerical codes and other patterns. The strategy and tactics of taxonomy in data classification have aroused the interest of biologists and of many other investigators now active in such new scholarly domains as information systems, data processing, and computer methodology. Far from both the bedsides and laboratories of today's clinical biology, many alert minds are exploring the challenges of taxonomy as a basic problem in scientific thought.[51-54]

The subject of taxonomy is hardly ever considered in contemporary medicine, however, either because the term *taxonomy* is usually reserved for botanical or zoological classifications, or because of the general belief that medicine—having entered the era of "molecular biology"—has been liberated from the classificational problems that were a primary concern of the past. To many modern clinical scientists, the very word *taxonomy* conjures up the image of an ancient biologist, passively observing the forms of nature, conceiving *schemas* and *rubrics* to categorize them, pedantically debating the merits of minutiae in different systems of classification, and speculating—without experimental proof—about the causes of what he saw and classified. Content to have advanced from the age of morphologic taxonomy to the age of experimental technology in medicine, a modern clinical scientist tends to regard attention to taxonomy as retrogression to an archaic past whose scientific defects lingered all too long. Besides, the problem of taxonomy in clinical medicine was presumably settled long ago when pathologists investigated and classified the morbid anatomy of disease.

These two beliefs—that medical taxonomy is too archaic a topic for intellectual concern, and that there are no taxonomic problems requiring solution—are the source of the fifth, and perhaps most important, of the major contemporary conceptual barriers to clinical science. What is archaic in clinical medicine today is not the idea of taxonomy, but the idea that the complex natural phenomena occurring in diseased people can be adequately classified by a taxonomy devoted only to disease. This concept—so well established, so pervasive in clinical thought, and so enormous a barrier to science in every ramification of clinical medicine—will be the last main topic for discussion in completing the "diagnosis" of intellectual infirmity in our current state of clinical science.

5. The Diagnostic Taxonomy of Disease: Past and Present

In his lucid discussion of patterns of scientific discovery, Bronowski[55] has made the remark, "A science which orders its thought too early is stifled." He illustrates the point by referring to ancient theories of taxonomy that long hindered the development of modern physics and chemistry, because a science "cannot develop a system of ordering its observations . . . until . . . [it] has passed through a long stage of observation and trial."

Despite the venerable traditions of clinical medicine, the observations and experiments of the modern era of clinical therapy are generally less than 50 years old. Before the technologic revolution of the past half century, a clinician could seldom confirm his diagnoses of disease until necropsy, and could seldom modify diseases by treatment with specific, potent agents. Today, with modern diagnostic and therapeutic techniques, a clinician can usually identify diseases early and accurately, and can often treat them effectively. This transition from passive observation to active experimentation has produced the new therapeutic domain of clinical medicine—an experimental discipline with novel data and procedures that are strikingly different from clinical activities of the past.

The development of science in this young therapeutic discipline is being stifled by an ancient taxonomy. The organization of data and thought in modern clinical therapy is still based on a diagnostic classification of disease—the taxonomy of morbid anatomy—that was initiated almost 200 years ago. In preserving the diagnostic nomenclature of pathologic anatomy as the main contemporary system of identifying human ailments, clinicians perpetuate a mode of thinking that classifies morphologic form, but not clinical function; that classifies disease, but not people or illness; and that classifies clinical inferences, but not clinical observations.

Diagnosis is the focal point of thought in the treatment of a patient. From diagnosis, which gives a name to the patient's ailment, the thinking goes chronologically backward to decide about pathogenesis and etiology of the ailment. From diagnosis also, the thinking goes chronologically forward to predict prognosis and to choose therapy. As the main language of clinical communication, diagnostic labels transmit a rapid understanding of the contents of the package; diagnostic categories provide names for the intellectual locations in which clinicians store the observations of clinical experience. The taxonomy used for diagnosis will thus inevitably establish the patterns in which clinicians observe, think, remember, and act. Yet the main diagnostic taxonomy used by clinicians today depends on the concepts and nomenclature of morbid anatomy observed by pathologists.

Clinicians have become so accustomed to using anatomic phrases as diagnostic nomenclature that we may fail to notice that morbid anatomy, rather than clinical observation, is the principal language of most clinical discussions. Consider some of the many different terms clinicians use as diagnoses:

> *myocardial infarction, phlebothrombosis, lobar pneumonia, duodenal ulcer, carcinoma of the stomach, cholelithiasis, cerebral arteriosclerosis, multiple sclerosis, hepatic cirrhosis, pseudocyst of the pancreas, atrial septal defect,* and the various *-itises—nephritis, diverticulitis, colitis, cystitis,* and many others.

Not a single one of these diagnostic terms represents an entity that is ever actually seen, heard, or touched in the ordinary bedside observations of a clinician. Every one of these entities is an abnormality of internal anatomic structure. The clinician at the bedside never observes these abnormal structures directly; he observes the symptoms and signs that are their clinical effects. With roentgenography, a clinician may see the silhouettes and shadows of these abnormal structures; with endoscopy, he may see those portions of an abnormality visible in the accessible lumen; with laboratory tests, he may note the associated disorders in physiologic and biochemical function; with surgical exploration in suitable situations, he may see a larger view of the abnormal structure and of its anatomic relations. But the only doctor who regularly witnesses the actual, complete appearance of all these anatomic entities—the only doctor who can regularly see them, feel them, and even cut them—is a pathologist.

Clinicians, however, work as clinicians, not as pathologists. A clinician's nomenclature must classify a host *and* an illness *and* a disease; a pathologist's nomenclature classifies only a disease. The taxonomy of a clinician must classify the patient's abnormalities in physiologic function, in biochemical function, and in clinical function as well as the abnormalities in structure; the taxonomy of an anatomic pathologist classifies only the structural lesions. A clinician must have a language that will categorize the living phenomena of the bedside, the variations in human clinical behavior, and the nuances of human response to sickness and to therapy; the pathologist's anatomic language provides categories for the morphologic entities of the operating room and morgue.

Clinicians, for example, often infer or diagnose the existence of myocardial infarction, but they do not observe a *myocardial infarction* clinically. Clinicians, instead, observe patients with or without chest pain, shock, dyspnea, edema, arrhythmias, or rubs. Clinicians see roentgenographic shadows, electrocardiographic tracings, and the data of other laboratory tests. But only a pathologist sees the myocardial infarction. In treating a patient's myocardial infarction with narcotics, vasopressors, or digitalis, clinicians choose, change, and evaluate the therapy not for what it does to *myocardial infarction,* but for its effect on pain, shock, or arrhythmias. When clinicians estimate prognosis or plan future management for a patient with myocardial infarction, the major ingredients of the judgmental decisions include clinical features of the illness and personal features of the host, and not just the pathologic diagnosis of disease.

The current concepts and nomenclature of "disease" are but the most recent of many different approaches used throughout medical history to classify human ailments. The classification of disease is called *nosology,* and nosology, like clinical activities, has undergone many changes before arriving at its present state. The changes have been well described by Faber[56] and by King.[57]

The nosologists of the past and present have used at least two different approaches for identifying "disease", and have classified at least three different types of data. In the *empirical* or observational approach to classification, the classified entity is a substance or phenomenon that has actually been witnessed; in the *hypothetical* or inferential approach, the classified entity is a deduction or speculation about the cause, "essence", or some other inferred attribute of what was observed. In an empirical classification of "disease", the categorized data can be the clinical manifestations (signs and symptoms) that are observed at the bedside, or the anatomic manifestations (in organs, tissues, and cells) that are observed in the necropsy room and laboratory. In a hypothetical classification, the categorized data can be the etiologic inferences contained in old or new iatrochemical theories—such as black bile or cholesterol metabolism, and deranged humors or endocrine imbalance—and in ancient or modern notions about infectious disease—such as miasmas or microbes.

In the days of Hippocrates, nosology was generally empirical, and many of the "diseases" were individual clinical manifestations, observed at the bedside as subjective symptoms and physical signs. The diagnostic terminology contained such "diseases" as *fever, cyanosis, consumption,* and *asthma.* This observational system of diagnostic nomenclature persisted for many centuries, although augmented (and sometimes replaced) by various etiologic nosologies based on chemical, infectious, or other hypothetical theories of "disease".

By the 17th century, inference rather than observation had become the prevalent basis for nosology. The nomenclature of individual symptoms and signs had proved unsatisfactory as a general means of classifying "disease", and morbid anatomy had not yet been studied well enough to provide an alternative empirical system. The existing knowledge of morbid anatomy in the 17th century had produced only

> ... disconnected observations, curiosities and abnormalities, from which were drawn no conclusions of importance for general pathology. ... Scientists revelled in theories and systems, more particularly in the hazy chemical theories ... which had been disseminated among the physicians throughout Europe by Paracelsus. These theories form the earliest beginnings of chemical physiology and the chemical conception of pathologic phenomena.[58]

The iatrochemical school of nosology was further advanced on the European continent during the 17th century by Sylvius and van Helmont, who developed many chemical concepts of "disease". Boyle's, Hooke's, and other early experiments in the physiology of respiration gave further support in England to the British iatrochemical theorists, then headed by Willis.

It was also in 17th century England, however,

> ... that the man lived and worked who was the severest opponent of the speculations of the iatrochemists, and who first consciously and clearly gave clinical observation its place of honor as a scientific method—Thomas Sydenham.[59]

Sydenham, trying to reject speculative hypotheses and philosophical systems, insisted that clinical reasoning be founded on direct bedside observation and on descriptions of what is now called the "natural history" of disease. He repudiated the general supposition "that diseases are no more than the confused and irregular operations of disordered and debilitated nature, and consequently that it is a fruitless labor to endeavour to give a just description of them".[60] Instead, Sydenham maintained that "Nature, in the production of disease, is uniform and consistent. . . . The selfsame phenomena that you observe in the sickness of a Socrates you would observe in the sickness of a simpleton".[61]

To Sydenham, "disease" was still a clinical rather than an anatomic abnormality, but he improved the existing clinical nosology by reviving and developing two taxonomic concepts that today might be called *cluster* and *temporal correlation.* In the concept of *cluster,* which is often used medically to designate a "syndrome", several individual manifestations are combined to form a single entity of "disease". In the concept of *temporal correlation,* a "disease" is named not just according to its immediate manifestations, but according to the correlated pattern of its evolving clinical course, or "natural history". Using these concepts, Sydenham descriptively separated the clustered temporal pattern of *gout* from the individual entities that had been called *rheumatism,* and the clusters of *measles* and *scarlatina* from what had been called *exanthemata;* he identified many other cluster entities, replacing their individual symptomatic designations by such titles as *St. Vitus dance* (chorea minor) and *quartan ague* (malaria). As King points out,[62] Sydenham "did not concern himself with the higher echelons of classification. He was content to bring precision into a few disease species, leaving more sweeping classification to his successors."

Relying on clinical manifestations alone, Sydenham's successors in the 18th century developed elaborate nosologies to classify "diseases" according to arbitrary clusters of symptoms and signs. Linnaeus, after creating an effective observational taxonomy for botany and biology, produced a medical classification system that had 11 major categories and 325 subdivisions of clinical "disease". Sauvages, using a similar approach, devised 10 major classes of "disease", subdivided into 44 orders, 315 genera, and 2400 species—all of them based on symptoms and signs. Cullen and others later tried to simplify these clinical nosologies by giving greater attention to internal logic in selecting categories, and by making a Sydenham-like attempt to distinguish individual symptoms and signs from "diseases".

The main defect of these 18th century nosologies was an intellectual construction that depended on cluster but not on correlation. The 18th century nosologists, King notes, "loaded themselves down with cumbersome nomenclature and an inadequate philosophy of science . . .".[63] The categories of the nosology were chosen as seemingly logical groupings of the observed clinical data, but no significant effort was made to select categories that would correlate with either the course of the defined "diseases" or with the underlying morbid anatomy. Sydenham's concepts of temporal correlation had been overlooked, and the morphologic concepts of pathology had not yet been fully developed. Consequently, the 18th century nosologies were uncorrelated catalogues of clinical manifestations—classifications prepared for the sake of classification, but lacking the prognostic or anatomic significance that would make the results practical and useful.

Although pathologic anatomy had been investigated sporadically during the 18th century and earlier, and had been advanced by the publication of Morgagni's *magnum opus* in 1761, a consistent system of anatomic correlations for "disease" was not provided until the 19th century. Begun by Pinel and Bichat, developed by many other French clinicians, and later augmented by workers throughout Europe, the characterization of "disease" as an entity of morbid anatomy produced a revolution in clinical thinking and a diagnostic taxonomy that has endured to the present.

A diagnostic nomenclature based on pathologic anatomy immediately removed two of the many obvious scientific disadvantages—in evidence and vocabulary—of the preceding "etiologic" and "clinical" classification systems:

1) The "etiologic" concepts of classification were speculative, unaccompanied by observational evidence. The "clinical" concepts were based on observation, but the evidence was transitory, not preserva-

ble, and often consisted only of a patient's subjective feeling. The organs and tissues of pathology, by contrast, were overt evidence that could be preserved and reviewed objectively.

2) The vocabulary of clinical descriptive language was a polyglot of observations made with different human sensory organs: the phrases described sights, odors, noises, palpatory sensations, discomforts, incapacitations, and many other sensory or intellectual perceptions. The descriptive vocabulary of morbid anatomy, although occasionally olfactory or tactile, required mainly the language and discipline of visual observation. In dealing with clinical evidence, the clinician had to look, talk, listen, smell, touch, and sometimes taste. In dealing with organs and tissues, the pathologist had mainly to look, and could concentrate on developing precision in the vocabulary for describing what he saw.

With these advantages for preserving objective evidence and for confining descriptions to a comparatively simple sensory vocabulary, anatomic pathology offered clinical medicine a basic taxonomy that was clearly preferable to the old "clinical" or "etiologic" diagnostic nomenclature. By correlating what was observed clinically with what was found in morbid anatomy, clinicians began converting their classifications of "disease" from clinical into anatomic terminology. The very word *disease,* which had originated as an expression of a patient's abnormal sensations (his *dis-ease*), now often became used to designate an abnormality of gross or microscopic structure. The old "clinical" diagnoses were replaced by the types of modern pathologic terms already cited in the earlier examples (on page 73), and by many other morphologic phrases that classified diseases as inflammations, degenerations, tumors, congenital abnormalities, and other structural aberrations.

The change in taxonomy gave a firm, consistent histopathologic basis to clinical diagnosis. Such heterogeneous entities as *fever, cyanosis,* and *consumption* were removed from their previous status as names of disease, and were converted to clinical manifestations. (With successive changes in nomenclature, many leading historical figures of clinical medicine were deprived of their commemorative eponyms. *Bright's disease,* for example, became *nephritis,* and one of Von Recklinghausen's many diseases became *neurofibromatosis.* The medical penchant for eponyms continued, of course, only now the commemoratees were often pathologists, e.g., *Aschoff body* and *Virchow node.*)

Moreover, the taxonomy of anatomic pathology provided clinicians with a new and fundamental scientific challenge. Before anatomic pathology, the clinician's adventures with empirical therapy seldom had scientific quality, and he had no opportunity for experimental confirmation of his "scientific" speculations about causes of disease. With the advent of the new pathology, the clinician's anatomic diagnosis became an act of experimental reasoning. Until that moment in the history of science, the astronomer had been one of the few scientists who could confirm his experimental reasoning merely by observing nature. He could predict the orbital path of a planet, and, by observing the planet's course, determine the accuracy of his prediction. Now, too, the clinician could enjoy such a challenge. His diagnosis was a scientific prediction, made during life, of what the pathologist would find after death.

For the clinician of that era, who had few ancillary diagnostic tests beyond clinical examination and few effective therapeutic agents beyond compassion, a correct histopathologic diagnosis became the main goal that could be scientifically tested. After observing symptoms and signs at the bedside, the clinician reasoned with the evidence, as an act of art, to comfort the living patient, and, as an act of a science, to infer what the pathologist would find *post mortem* in the organs, tissues, and cells of the corpse.

This pathologic diagnostic challenge has become a standard part of the clinician's activities in patient care. The challenge has been amplified and made traditional by the popularity of the clinico-pathologic conference (CPC), conducted regularly in medical centers, both for its value as an effective teaching procedure and for the intellectual entertainment afforded the audience as the clinician-detective tries to "find the killer" in a "who-dunit" mystery that will shortly be "solved" by the pathologist.

During the past few decades, the CPC has lost some of its original intellectual attraction because the old disparity between "clinical" and necropsy evidence has been markedly reduced. The clinician's *pre-mortem* evidence now includes not only the traditional clinical observations, but also all the results of modern adjunctive diagnostic tests, providing many morphologic details that formerly could not be discerned until necropsy. With the increasing availability of biopsy for many anatomic structures, the clinician (and surgical pathologist) can now even see, during life, the very tissues that were formerly observable only after death. Consequently, in selecting CPC topics, the necropsy pathologist has fewer "interesting" cases to choose from, because a high percentage of diagnoses were already adequately established during life, and because many tissues were already examined *pre-mortem*. The clinician now finds the proceedings somewhat less instructive than formerly, because the many diagnostic tests performed while the patient was alive have often already demonstrated what used to be shown only by the necropsy pathologist.

Without (and sometimes even with) the aid of these adjunctive diagnostic procedures, however, a clinician's attempt to deduce an anatomic diagnosis is an extraordinary feat of intellectual virtuosity. Relying only on bedside observations, the clinician must traverse a maze of multiple sequential inferences before his clinical evidence is converted into an anatomic diagnostic deduction.

Consider the different ways in which a pathologist and a clinician perform anatomic diagnostic reasoning. The pathologist observes organs, tissues, and cells. To classify them, he needs criteria for deciding their normal range in morphologic structure, and for deciding when a structural abnormality is an inflammation, neoplasm, degeneration, or other derangement. But all of his classificational criteria deal with what he observes. To arrive at a diagnosis of morbid anatomy—such as *myocardial infarction, epidermoid carcinoma of the lung,* or *hepatic cirrhosis*—a pathologist makes no deductions or inferences. He classifies what he sees.

The pathologist often engages in many deductions, inferences, and speculations, but they deal primarily with causes of disease, not diagnosis. He may infer that the myocardial infarction was due to coronary atherosclerosis caused by abnormalities in lipid metabolism; that the carcinoma of the lung was caused by cigarette smoking, urban fumes, or other agents; and that the hepatic cirrhosis was possibly attributable to gallstone obstruction, poor nutrition, alcoholism, or previous hepatitis. In all of these etiologic decisions, the pathologist classifies what he infers; in all of his diagnostic decisions, he classifies what he observes.

Now consider the clinician's pathway to an anatomic diagnosis. At the bedside, a clinician makes certain direct observations of a patient's illness, manifested in the patient's story of his sensations, in the information sometimes obtained from conversation with other people, and in the findings noted by physical examination. These observations, made by both patient and clinician, are the actual direct "clinical" evidence. The clinician's first-order classification of this evidence is to designate certain entities with the names of different *symptoms* and *signs*. For example, the patient's description of a certain type of respiratory discomfort may be designated, by first-order classification, as the symptom of *dyspnea*. On examining the patient's legs, the clinician may observe a type of subcutaneous swelling that he designates, by first-order classification, as the sign of *edema*.

After these first-order classifications are completed, the clinician has essentially finished categorizing his observed evidence. If he gets no additional help from biopsies, roentgenograms, or laboratory tests, almost all of the remaining activities in classification are purely intellectual rather than observational. To achieve an anatomic diagnosis, the clinician must make a sequential series of deductions, classifying each new deduction, proceeding to the next deduction, classifying it, engaging perhaps in several additional inferential steps, and then finally reaching the ultimate inference that constitutes the anatomic diagnosis.

Let us assume, for the sake of example, that the clinician's diagnostic reasoning is purely "clinical", without the aid of adjunctive tests. His next step with the patient just described might be to combine some of the first-order classifications into a "cluster" or "syndrome". The "cluster" or "syndrome" may be a designation that arbitrarily combines a particular set of manifestations, or it may represent an abnormality in the physiologic function of some organ of the body. For example, the patient's pair of manifestations (dyspnea and edema) is often found as a clinical cluster in the functional disorders that are called *congestive heart failure, nephrotic syndrome,* and *hepatic decompensation.* The dyspnea and edema, of course, might not be caused by a single disorder. They might merely co-exist, each due to a separate cause. The dyspnea might be due to some local disorder in the lungs; the edema might be due to a local hydrostatic disorder in the veins of the legs.

At this point, the clinician must engage in at least three distinct acts of classificational decision. The first deals with his criteria for the designation of one of these cluster disorders. How many of the symptoms and signs that might occur in a total cluster does he require for designating that "disorder" as present? For example, is he willing to use the term *congestive heart failure* if a patient has dyspnea or edema but not both, or if a patient with dyspnea and edema does not have tachycardia or pulmonary signs? Will the clinician demand that ascites or jaundice be present in addition to dyspnea and edema before applying the designation of *hepatic decompensation?* Second, having decided about his general criteria for categorizing cluster disorders, the clinician now must decide whether to attribute the dyspnea and edema to two separate disorders or to one. Let us assume that he decides to consider only one disorder. His third step in this sequence of categorization is now to decide which one of the three cited disorders (in heart, liver, or kidney) is present. With this inferential decision, he thus converts his first-order classification choices (*dyspnea* and *edema*) into a second-order classification choice. Let us assume that his choice was *congestive heart failure.*

He is now ready for his third-order classification, an inference about the structural abnormality responsible for the congestive heart failure. He can choose among such categories as congenital, rheumatic, hypertensive, arteriosclerotic, or other forms of heart disease. To make this decision, he assesses some additional clinical evidence. The evidence may include such items as a history of previous childhood illness, the findings reported at prior physical examinations of the patient, the current dimensions of the blood pressure, the location of the apex beat of the heart, and the presence or absence of certain types of chest pain, murmurs, thrills, heaves, and cyanosis. To all this clinical evidence, the clinician now applies new criteria for inferring the type of cardiac structural lesion, thus completing his third-order classification.

And he may not be finished yet. Let us assume that he designated his third-order inference as *congenital heart disease.* He now must go on to a fourth-order inference and must sometimes go even higher. His next step here is to decide in which wall, valve, or associated vessel of the heart the congenital lesion is located. For this decision, he needs additional inferential criteria, based on clinical evidence that he may or may not have used until now.

Let us assume that the clinician, after applying his fourth-order criteria for this latest deduction, has now arrived at his final anatomic diagnosis, which he classifies as *atrial septal defect.* He may, of course, like the pathologist, want to go further into etiologic speculations about the cause of the atrial septal defect, deciding perhaps that it occurred because the patient's mother had rubella during the patient's gestation. But the clinician has now achieved an anatomic diagnosis, and, for the purposes of this example, he can rest.

Now recall, by contrast, how a pathologist makes the diagnosis of an atrial septal defect. He opens the dead heart and looks.

A taxonomy based on inference, rather than evidence, is bound to create many problems for its users. For any taxonomy to be used reproducibly by different people, each designation must be defined by comprehensive criteria. Such criteria are much easier to establish for observational than for inferential classifications.

When a taxonomic classification is based on observation, the criteria need only give descriptive specifications. When the classification is based on inference, the criteria must deal with all the various types of inclusions, exclusions, and probability decisions that occur in human deductive reasoning. For example, a simple verbal statement can be given for the criteria that enable a visible hole in the heart to be classified as an atrial septal defect, or that enable a certain type of respiratory sensation to be classified as dyspnea. It is much more difficult to state the criteria for inferring that an atrial septal defect is due to maternal rubella, or that dyspnea is due to congestive heart failure. When the endpoint of the taxonomic classification is reached after not one inference, but after a sequence of inferences, the problems of establishing reliable criteria and reproducible designations are enormous.

Clinicians already have many difficulties in clinical reasoning because good criteria are generally unavailable for even the first-order observational classifications of symptoms and signs. For example, no standard criteria exist for applying such symptom-names as *dyspnea* and *anorexia* to the respiratory or digestive sensations described by a patient; no standard criteria exist for applying the sign-names of *râle* or *third heart sound* to the auscultatory noises heard by a clinician. When clinicians advance from the first-order observational to the subsequent inferential classifications, the existing troubles are multiplied exponentially. With uncommon exception,* no consistent, generally accepted, and generally used clinical criteria exist today for *any* of the reasoning used in the sequence of second-, third-, fourth-, or higher-order inferential classifications that lead from clinical observation to anatomic diagnosis.

Every clinician has his own criteria for clinical diagnosis of *congestive heart failure, nephrotic syndrome, and hepatic decompensation,* but no criteria have been standardized and none are used uniformly. Every clinician has his own criteria for such clinical diagnoses as *hypertension* or *coronary artery disease,* but no definitive criteria

---

* At least one exception in anatomic diagnosis is *rheumatoid arthritis,* for which clinical diagnostic criteria were recently established.[64] Another exception, although the diagnostic name is not an anatomic entity, is *rheumatic fever,* a diagnosis whose uniformity has been markedly improved by the establishment[65] and subsequent modifications[5, 66] of the Jones criteria.

have been established. Every clinical textbook contains many remarks about diagnosis of disease, but none presents the rigorous delineations required of scientific criteria. Even a traditional textbook[67] devoted specifically to "nomenclature and criteria" for cardiovascular disease contains no instructions for the type of exclusions and inclusions that are required in inferential reasoning, and the editors of the most recent edition have purposefully eliminated the crucial first-order classification of physical findings as having "no rightful place in a nomenclature or in a set of criteria".[68]

With criteria absent, underdeveloped, ignored, or deliberately excluded for all of the intellectual acts that convert clinical observation into anatomic inference, every clinician has developed his own techniques of diagnostic reasoning. Some of the techniques are excellent and some are not, but all lack the standardization of science. Consequently, diagnostic controversies and misunderstandings are rampant in clinical medicine today—particularly for diseases whose diagnosis is not easily confirmed by the various adjunctive tests that supplement contemporary clinical examination.

The same diagnostic name may represent different clinical entities to different clinicians; conversely, different diagnostic names may be used for the same disease. For example, despite all the clinical studies devoted in the past 20 years to anticoagulant therapy of myocardial infarction, no consistent criteria have been uniformly used for all the different observations and inferences contained in the clinical diagnosis of *myocardial infarction*. Some of the studies have even included patients with *impending myocardial infarction,* but have not specified what is meant by "impending". Many of the current conflicts about anticoagulant therapy for this disease may be due to the difficulty of reproducibly identifying an experimental material repeatedly classified according to criteria that are diverse or unstated. Similar uncertainties and ambiguities exist for the clinical distinctions used in diagnosis of such anatomic diseases as *cerebral arteriosclerosis, diverticulitis, chronic nephritis,* and *ulcerative colitis.* A different type of illustration for this problem is provided by the discovery only recently[69, 70] that the *chronic bronchitis* diagnosed by clinicians in Britain and the *pulmonary emphysema* diagnosed by clinicians in the United States were essentially the same disease.

In no other branch of science is the main taxonomy so distant from the data. As a clinician's reasoning goes sequentially from one inference to the next before he finally reaches an anatomic diagnosis, each step in the sequence takes him farther from the observed evidence, and increases the difficulty of achieving reliable criteria for the total classification process. For the diagnostic reasoning of a pathologist, who observes the dead tissue that he classifies, the nomenclature of morbid anatomy gives the histologic evidence immediate vitality. For the diagnostic reasoning of a clinician, who observes the signs and symptoms of a living patient, the nomenclature of morbid anatomy encloses bedside evidence in a shroud of inference for the distant microscope and morgue.*

Before the end of the 19th century, Claude Bernard and many German pathologic physiologists had begun to reject the nosology of morbid anatomy for its failure to identify abnormal function in human "disease". If necropsy had remained the only way of confirming anatomic diagnosis, clinicians might also have begun to reject morphologic taxonomy for its requirement of too many inferences that could not be verified during the life of a patient.

At this stage in the long history of nosology, however, there occurred the technologic revolution of the 20th century. Roentgenography, endoscopy, biopsy, and unprecedented surgical operations became available, allowing clinicians to observe specific representations of morbid anatomy during life. With these new techniques of observation, the clinician could now classify evidence directly. For pathologic diagnosis alone, he could often abandon his purely clinical inferences and could sometimes abandon even his clinical observations. His anatomic conclusions after physical examination of the chest could seldom be as penetrating as those made with help of the X-ray; his palpating finger could neither reach as far into the rectum nor see as well as his sigmoidoscopically aided eye; his mind need not probe too deeply to identify a tissue amenable to biopsy with

---

* Not all branches of clinical diagnosis have fallen under the spell of the pathologist's vocabulary. Dermatology has continued to maintain its own taxonomy—a colorful cornucopia of concatenating cutaneous classification. Dermatologists, luckier than most other clinicians, can constantly see and touch the disease they diagnose in the skin, and so the dermatologist still makes diagnoses based on what he, rather than the pathologist, observes. The diagnostic vocabulary of dermatology is doubtlessly over-cluttered and sometimes seems strange to other clinicians, but the taxonomy is effective. Despite many problems in the appraisal of therapy, the domain of dermatology seldom suffers from the kinds of major controversies and misunderstandings that are particularly common about *diagnoses* in internal medicine.

needle or knife; and, should all these other maneuvers fail to achieve an anatomic diagnosis, he could now in relative safety take a surgical look at almost any part of the body.

The nosology of morbid anatomy had been rescued and enhanced by modern technology. The new adjunctive diagnostic procedures transfigured the pathologist's vocabulary into a language that was both effective and necessary for clinical communication. The pathologist's vocabulary was effective because clinical diagnoses could now often be empirical rather than hypothetical: a clinician could now frequently see a good or exact facsimile of the morphologic entity he diagnosed. The pathologist's vocabulary was also necessary because it became the *lingua franca* that provided a common mode of diagnostic expression for many new types of evidence perceived with different technologic procedures. Pathologic taxonomy could act as a unifying diagnostic language to co-ordinate the diverse forms of substance and shadow observed with the methods of such varied sites as the bedside, the X-ray chamber, the endoscopic table, the surgical operating room, the microscope bench, and the morgue.

These consequences of the technologic revolution have established the nosology of morbid anatomy as a permanent, valuable constituent of clinical diagnosis. The topographic and morphologic categories of the taxonomy are well organized; the classifications are generally accepted; there seem to be relatively few outstanding problems. Since the anatomic taxonomy has not recently created any basic dissensions and challenges, it has provoked relatively little intellectual excitement. The taxonomy thus seems archaic now as a subject of scientific attention.

The "diseases" that *have* required taxonomic attention in modern medicine are entities demonstrated by the new technology. The increasing array of modern laboratory tests has identified physiologic and biochemical disorders, etiologic agents, and many other aspects of "disease" that cannot be detected from observation of morbid anatomy. These new "diseases" can be discerned from observation of graphic tracings, microbial organisms, chemical measurements, cytologic preparations, fluoroscopy, cineroentgenography, electrophoretic patterns, and the results of various other laboratory tests. A new medical specialty, called "clinical pathology", has now evolved for dealing with many of these tests.

These "new" disorders have required, and received, new systems of classification based on the observations that cannot be described with conventional morphologic taxonomy. The new systems are now in use for classifying microbial organisms and for categorizing abnormalities in serologic antibodies and complement-fixation capacities; in protein, carbohydrate, lipid, and mineral metabolism; in cardiac and gastrointestinal motility; in pulmonary gas exchange; in intracardiac pressures; and in the taxonomic wonderland of blood groups, bleeding, and clotting.

(The "new" disorders discovered in the laboratory have even led to a new fashion in eponyms. Some of the "diseases" are still named after their discoverers, e.g., *Franklin's* disease and *Tamm-Horsfall* proteinuria, but the discoveries are now biochemical, rather than clinical or anatomic. In many instances, however, the research "team" of laboratory discovery contains too many people to crowd into an eponym, or the discovered abnormality has a jaw-breaking name. So the eponym goes to the city where the discovery occurred, e.g., *Philadelphia* chromosome; or, completing the full taxonomic circle in medicine, some discoveries have now been named after the patient in whom they were found, e.g., *Christmas* disease, *Hageman* factor.)

The many new supplements to pathologic taxonomy have recently been formally recognized. The College of American Pathologists has presented a "Nomenclature and Classification of Disease" [71] that may remove some of the deficiencies now present in the two main existing catalogs of diagnostic classification.[72, 73] In the new pathologic taxonomy, "disease" is classified according to four separate modalities called *topography, morphology, etiology,* and *function.* The topographic and morphologic sections of this new taxonomy contain the conventional terminology of morbid anatomy, but the etiologic and functional sections provide nomenclature and classifications for many abnormalities omitted in morbid anatomy. The new sections give names for almost all the disorders detected with modern laboratory tests, for many states of disordered physiologic function, for the old "clinical" diagnoses that still persist as names of "disease", and for a few surviving eponymic entities. With this new expansion of its contents, pathologic taxonomy provides diagnostic categories for almost every "disease" known in contemporary medicine.

With a variety of diagnostic names available, and with adjunctive tests to provide appropriate morphologic and other evidence, the modern clinician can often diagnose "disease" accurately, early, and empirically. Moreover, since a single well-selected adjunctive test may disprove a unanimity of expert opinions based only on bedside evidence, many modern clinicians have begun, quite understandably, to depend more on adjunctive tests than on clinical observation in diagnostic reasoning.

The adjunctive evidence acquired in the laboratory and in other para-clinical sites has made the clinician a more reliable diagnostician than he used to be. The transition of "clinical" observation from bedside to laboratory has also, however, given him many new problems in diagnostic criteria, while distracting his attention from critical old problems that remain unsolved. The clinician still lacks criteria for many of his old as well as his new diagnostic classifications of "disease". Most importantly, he continues to treat sick people while classifying "disease" but not human illness.

6. The Diagnostic Taxonomy of Disease: Problems in Criteria

Before the 20th century revolution in technology, a clinician's main scientific problem in diagnostic reasoning was the selection of criteria for converting his clinical observations into anatomic inferences. Many of these inferential criteria are no longer necessary today, because the clinician, aided by technologic assistance, can now make many anatomic diagnoses by directly observing the affected structure or its silhouette. He can now also obtain direct para-clinical evidence of "diseases" that are not anatomic entities.

By eliminating the need for inference in many clinical diagnostic decisions, these new observational adjuncts have greatly improved the clinician's diagnostic accuracy. Like other advances of modern technology, however, the improvements have brought many new problems of their own, while diverting attention from many old difficulties that still persist.

DELEGATION OF DIAGNOSTIC CRITERIA

Since many contemporary diagnostic questions receive precise answers away from the bedside, the clinician has transferred many of his old criteria problems to other diagnosticians—radiologists, surgical pathologists, clinical pathologists, and laboratory technicians. In their morphologic and non-morphologic activities, all of these people need criteria: the radiologist, for converting his observed roentgenographic images into anatomic inferences; the surgical pathologist, for making diagnostic decisions from samples of tissue smaller than those obtained at necropsy and often representative of different stages of disease; the clinical pathologist, for maintaining the standardization and accuracy of laboratory tests in the midst of technologic proliferation; and the laboratory technician, for performing the tests reliably while deluged with new specimens and new procedures.

Having delegated these diagnostic problems, the clinician often assumes they have been solved by their new recipients. He may give too much scientific credence to reports or opinions received from human and technologic sources that contain—in observation and interpretation of evidence—all the potential errors of people, machines, or people using machines. Many defects may still be present in either the tests or the diagnostic criteria of the clinician's para-clinical colleagues, and all of their diagnostic results must still be co-ordinated with the clinical ailments present in the patient.

OBSERVER VARIABILITY IN MORPHOLOGIC DIAGNOSIS

The radiologist and histopathologist are just as human as the clinician, and may be just as prone to err in their subjective interpretations of observed evidence. The radiologist's conclusions are often checked by the histopathologist, but the histopathologist is usually a policeman without a "civilian" review board. Seldom exposed to a reversal of the interrogative direction of the clinico-pathologic conference, the histopathologist may not have the frequent opportunity or incentive to suspect, discover, and correct his human fallibility.

Histopathologists are not always consistent in the criteria used to distinguish inflammation from neoplasia, "benign" from "malignant" tumors, and one histologic type of cancer from another. The criteria for diagnosing histologic types in lung cancer, for example, have been frequently disputed[74, 75] and frequently altered[76-78]—making uncertain the current prevalence of "epidermoid", "bronchiolar", "carcinoid", and other forms of pulmonary neoplasia. Because of observer variability among surgical pathologists, the "tumor" removed in occasional cases of gastric or pancreatic "carcinoma" may have been benign or merely inflammatory.[79, 80]

TECHNOLOGIC VARIABILITY IN NON-MORPHOLOGIC DIAGNOSIS

Although the numerical expression of laboratory tests can avoid the subjectivity of a verbal morphologic description, the tests still produce many problems in method, in standardization, and in criteria for range of normality. The test itself may be inaccurate (e.g., measurement of hemoglobin by gross visual colorimetry), or an accurate test may be impaired by associated clinical events (e.g., falsely high elevations of serum protein-bound iodine after roentgenographic use of iodinated contrast media). The same entity may be tested by different methods or expressed in different units. For example, the gravitational fall of an *erythrocyte sedimentation rate* can be assessed by at least three different methods; serum or urinary *calcium* can be measured by flame photometry or by at least two different chemical procedures; *serum alkaline phosphatase* can be expressed in two different types of units; and a *group A streptococcal infection* can be diagnosed on the basis of a blood agar culture, a fluorescent stain, or an antibody titer.

When the same test is done by the "same" method and expressed in the same units, the actual performance of the method may not be standardized among different laboratories or among different technicians. Even when the tests, units, methods, and performances are all standardized, different laboratories may still have different criteria for interpreting range of normality in the results. Two laboratories that do the same test in exactly the same way may nevertheless have a marked difference in their dimensional concept of normal range for such entities as *blood urea nitrogen, serum uric acid,* and *prothrombin time.*

CO-ORDINATION OF CLINICAL AND PARA-CLINICAL FINDINGS

Although a diagnosis may sometimes be "established" or "ruled out" by a para-clinical test, the clinician must still co-ordinate the diagnosed entities with the clinical findings. The "diseases" detected in roentgenographic and other procedures often do not account for the patient's symptoms. For example, many digestive or abdominal symptoms unrelated to gall bladder disease have been erroneously attributed to the *cholelithiasis* found at roentgenography. Many low back pains have, by similar error, been ascribed to *osteo-arthritis.*

A biopsy may be "positive" because of an error in the pathologist's interpretation; a negative result does not always exclude the suspected disease. In a patient with an anatomic disease susceptible to biopsy, the biopsy specimen can be falsely negative for many reasons: the "disease" may not yet have produced morphologic changes in the examined tissue; a blindly inserted biopsy needle may have failed to reach the involved location; a small focus of tumor may have been missed either because the surgeon excised an adjacent unaffected lymph node or because the technician did not cut the section through a plane that included the tumor.

When a diagnosis is "established" by a non-morphologic laboratory test, the clinician must also constantly beware of "false positive" and "false negative" results. The pathologic diagnoses made from these tests are often just as inferential (and erroneous) as the conclusions drawn from purely clinical evidence. An elevated serum uric acid does not necessarily imply *gout,* for example, nor a positive latex fixation test, *rheumatoid arthritis.* An elevated anti-streptolysin O titer does not prove the existence of *rheumatic fever,* and an abnormal cephalin flocculation test does not mean *infectious hepatitis.*

(Another tragic chapter in the history of therapy in "modern clinical science" was produced by the long courses of arsenical treatment given to patients erroneously diagnosed as having *syphilis* because of a false positive Wassermann test. The positive result was later discovered to be due to a disease sometimes no more serious than *infectious mononucleosis.* The incorrect diagnosis itself must have been severe psychologic trauma for many people; the unnecessary arsenical therapy, in adding injury to insult, gave some of them severe cutaneous or systemic reactions, and a few patients died.)

A clinician's primary job is to discover what ails the patient, not merely to diagnose disease. No matter how scientifically precise or interesting, a diagnosis that does not account for the ailment may be clinically worthless.

CHOICES OF ADJUNCTIVE TESTS

A different problem in diagnostic criteria arises from the many tests that have become available as diagnostic adjuncts. The clinician must now develop scientific criteria and judgment not for his choice of diagnosis, but for his choice of diagnostic tests. Which ones, and how many, should he get, and in what sequence? If he orders too many tests indiscriminately, he wastes everyone's time, effort, and money. The costs may bankrupt the patient (or the health insurance program), and the multitude of tests may overwhelm the laboratory's capacity for accurate results. If the clinician orders too few tests, believing that his purely clinical reasoning needs no supplementation or confirmation by precise para-clinical aids, he runs the risk of making major diagnostic and therapeutic blunders.

Of greater clinical importance, however, is the danger of the tests themselves. Many patients develop unexpected, untoward, severe reactions to either the agents or the manipulations of the diagnostic procedures. In general, the more revealing a new procedure, the greater are its risks to the patient during the "hazards of hospitalization", whose current prevalence Schimmel[81] has described. As Schimmel points out, *primum non nocere,* an old clinical maxim in making therapeutic decisions, now applies equally well for decisions regarding the choice of diagnostic tests.

Despite the obvious necessity for criteria, no formal collection of strategy and tactics in selecting these tests has yet been clinically developed or promulgated. Thus, the clinician's para-clinical diagnostic colleagues, in exchange for some of the criteria problems he has given *them,* have left *him* with new problems about when and how often to ask for adjunctive diagnostic help.

INTER-DISCIPLINARY PROBLEMS IN DIAGNOSTIC CRITERIA

When the histopathologist, the clinical pathologist, the radiologist, and the clinician all use a common vocabulary for diagnosis, they may confuse one another with different connotations for the same name, and with inadequate or unstandardized specifications of the different "diseases" that may be present in the same patient.

AMBIGUOUS NOMENCLATURE

Different observers may use the same "disease" name for diverse structural or functional abnormalities. For example, the diagnosis of *pulmonary edema* may mean, to a histopathologist, fluid in the alveolar or interstitial spaces of the lung; to a radiologist, a prominence of certain vascular markings; and, to a clinician, a patient with inspiratory crepitations who is gasping for air. Yet a patient may have *pulmonary edema* clinically but not roentgenographically, and the histopathologic diagnosis of *pulmonary edema* is often made in patients who showed no acute respiratory distress.

Comparable inter-disciplinary problems in ambiguous nomenclature exist for such diagnoses as *gastritis, diverticulitis, pericarditis,* and many others, including the illustrations cited earlier (pages 67–69) in which clinicians connote function with the same diagnostic term used by histopathologists or radiologists to denote form.

INADEQUATE ABRIDGEMENT

In the modern zest for compressing complexity into brevity, many diagnoses are condensed into short phrases that fail to identify distinctive variations in the condition of the "disease". When a single site is affected by several different aspects of "disease", the abridged diagnosis may identify an abnormality in form but not in function, or in function but not in etiology, or in etiology but not in form.

For example, a patient's lungs may be simultaneously affected by *interstitial pneumonitis,* a morphologic lesion; *alveolo-capillary block,* a physiologic dysfunction; and *active tuberculosis,* an etiologic state. Yet only one or two of these three distinctive "diseases" may be specified as *the* "diagnosis". Some of the confusion already described (page 84) for *pulmonary emphysema* and *chronic bronchitis* occurred because American and British clinicians were using abridged single diagnoses for a "disease" affecting two different parts of respiratory anatomy.

In its pioneering efforts three decades ago to improve clinical diagnostic nomenclature, the New York Heart Association[82] established a system for classifying etiology, anatomy, physiologic function, and clinical consequences in the diagnosis of heart disease. Such a system is obviously applicable and necessary for gastrointestinal, metabolic, neurologic, renal, respiratory, and many other "diseases"—but no such classifications have been constructed. Even the system of distinctive multiple categories for classifying cardiac disease is not yet used universally or consistently.

As a result of excessive abridgements in specification of disease, many contemporary single diagnoses are arbitrary, inadequate, and misleading. Many errors are thereby produced in the "vital statistics" of morbidity or mortality rates for various "diseases", and in clinical or therapeutic activities that depend on reproducible identification of the total state of a patient's "disease". For example, the response of *active tuberculosis* to antibiotic therapy may vary greatly according to whether a patient also has *interstitial pneumonitis, alveolo-capillary block,* both, or neither. If the presence or absence of these two and other pertinent disease states is omitted, and the patients receive only the diagnosis of *active tuberculosis,* the author (and reader) of an analysis of treatment for tuberculosis may have great difficulty deciding why certain patients were "resistant" to the drugs while others were "cured".

CLINICO-STATISTICAL DIFFICULTIES

The enthusiasm for a diagnosis of morbid anatomy is often carried to excess in situations where neither the clinician nor the histopathologist observes good evidence of the diagnosed anatomic entity.

In many clinical situations, the anatomic diagnosis is an inference unconfirmed during the life of the patient, if at all. Such situations are particularly common for diseases in heart, brain, and other regions in which surgery is infrequent, biopsy dangerous, and roentgenography inconvenient, hazardous, or unrevealing of adequate morphologic detail. *Myocardial infarction, rheumatic carditis,* and *diabetic retinopathy* are all examples of anatomic diagnoses that often cannot be morphologically verified by microscopic examination of tissue while the patient is alive.

Perhaps the most common of the unverified morphologic diagnoses occurs in the clinical situation that is sometimes called a "cerebrovascular accident" or *stroke.* What the clinician observes is the story and effects of an episode in which the patient, transiently or permanently, develops disorientation, aphasia, paresis, or other clinical manifestations. If the episode is transient enough and mild enough, it may never enter the morbidity or mortality statistics because the patient is not hospitalized. The clinician's private files may record the diagnosis as *stroke* (or *small stroke*), and no further diagnoses or tabulations may be made.

If the episode is more severe, however, the patient is often admitted to a hospital; adjunctive tests are obtained; and an "institutional" diagnosis is made for the assembled statistics of "disease". The adjunctive tests do not often include cerebral arteriography, however, and cranial surgery is seldom necessary. If the cerebrospinal fluid is bloody, a hemorrhage may be inferred. If the fluid is not bloody (and even if it is), a clinician cannot be sure whether the stroke was due to rupture of a blood vessel; occlusion of a blood vessel by atheroma, thrombus, or embolus; or derangement of cerebral function by tumor or other space-occupying lesion.

For most strokes, therefore, the clinician does not get to see either the involved vessels or the involved tissue, and must make anatomic diagnoses as generally unverified inferences. If surgery is not done during life, the only way he can observe the anatomy of his diagnosis is after necropsy, provided that the cranial contents can be examined. Thus, a clinician sees most strokes as strokes, and calls them *strokes* in his everyday practical clinical vocabulary. When he performs the important institutional exercise known as "signing out the chart", however, he may write *cerebral arteriosclerosis, encephalopathy,* or other anatomic designations.

If his hospital's disease taxonomy is the *Standard Nomenclature of Diseases and Operations* (SNDO),[72] the clinician can not diagnose *stroke* even if he wishes; the term is not contained in the index or categories of the SNDO. If the hospital's diagnostic taxonomy is the *International Classification of Diseases, Adapted* (ICDA),[73] the clinician can diagnose *stroke* only by risking the opprobrium of his colleagues. According to the ICDA, the diagnosis of *stroke* "connotes vagueness, and should not be used, if more specific diagnoses can be determined". Anxious to sign out the chart, and reluctant to write things that suggest he is ignorant, the clinician makes an anatomic guess. A guess that is often thoughtful, educated, and accurate—but a guess.

William Farr, who is often regarded as a founder of "vital statistics", was vigorously opposed to such excessive refinements in nomenclature. Said Farr, "The refusal to recognize these terms that express imperfect knowledge has an obvious tendency to encourage reckless conjecture." [83] Nevertheless, the morphologic taxonomy of contemporary "disease" discourages the clinician from an accurate expression of imperfection. Instead, he makes a guess that leaves everyone happy. He is happy because the chart is signed out; the medical record librarian is happy because she can now code something specific, like *thrombosis of lenticulostriate artery;* and the collector of morbidity and mortality rates is happy because he can tabulate this guesswork and call it "vital statistics".

The deficiencies of a falsely morphologic designation for *stroke* create confusion in clinical as well as in statistical literature. Many patients with *cerebral arteriosclerosis* are asymptomatic; many cases of *encephalopathy* are due to non-arteriosclerotic causes; and many strokes are associated with neither *arteriosclerosis* nor *encephalopathy*. Consequently, when a cerebrovascular accident is reported only in inferential anatomic terms, a clinician has no idea of what kind of *stroke,* if any, was observed. Since different kinds of strokes have different prognoses and respond differently to treatment, an intelligent clinician may have great difficulty contemplating how to apply the morphologically reported information of medical literature when he makes decisions in the treatment of individual patients. An intelligent patient[84] may have great difficulty trying to find a coherent discussion of his *stroke* in clinical textbooks.

A separate problem in clinical and statistical aspects of diagnosis arises because certain diseases occur in anatomic locations, such as temporal bone or calf veins, that are usually prohibited from postmortem exploration and are hence often left unexamined in a routine necropsy. A *pulmonary embolus* may be falsely attributed at necropsy to a small clot found in the uterine or prostatic venous plexus because the true source was not found in the unexamined leg veins. Such clinical diagnoses as *phlebothrombosis* and *thrombophlebitis* are often used interchangeably or erroneously because good anatomic data are not available to correlate the clinical and morphologic manifestations. Finally, the prevalence and consequences of these venous disorders and of other diseases, such as *otosclerosis,* may be distorted because the appropriate regions cannot be routinely examined at necropsy.

"CLINICO-TECHNO-MORPHIC" CRITERIA

For many diseases that cannot be identified by direct inspection or biopsy of affected tissue, contemporary diagnosis requires an integrated appraisal of different components of clinical and para-clinical evidence. Some of the non-morphologic diagnoses represent a straightforward classification of observed para-clinical evidence; for example, the "chemical" diagnoses of *porphyria, hyperglycemia,* or *proteinuria* and the "physiologic" diagnosis of *atrial tachycardia with 3:1 block.* Other non-morphologic diagnostic terms represent a classification of various combinations of clinical, laboratory, and radiographic evidence; for example, *gout, syphilis, rheumatic fever, influenza, hyper-thyroidism,* and *hemophilia.*

In the examples just cited, the name of the disease is not anatomic, and the diagnosis represents an empiric classification of observed clinical and laboratory evidence. When the disease is a "non-biopsy" anatomic entity, however, the diagnosis is made as an inference from combinations of different types of clinical and para-clinical evidence. Such diseases as *myocardial infarction, lobar pneumonia, duodenal ulcer, cholecystitis,* and *encephalitis* are anatomic entities, not usually susceptible to biopsy, that may sometimes be diagnosed with clinical evidence alone, with para-clinical evidence alone, or with combinations of both. The para-clinical tests, even when not "diagnostic" in many of these anatomic diseases, may provide confirmation of diagnosis or help rule out alternative causes for the clinical manifestations.

With the rare exceptions already cited for *rheumatic fever* and *rheumatoid arthritis* (page 83), no standardized rigorous criteria exist today for any of the classifications and inferences that convert various combinations of "clinico-techno-morphic" evidence into diagnostic designations. Criteria established by authoritative committees have been issued for the diagnosis of cardiovascular diseases[67] and of pulmonary diseases,[85] but the statements are often discursive rather than precise; the distinctions of inferential inclusion and exclusion are omitted; and the discussions are frequently based mainly on morphologic details that are not available during the life of the patient.

Despite their deficiencies, such criteria are better than none. Metabolic, renal, hematologic, and many other major diseases today still lack any authoritative formulation of standard diagnostic criteria. For example, what are the classificational criteria for separating "primary" from "secondary" *gout,* and for distinguishing *gout* from other causes of joint pain in a patient with hyperuricemia? Of the many procedures available for appraising glucose metabolism— urinalysis, measurement of fasting blood sugar or post-prandial blood sugar, performance of oral or intravenous glucose tolerance tests— which is the accepted standard for the diagnosis of *diabetes mellitus,* and what are the quantitative requirements? How do we decide that an L.E. cell preparation is "false positive" in a patient with *rheumatoid arthritis* or that a serologic test for syphilis is "false positive" in a patient with *lupus erythematosus?* Every good clinician can answer these questions, but no two answers might be the same. No general criteria exist.

The deficiencies due to absence of such "combined" criteria for inferential anatomic diagnosis are magnified by the failure, in modern medical literature, of many authors to state their own individual diagnostic criteria for the treated diseases. For example, in a recent survey[86] of 32 published reports of anti-coagulant therapy for myocardial infarction, it was found that 16 reports contained *no* statement of the various clinical, electrocardiographic, and laboratory manifestations that were used as diagnostic criteria for *myocardial infarction*. In nine other reports, the statements of diagnostic criteria were worded too vaguely for the authors' techniques to be reproducibly applied elsewhere.

PERSISTENT OMISSIONS IN OLD "CLINICAL" CRITERIA

Despite the profusion of diagnostic terms derived from morbid anatomy and from the laboratory components of pathologic taxonomy, many old "clinical" veterans have lingered as names of "disease". Some of these names (*diabetes mellitus, gout, hemophilia, influenza, lupus erythematosus, rheumatic fever,* and *syphilis*) have already been mentioned (page 98). Other clinical patriarchs of modern nosology are the diseases cited in such "cluster" designations as *cerebral palsy, delirium tremens, epilepsy, goiter, heat exhaustion, measles, migraine, pemphigus, psoriasis, smallpox, sprue,* and many other titles in the taxonomic plethora of dermatology and infectious exanthemas. Sydenham and Huntington have managed to maintain eponymic survival in their respective forms of *chorea,* and many other old or more recent clinicians (e.g., Adams, Cheyne, Downs, Klinefelter, Morgagni, Paget, and Stokes) are still commemorated in the names of "diseases" or "syndromes".

Not all "clinical" diagnoses represent a "cluster" of manifestations. Certain individual symptoms, signs, or personal attributes of patients are still in good nomenclatural standing as diagnoses. The "diseases" of *pruritus ani* and *myasthenia gravis* are the names of symptoms; *erythema nodosum* and *hypertension* are the names of signs; *chronic alcoholism* and *narcotic addiction* are the names of personal habits. After the onset of anatomic nosology, *angina pectoris* continued to be a "disease" for many years until ultimately correlated with *coronary atherosclerosis* and relegated to its current status as a mere symptom.

Among Wunderlich's revelations with clinical thermometry was the conversion of *fever* from a "disease" to a symptom.[87]

Some of the antiquarian "clinical" nomenclature has survived by chameleon-like stealth: *asthma* is now sometimes a "disease" (bronchial asthma), sometimes a clinical state (status asthmaticus), sometimes a symptom (cardiac asthma), and sometimes a sign (asthmatic breathing). A few seasoned clinical campaigners have resisted vigorous efforts at replacement. The *common cold,* for example, a diagnosis accepted by both SNDO and ICDA, has not yet been successfully supplanted by the morphologic *rhinitis* or *nasopharyngitis,* by the "fancy" topographic-etiologic substitute of *upper respiratory infection,* or by the sesquipedalian *acute undifferentiated viral illness.* Some good clinicians prefer to designate this ailment with the ancient but still eloquent diagnosis of *coryza.*

Since no specific anatomic abnormality is involved, all of the "clinical" entities just cited are "diseases" diagnosed by empirical classification, not by inference, and almost all of them antedate the modern "diseases" of contemporary pathologic taxonomy. Several newer "diseases" are "modern" clinico-physiologic states diagnosed by partial inference. Among such "diseases" are *congestive heart failure, renal failure, nephrotic syndrome, hepatic decompensation,* and *irritable colon.* These diagnoses imply a physiologic dysfunction, but the inference remains purely clinical. The diagnoses cannot be confirmed by any combination of morphologic or adjunctive tests, since the "diseases" have no pathognomonic counterpart in para-clinical evidence.

All these examples of "clinical" diagnoses persist today because the names are necessary. No alternative morphologic, physiologic, or biochemical designations have been adequate to include the wide spectrum of clinical manifestations covered by the "clusters", or to provide a consistent specificity in identifying the affected patients. In addition to these names for "organic diseases", the terms of nosology are almost entirely "clinical" for the ailments found in psychiatry, the one medical specialty whose "diseases" have little or no correlation with morbid anatomy or with the results of conventional para-clinical tests. Psychiatry must classify all of its "psychopathology" by means of non-morphologic designations, and is still in search of a satisfactory diagnostic taxonomy. The current psychiatric debates about systems of classification, the many hypothetical and unconfirmed schemas of "psychodynamic mechanisms", and the concern with etiologic inference rather than observational evidence are noso-logic activities sometimes reminiscent of those conducted by the medieval taxonomists.

Except for the many psychiatric designations and the few clinico-physiologic states that are diagnosed by inference, all of the old "clinical" diagnoses represent classifications of observed evidence. The evidence for some of the "diseases" is purely clinical, and for others comprises the "clinico-techno-morphic" features discussed earlier. Yet, even for those diagnoses that have depended for years on exclusively clinical evidence, no rigorous criteria exist for diag-nostic classification. For example, how often would two clinicians independently cite exactly the same criteria for differentiating *chorea* from hyperkinetic movements or habit spasms; Sydenham's *minor* variety of *chorea* from Huntington's *major; psychomotor epilepsy* from other epilepsies and neuropsychiatric states; and the three varie-ties of *measles* that can receive the Latin designations of *rubeola, ru-bella,* and *exanthem subitum?* The distinctions of such criteria will vary not only with each clinician, but also with each clinical textbook.

Many aspects of medical science have had the benefit of criteria established by meetings of international commissions. The meetings have attempted to standardize nomenclature and criteria in such domains as gross normal anatomy, the morphology of cancer, the designation of the "new" hemoglobins, and of many chemical and other entities in modern medicine. Never has an authoritative group of clinical experts assembled to standardize the rational formulation of the hundreds of diagnoses for which no specific criteria exist.

No other branch of natural science is so imprecise in defining the material exposed to experiment. Although all the diagnoses are made differently, although no uniform standards have been ratified and disseminated, it is commonly believed that rigorous criteria are in-variably present. The clinician's capacity for intellectual self-deception is illustrated by the widespread acceptance of this illusion. For most of the "established" diagnoses of modern "disease", standardized criteria do not exist, but are necessary, and must be established for true scientific progress in clinical medicine. For clinicians to improve scientific quality in the treatment of "disease", a basic demand of science is an accurate, reproducible identification of "disease". Such identifications will require clinicians to establish and disseminate the specific details of suitable criteria for diagnosis of each "disease" subjected to therapy.

The human and logistic problems of establishing such diagnostic criteria are difficult. Appropriate delegates from different parts of nations and hemispheres will have to assemble, argue, debate, reach a consensus, and then proselyte their colleagues and students. The problems are not insurmountable, however. The same age of technology that helps create such problems also provides the automobiles, jet airplanes, closed-circuit television networks, and long-distance telephone or radio group-communications with which the necessary "workshops" can be arranged and conducted.

*   *   *

The clinician has all these problems in his diagnostic and technologic activities because he continues to use the nomenclature of pathology as his basic system of diagnostic taxonomy. There is nothing really wrong with the system, however, that cannot be overcome if clinicians apply themselves adequately to its problems. Moreover, in our current state of medical knowledge, there is probably no better *single* system for the diagnostic nomenclature of disease.

Because major elements of disease are manifested by morbid anatomy, histopathologic designations will remain necessary to identify the abnormal anatomic structures. Supplemental "clinical", etiologic, and "functional" designations will also be needed to identify types of disease undetected in morbid anatomy. All of the distinctive "clinical", topographic, morphologic, etiologic, and "functional" components of contemporary pathologic taxonomy should be preserved. They designate different evidence, different "causes", and different effects in human disease—and they are all basic ingredients of clinical diagnosis.

The main defects of the pathologist's diagnostic taxonomy are its omissions, not its contents. It is too incomplete for use alone as the taxonomy of therapy. Pathologic taxonomy identifies diseases, but not patients. The contemporary clinico-pathologic conference and pathologists present clinicians with a challenge in diagnosis, but a clinician's main scientific challenge in medicine today is treatment, not pathologic diagnosis.

7. The Diagnostic Taxonomy of Disease: Problems in Therapy

Because of all the diagnostic aid clinicians get from para-clinical sources, the clinician's pathologic diagnosis is much more accurate now than it used to be—despite the many problems cited in the preceding chapter—and is no longer accomplished exclusively or frequently by the intuition, *augensblick,* educated guess, or professorial fiat of the past. A clinician at major medical teaching centers can no longer expect his colleagues and students to accept diagnoses proposed only with the inspiration of faith and supported only by the dogma of authority. There are too many other people checking him now besides the pathologist.

Superseding diagnosis as the clinician's main problem in modern science is the challenge of therapy, an experimental activity that is designed mainly by clinicians, rather than by pathologists or by other colleagues who give a clinician assistance in diagnosis. For these experiments in treatment, the clinician today has an opulence of agents and opportunities. Instead of the non-specific, often ineffective therapeutic remedies of the past, physicians now use potent drugs that can eradicate bacteria, thwart viruses, imitate glands, alter heartbeat, change consciousness, or affect emotion; surgeons perform operations that can remove, reconstruct, replace, or transplant many parts of the human body.

Today a clinician can no longer select the name or "cause" of a disease and feel that he has completed his obligation to clinical science; the clinician's main scientific responsibility is to decide when and how to use the available modes of treatment. Pathologic diagnosis is a "passive" experiment in which the answers are often found in the inanimate substances observed by the clinician's para-clinical colleagues; treatment is an "active" experiment in which most of the answers are found in the living patient observed by the clinician himself.

For the classifications and reasoning of scientific clinical *therapy,* the taxonomy of pathology, and particularly the nomenclature of morbid anatomy, has many inadequacies beyond the problems it creates in clinical *diagnosis.* Some of the defects to be cited—particularly, the restricted morphologic emphasis of the clinico-pathologic conference (CPC)—arise as errors of commission. All the major faults, however, are errors of omission, inevitable in any system of diagnosis that classifies "disease" pathologically but not prognostically.

The lessons that Hippocrates and Sydenham taught about correlating the "natural history of disease" have been generally forgotten in current nosology. For more than a century, the diagnostic reasoning of clinicians has been an attempt at simultaneous correlation of anatomic form and clinical function. This type of diagnosis is a uni-temporal correlation between bedside manifestations and concomitant anatomic or laboratory manifestations; it provides a pathologic name of "disease" for a clinical ailment at a single moment in time. The nosology is based on concepts of "disease", not on concepts of "natural history of disease"; it depends on what ails the patient now, but not on what is going to happen later. The diagnostic categories contained in contemporary pathologic taxonomy were generally derived without reference to prognosis of the cited diseases.

In the 17th century, Sydenham had made multi-temporal prognostic correlations in identifying new "diseases". He used the repetitive self-limited episodes of *gout* as a way of separating it diagnostically from other forms of rheumatism, and the non-repetitious transiency of *measles* to distinguish it from other cutaneous eruptions. In modern nosology, however, a carefully studied prognosis has not been a constituent of the reasoning used to define or delineate the many anatomic, chemical, microbial, and other "diseases" whose designation represents a single state in time. The subsequent course of patients with carcinomas, infarctions, inflammations, degenerations, congenital abnormalities, and other "diseases" was generally not considered in arriving at the diagnostic designations.

Such uni-temporal concepts of a patient's ailment may be satisfactory for a pathologist, who sees the "disease" usually only once, but not for a clinician, who may treat a "disease" for a lifetime before it reaches the pathologist. The clinician has had to add such chronologic terms as *acute, subacute, chronic, impending, paroxysmal,* and *relapsing* to diagnostic nosology, and is still in need of many other specifications that will help him deal with temporal and prognostic distinctions. Attempting to cope with the mosaic spectrums and moving pictures of human ailments, contemporary clinicians are severely restricted by the views of "disease" provided in the still photographs of the camera of pathology. Some of the many defects of pathologic taxonomy in the *treatment* of human illness are noted in the sections that follow.

LIMITATIONS OF CONTEMPORARY MORPHOLOGIC EMPHASIS

If clinicians are suffering today from a "crisis of identity" or an uncertain "corporate image", pathologists have an analogous problem. A clinician, pursuing morbid anatomy, may forget that his name comes from κλινικος, the word for *bed,* and may sometimes neglect adequate attention to the patient who occupies the bed. A pathologist, also pursuing morbid anatomy, may forget that *his* name comes from παθος λογος, the *study of disease.* He may arbitrarily restrict the boundaries of "disease" to morphologic entities, and may restrict the "study" mainly to causes, development, and visual diagnosis of disease, while disregarding other types of diagnosis, the problems of treatment, and prognostic correlations of the clinical *dis-ease* whose morbid anatomy he observes.

Because pathology is the intellectual domain that co-ordinates manifestations of human disease at every level from isolated cell to intact man, it has long held a central role in medical education. The pathologist no longer performs this role as well as he did in the past, not merely because so many academic pathologists now emphasize the artificial diseases induced in animals rather than the natural ones of man, but because the pathologist has not fully adapted to the new complexities of human disease that have been found during the past half century. To maintain his fundamental role in medical science, the pathologist may need to make many changes in his current activities—changes that will restore his domain as an intellectual beacon for attracting clinical visitors, and that will move him and his beacon, from their remote location in the necropsy room and microscope bench, to a position of greater illumination in the wards and pavilions of the clinician.

THE CLINICO-PATHOLOGIC CONFERENCE

The CPC was originally intended to be a conference of co-ordination. The pathologist's role was that of a scientific watchdog on the clinician, checking his reasoning and making him justify his clinical decisions. This function is no longer performed effectively during the morphologic type of CPC conducted at many modern medical centers. Many of the clinician's contemporary diagnoses are not anatomic, and cannot be checked morphologically; many other diagnoses that *are* anatomic have been already checked adequately before necropsy. As for justification of clinical decisions, the most important decisions to be justified today are the strategy of the diagnostic "work-up" and the tactics in therapy, not merely the anatomic conclusions of diagnostic reasoning.

Despite these many changes in contemporary medicine, the CPC continues generally to be a purely histopathologic exercise based on necropsy or sometimes on surgical material. No longer a donor of the ultimate word on "disease", the histopathologist may use the new technology to enhance his morphologic views with new sections, stains, and magnifications—but his focus has remained morphologic. He continues to classify morbid anatomy, but he often does not correlate the diverse clinical and temporal manifestations of disease; he continues to be a watchdog on diagnosis, but he often does not extend his critical talents to police the choices of diagnostic tests and treatment. Surrounded by major revolutions in techniques of diagnosis, alternatives of therapy, and spectrums of epidemiology in "disease", the histopathologist persists in keeping the traditional morphologic format of the CPC intact and essentially unchanged.

The contemporary routine CPC has often become an exercise mainly for medical students, and fails to attract the attendance of many knowledgeable clinicians, who may not find the performance rewarding enough to relinquish the time it takes. Confronted with the realities of modern medicine, a clinician may find the conventional CPC somewhat irrelevant: it often contains "museum pieces", rather than common problems; it often presents histologic esoterica for which treatment would have been the same even if an errant diagnostician had known the correct diagnosis; and it deals mainly with morphology, not with non-morphologic disease and not with treatment. A clinician has learned that he will almost never encounter, at CPC, a case in which the primary diagnosis is chemical or "functional" rather than anatomic. Such "diseases" as *porphyria, hyperthyroidism, hypogamma-globulinemia, ventricular tachycardia, hyperventilation syndrome, irri-*

table colon, schizophrenia, and many other major ailments found in modern medicine cannot be cut and shown through the pathologist's slide projector. A clinician has learned that the pathologist, at CPC, may seldom stimulate discussion or provoke debates about choice of diagnostic tests and therapeutic strategy. Immersed in morphology, or reluctant to ask probing questions about the new diagnostic and therapeutic procedures, the histopathologist may confine himself merely to being a critic or censor of anatomic diagnosis alone.

Although clinicians may attend less often than formerly, the CPC continues to attract the minds of the young—medical students—and on these minds the CPC may have its most striking effects. An experienced clinician has learned that the "detective story" of the CPC is, like other detective stories, an often entertaining escape from reality. The young medical student, however, may come to regard the frequent esoterica, the pathogenetic speculations, and the restricted morphologic focus of the contemporary CPC as reality. The experienced clinician has learned that most of the ailments that bring patients to doctors are not primarily morphologic, and that treatment of functional as well as structural disorders is a fundamental problem of clinical medicine. A young medical student, however, may get the impression from CPCs that "disease" is mainly a morphologic entity and that diagnosis of morbid anatomy is the clinician's only or main scientific challenge. Because the anatomic emphasis of CPCs may inculcate the belief that a *real* "disease" is always an "organic" entity, and because clinical teachers often fail to overcome this belief, many young doctors today have great difficulty in understanding and treating patients with "functional" disorders.

Another intellectually deleterious aspect of the contemporary CPC is its occasional conversion into a competition, rather than a collaboration, between two different medical disciplines. The "detective story" CPC sometimes gives the impression that it is a comparative test of the *reasoning* done by the clinician and by the pathologist. The pathologist always wins the competition, of course, since he begins with the answers; moreover, he can greatly increase his margin of victory by selecting, as he sometimes does, a case impossible to diagnose with any valid form of clinical logic. The fallacy of this spirit of competition is that the CPC is not at all a comparative test of reasoning in the two disciplines. A clinician must go through a complex system of deductions to achieve anatomic diagnosis in a living patient, but a pathologist does almost no reasoning to make a "correct" diagnosis at necropsy; all he has to do is look. Because the pathologist is always "right" at CPC, however, he and his audience may begin to believe that his reasoning is as good as his observations. When he does engage in reasoning to make etiologic inferences and pathogenetic conjectures, a false aura of his omniscience may becloud the mind of his audience, and may often affect his awareness of his own potential for human fallibility.

The CPC is an extraordinarily valuable teaching procedure for doctors young and old, but it should be an exercise in correlation, not just diagnosis; in mutual education, not just unilateral revelation to the clinician; and in the study of disease, not just the immediate morphologic interests of the pathologist. The CPC need not always be a "detective story"; its outcome need not always be expressed in morbid anatomy; and its ultimate "expert" need not always be a pathologist. To be a student of *disease* and *dis-ease,* the pathologist can sometimes present an "open book" conference in which the main point is not to answer a diagnostic riddle, but to demonstrate the correlation (or lack of correlation) for particularly interesting clinical and morphologic findings. To be a co-ordinating watchdog on diagnostic procedures while still maintaining a "detective story" CPC, the histopathologist can occasionally invite the radiologist or the clinical pathologist to discuss choices of tests and to present the endpoint data in cases where the microscopic findings were unimportant. Another clinician (or pathologist) might sometimes be invited to discuss selected cases in which the ultimate diagnosis was purely "clinical", with all the ancillary tests being unnecessary or worthless. To be a watchdog on therapeutic choices, the pathologist might ask an appropriate statistician, epidemiologist, clinician, or pathologist to criticize and evaluate therapeutic rather than diagnostic maneuvers in pertinent cases.

An academic pathologist may protest that many such conferences will be difficult to arrange. To find suitable cases for the conferences, he would not be able to wait for patients to reach necropsy, and he would have to leave the laboratory and morgue to see what is happening to "disease" on the wards, pavilions, and diagnostic chambers of the medical center. If the clinician of the 19th century could travel to the necropsy room to learn about "disease", the pathologist of the 20th century may need to reverse the direction of migration in order to maintain his central co-ordinating role in the study of "disease".

THE IMPORTANCE OF NECROPSY

Although the necropsy, the ordinary microscope, and histologic abnormalities are still venerated at CPC, they are often depreciated when the pathologist leaves the conference and returns to his own domain. The pathologist at most community hospitals today, away from the medical center, is often no longer the connoisseur that he used to be of morphology, because he is occupied mainly as a clinical pathologist, directing the hospital laboratories. At many academic medical centers, the young pathologist or the graduate trainee has—like his clinical counterpart—become diverted from the classical heritage of his discipline. Rejecting morbid anatomy and "clinical" types of research, the young investigator in pathology may prefer to work with animals as part of "experimental" pathology, or to apply ultra-morphologic vision in looking through an electron microscope.

In the histopathologic activities of certain modern medical centers —notably in the interpretation of biopsy specimens of liver, kidney and, particularly, bone marrow—clinicians have sometimes begun to rely on the readings made by clinical specialists, rather than by pathologists. Even the value of the routine necropsy itself has come into question with occasional accusations that it may be administratively over-rated, interfering with the busy pathologist's other tasks in chemical and animal laboratories. Suggestions are sometimes made that the necropsy is not always performed thoughtfully[88] or competently;[89] and that it may even be scientifically unnecessary,[90] replaceable by a selection of chemical tests, roentgenograms, and diverse *post-mortem* "biopsies".

If the clinician cannot understand man merely from studying man's parts, the pathologist surely cannot understand diseased human tissue merely from studying animals, molecules, or infracellular fragments. Histopathology, like gross anatomy, will always be a fundamental constituent of medical science. Moreover, a careful necropsy will always be just as essential, at the end of "disease", as a careful history and physical examination were at the beginning. The histopathologist cannot be replaced by the chemist, the immunologist, or the electron microscopist, and the invaluable information of the complete routine necropsy cannot be abandoned in favor of the uncertain aliquots and directions of *post-mortem* "biopsies", or the chiaroscuro inferences of roentgenography. The necropsy is, and remains, the final, crucial, common pathway in "disease".

In defending the value of the routine necropsy, pathologists rightly point out its importance in diagnostic and other confirmations of disease,[91, 92] its proper role "as an element of medical care rather than something which merely satisfies professional curiosity",[93] and its failure to thrive in an age of science that often allocates prestige and large sums of money to investigators who study animals and molecules rather than man.[91, 94] Pathologists also cite the general educational importance of the necropsy as a point in its defense, and may sometimes note[95] the clinician's failure to attend the actual necropsy procedure as a factor contributing to its decline.

The educational value of necropsies can be greatly improved, but not by making the clinician watch the pathologist at work. Since a busy pathologist does not usually attend the physician's routine clinical examinations or the surgeon's routine operations, it is not clear why a busy clinician must be present at the pathologist's usual labors. What necropsy should have to increase its educational value is better methods of communication. Pathologists might improve their notorious lateness in completing their written reports; at many medical centers today, the "referring" clinician does not receive an account of the microscopic findings until almost a year after the necropsy, when his recollections and interest may have vanished. Pathologists could also devote more care to maintenance of the necropsy data; new techniques for coding and processing data have not yet been established at most departments of pathology, and the total results often lie fallow as sources of potential research because they are not appropriately tabulated and assessed. The contents of the standard necropsy report might also be expanded to contain a section on "correlation", which is absent from the written "protocols" at many institutions. The final "protocol" often states only the anatomic findings, or the anatomic findings plus a dissociated summary of the antecedent clinical and laboratory data, but does not provide a specific correlation (or explanation) of the various manifestations noted during life and afterward.

These efforts at correlation will require co-operation and interest by clinicians, but the clinician need not be present at the necropsy itself. What is important to a clinician about the routine necropsy is not how it is done but what it shows. As long as the findings can be demonstrated later, the clinician need not take the time to watch the pathologist's operative technique. The post-necropsy demonstration conferences, if scheduled suitably and conducted well, can be one of the most valuable ways of advancing education, knowledge, and research in medical science. But the conference must be a true collaboration, not just a unilateral demonstration; a symphony of intellectual harmonics, not just a soloist's "organ recital". The clinician should come prepared not just to look, but to contribute information that may be absent from the medical record and to ask for explanations of all hitherto unexplained clinical findings. The pathologist should come prepared not just to demonstrate, but to solicit absent clinical information and to provide whatever explanations are possible. The conference should be a conjunction of diverse observers correlating their data, not just a visual display of diagnostic anatomy. The questions asked and the information exchanged at these conferences can provide many of the intellectual correlations now absent in both the clinician's and the pathologist's work, and can lead to many fruitful collaborations in subsequent research.

Instead of instituting such conferences or improving their performance to attract the absent clinicians who can provide stimulation and data, the necropsy pathologist may accept a hermit's role. He may confine himself, in performing the necropsy and its written sequels, to an isolation that is stultifying intellectually and deficient scientifically. Confronted with doing a necropsy, he may lament his relative solitude in the morgue, scan the patient's medical record, grumble about its deficiencies, do the necropsy, omit any further effort to get additional clinical information or explanation, and write a report that is anatomically complete but scientifically defective because the anatomic diagnoses have not been adequately interpreted or correlated with the patient's clinical findings and clinical course. The situation is often made worse, of course, by the clinician's frequent neglect of suitable oral or written instructions to the pathologist before the necropsy begins, and by the clinician's frequent failure to provide suitable information when the pathologist asks for it.

Recognizing that the necropsy is of fundamental importance and irreplaceable in medical science, clinicians should join pathologists in helping to improve its value in education and research.

RESEARCH IN HISTOPATHOLOGY

Just as many clinicians in modern "science" have developed the false belief that science cannot come from the direct study of patients, many pathologists have concluded that nothing new can be learned from the necropsy or from conventional histopathology. Yet, like the clinician, the pathologist is still offered many investigative scientific challenges in the precise observation, verification, and quantification of the phenomena of nature detectable in his traditional objects of observation. Without elaborate colonies of animals, esoteric histochemical stains, or ultramicroscopic vision, the research pathologist still has much to learn from his surgical and necropsy material by using his naked eye, his customary stains, his standard magnifications, and his brain.

He has yet to solve the many problems already discussed (pages 90–91) in observer variability. He has yet to quantify many structures that have hitherto been described only qualitatively, or measured in two dimensions but not three. For example, histopathologists have not yet developed ways to appraise the total number and size of diseased islet cells in the pancreas, to determine the proportions of diseased and non-diseased renal glomeruli, and to give a *volumetric* assessment for fibrotic or neoplastic lesions in the liver. The pathologist has yet to study many tubular structures in longitudinal views, rather than cross sections, and to study many derangements of an organ as a whole rather than the abnormalities in isolated parts. For example, histopathologists have recently advanced our knowledge of emphysema by making sections of a whole lung rather than by looking at scattered segments of parenchyma.[96] Similar total-structure and longitudinal studies may be necessary to understand the distribution and function of diseased coronary vessels in the heart, of the diverse channels in diseased kidneys, and of various other relationships that will clarify the way that a whole organ comprises its parts. Starr[89] has shown how the cadaver, despite its absence of life, can be used to study the physiology of the cardiovascular system.

As the pathologist augments his perspectives of morbid anatomy, he might particularly consider extending his scope to epidemiologic as well as to better clinical and therapeutic correlations. The epidemiologic aspect of the necropsy is actually one of the best reasons for maintaining interest and quality in its routine performance. The "epidemiology" of the necropsy is provided by its unexpected ancillary findings, which are now a generally unquantified territory of pathology. The main disease that "caused" death has generally, at most good medical centers, been well identified and studied during life; the necropsy usually confirms the diagnosis or occasionally demonstrates a significant, instructive error. Pathologists and clinicians, however, when interested primarily in the "main" disease, may give little attention to all the other "diseases" that are present at necropsy. A topic that often receives no further investigation is the "surprise discovery" of major ancillary diseases that were unsuspected or undetected during life: a non-lethal carcinoma in a patient who died of a heart attack; multiple old myocardial infarctions in an asymptomatic person who was killed in an accident; extensive vascular sclerosis in a patient, dead of pneumonia, who never had any difficulties attributable to the sclerosis; and many other examples.

Such "surprises" are often noted at necropsy, but their specific incidence is seldom tabulated, and their biologic significance is seldom further contemplated. The pathologist may dismiss the unexpected finding by assuming that the disease was not suspected during life because the clinician was too inept to make the diagnosis. The clinician, knowing that the patient had not complained of any symptoms that might arouse suspicion of the unexpected lesion, may dismiss the "surprise" by assuming that the patient was too stoic or ignorant to seek attention for the symptoms that must have been present.

The lesions discovered unexpectedly at necropsy are of fundamental importance in understanding the epidemiology and natural history of disease. Such "silent" lesions help indicate the amount of latent disease in the community beyond the hospital and doctor's office. In a disease's natural history, such lesions demarcate the portion of the spectrum that can exist without affecting clinical function or without making the patient feel sick enough to seek medical attention.

Because of this apparent biologic dissociation of form and function, a lesion that was asymptomatic and detected unexpectedly at necropsy may be an important clue to the complexity of nature, not an indictment of a clinician's competence or of a patient's perception. How do these undetected lesions differ in structure from otherwise comparable but detected instances of apparently the same "disease"? What distinction of their structure (or function) allows them to escape detection during life? What topographic and morphologic features make the "same" lesion distressing or incapacitating for one patient but not for another? By attributing these distinctions of disease to vicissitudes in the human psyche or intellect, pathologists and clinicians may overlook an important manifestation of biologic variability in the natural course of human ailments.

Finally, and perhaps most importantly, the pathologist needs an expansion of his scope to include an extra dimension: time. Some of the many existing defective clinico-pathologic correlations in natural history of disease may arise because clinicians and pathologists fail to appreciate epidemiology, but most of the problems arise from the temporal restrictions of a diagnostic concern that often omits prognosis and therapy.

PROBLEMS IN CLINICO-PATHOLOGIC CORRELATION

Because contemporary concepts in pathology frequently lack suitable clinical correlations, the clinician encounters at least four major difficulties in dealing with the natural history and treatment of disease.

SPECTRAL LIMITATIONS

Necropsy pathologists and clinicians have created major errors in comprehension of natural history by extrapolating inappropriately from the boundaries of necropsy material to the entire clinical spectrum of a disease. In many acute and chronic diseases, necropsy pathologists see only the fatal end of the spectrum, and their interpretations cannot always be applied to the opposite end. Nevertheless, pathologists and clinicians have sometimes developed the mistaken concept that *all* of a human disease resembled the partial view seen in the morgue. For example, patients who have acute rheumatic fever *without* carditis do not die *of* acute rheumatic fever. The only patients who die *of* acute rheumatic fever have severe carditis. Yet, on the basis of the carditis constantly noted at necropsy in the acute rheumatic deaths, pathologists and clinicians believed for years that acute rheumatic fever always produced carditis. Similarly, if necropsy had been the sole source of epidemiologic data on acute infection with poliomyelitis virus, bulbar involvement would be universally anticipated because it is always found in patients who die *of* the acute disease. At necropsy, pathologists would not encounter, and hence would not know, acutely ill patients without bulbar involvement who survive paralytic or non-paralytic attacks.

TEMPORAL UNCERTAINTIES

In coronary, cerebrovascular, neuropathic, and other protracted diseases not currently susceptible to biopsy, the original diagnosis, therapeutic plans, and subsequent clinical observations must all be carried out before the confirmatory pathologic evidence of diagnosis can be obtained at death. Because the lesion is not seen until long after it was treated, the pathologist's findings in these chronic diseases must always be correlated with great care. When necropsy is performed months or years after the original therapeutic decisions were made, the anatomic situation may be quite different from what it was initially.

Only with the recent advent of frequent biopsy for kidney and liver disease have clinicians discovered the difficulties and errors involved in applying, at the bedside of the acutely ill patient, the old morphologic concepts of the *chronic nephritis* and *cirrhosis* observed at necropsy.

THERAPEUTIC INSUFFICIENCIES

The language and lesions of pathologic anatomy cannot be used effectively for evaluating the results of treatment in any "disease" that is not susceptible to *repeated biopsy*. For example, we assess the treatment of *myocardial infarction* by evaluating clinical, radiographic, electrocardiographic, and laboratory evidence; the morphologic evidence of a myocardial infarction is not observed unless treatment has been a total failure. Comparable problems exist for evaluating treatment of other "non-biopsy" diseases (such as *multiple sclerosis, diabetic retinopathy,* and *stroke*) and for many other anatomic enties (such as *acute hepatitis, regional ileitis,* or *glomerulonephritis*), in which biopsy may be applied for the original diagnosis, but may be too hazardous or inconvenient to be used repeatedly thereafter as a morphologic index of response to treatment.

This defect of pathologic taxonomy is probably irremediable. Although a specimen of morbid anatomy can often be observed for a satisfactory initial diagnosis of disease, the difficulties of obtaining repeated specimens during and after therapy are too great for most diseases that are morphologic entities. At present, the only non-dermatologic clinician who can easily obtain repeated "biopsies" of the "disease" he treats is a hematologist, who studies the cytopathology of blood, rather than the histopathology of organs and tissues.

The absence of satisfactory indexes for evaluating therapeutic accomplishment is a profound deficiency in contemporary clinical science. (See subsequent discussion in Chapter 14.) The problem cannot be solved merely by improved clinico-pathologic correlations, however, and requires that the clinician develop new approaches and new techniques in the taxonomy of treatment.

PROGNOSTIC INADEQUACIES

Perhaps the greatest problem of pathologic diagnostic taxonomy is its frequent failure to correlate with the subsequent course of the diagnosed disease. Some patients with *epidermoid carcinoma of the lung, rheumatic carditis,* and *pneumococcal meningitis* may die quickly after diagnosis, while others survive a long time, or are "cured". Some patients with *diabetes mellitus, duodenal ulcer,* and *multiple sclerosis* lead relatively normal lives, while others are harassed by multiple complications and incapacitation. Yet these variegated courses of disease in different patients are designated by the same diagnostic label.

Although contemporary diagnosis has become an act of extraordinary and often quantified biologic precision, prognosis remains a vague and often inaccurate generality. Despite the development of an anatomic staging system for cancer, surgeons, radiotherapists, and chemotherapists may have major dissents about the results of treatment for patients in the same anatomic stage, because the morphologic data are alone inadequate to demonstrate subtle prognostic distinctions.[25] Cardiologists may engage in vigorous public controversy about the life expectancy of a President who has had a myocardial infarction, because the diagnosis and general statistics of *myocardial infarction* do not adequately specify the prognosis in different subgroups of patients. Polemical debates may rage[33] about how to treat diabetes mellitus, pulmonary emphysema, urinary tract infections, and many other ailments of man, because the diagnostic names are inadequate both for indicating the nuances of current clinical state and for predicting subsequent developments.

The contemporary absence of such prognostic distinctions is partly due to the taxonomic transformations that converted medical ailments from the clinical *dis-ease* of the bed to the anatomic *disease* of the morgue. But the absence is also attributable to changing intellectual fashions that affect the medical focus of both the clinician and the pathologist. Santayana[97] has said that "those who forget the lessons of history are condemned to repeat them." Clinicians and pathologists have forgotten the lessons to be learned from the history of nosology.

THE EVOLUTION OF PROGNOSTIC NOSOLOGY

In the old Hippocratic concepts of "disease", prognosis was an essential aspect of the reasoning used to identify certain symptoms and signs as "diseases". For example, the "Hippocratic facies", as a precursor of death, is one of the many prognostic indexes that has endured from ancient times. When Sydenham, in the 17th century, rescued nosology from the iatrochemists and re-instated the bedside as the major site for observing "disease", he indicated that "natural history", and not just isolated clinical manifestations, should be used in establishing diagnostic entities. He correlated his classifications with prognosis. Sydenham's followers in the 18th century, however, forgot his correlative proscription; they created elaborate nosologies in which clinical manifestations were generally classified arbitrarily, without specific regard to prognostic distinctions.

When Morgagni, Pinel, and particularly Bichat, in the late 18th and early 19th centuries, established morbid anatomy as a paramount consideration in "disease", their concern was to correlate the clinical manifestations of the bedside with the anatomic "diseases" of the necropsy room. Such correlations were particularly effective for the material studied in 19th century hospitals: the patients were often moribund, and the interval between the observation of clinical evidence and its anatomic correlation was often brief. During the early 19th century, the "patho-clinicians" who followed Bichat identified many of the ailments we know today. Corvisart correlated disease of the heart with its symptoms, and with signs discerned from Auenbrügger's method of percussion. Corvisart's pupil, Laënnec, made anatomic sense of sound, correlating the auscultatory findings in the chest with diseases of the lungs, recognizing tuberculosis as a single "disease", and identifying the abnormal hepatic anatomy that still bears his name. The great Irish and British "patho-clinicians" (among them Adams, Addison, Bright, Cheyne, Corrigan, Graves, Hodgkin, Parkinson, and Stokes) joined their French colleagues in providing the clinico-anatomic correlations for which their names are still remembered. Viennese, German, and other European "patho-clinicians" added to the outflow of observation and correlation that made the new nosology flourish.

As a result of these activities, Faber notes,

> an entirely new clinical medicine developed during the first part of the nineteenth century. . . . The violence with which clinical medicine

was completely revolutionized in the course of a few decades by these important and striking discoveries will always remain one of the wonders of medical history.[98]

A "disease" had become an entity in which specific clinical manifestations, caused by specific anatomic abnormalities, could evolve in a specific course and might even be cured by specific therapeutic agents.

The new clinico-anatomic nosology had many defects, however. The specific clinical manifestations of the bedside often did not correlate with the anticipated anatomic lesions, and often no distinct lesion of any type could be found to explain such functional disorders as diarrhea, fever, and various rheumatic pains. Moreover, a specific therapy could not generally be found that achieved consistent success in the treatment of each specific disease. And finally, even when a specific anatomic cause could be found for the bedside manifestations, what had caused the anatomic abnormality?

These obvious defects in the early clinico-anatomic nosology, and perhaps some national chauvinism, encouraged the German pathologists of the later 19th century to vigorously oppose the foreign doctrine —initially Greek (Hippocrates), later English (Sydenham), subsequently Italian (Morgagni), and now French (Pinel, Bichat, et al.)— of a specific correlation for clinical manifestation, disease, and outcome. Wunderlich and others denounced the concept of specific entities in disease, called it "ontology", pointed out its flaws, and urged that "pathologic physiology" be the true basis of medical science.

This rejection of "ontology" was probably the origin of the current separation between the "basic" and the "clinical" sciences of medicine. The doctors who had initially investigated "disease" anatomically were clinicians, correlating in one mind the observations made in the two localities of bedside and morgue. The rejection of "ontology" by the new pathologists, and the opportunity to apply new technologic methods in research, was accompanied by a rejection of concomitant activities at the bedside. Pathologists now began to work almost exclusively in the morgue and in laboratories, and began to engage in two different types of activity related to cause and function in disease.

One group of "pathologic physiologists", headed by Virchow, concentrated on delineating causes and mechanisms of disease, and soon developed a fundamentally morphologic approach. The earlier clinico-anatomic nosology had been a correlation of clinical manifestations with grossly visible anatomic lesions. Aided by the use of microscopes,

Virchow converted the gross lesions of organs and tissues into "diseases" of cells. Virchow's work was magnificent, laying the foundation on which modern histopathology still rests, and demolishing the erroneous doctrine of humoral causes for disease, an etiologic concept bequeathed to medicine by the Hippocratic school and maintained for centuries after the more valid Hippocratic concepts of prognosis had been forgotten. In developing pathology as a microscopic discipline, Virchow also laid the groundwork for intellectual beliefs that sometimes dominate the thought of many pathologists today: a pre-occupation with causes of "disease", a frequent lack of concern with therapy, and an absence of intensive clinical correlations. With "disease" defined by its "causes" and microscopic appearance, the pathologist became relatively absolved of the responsibility for determining whether a patient's clinical illness coincided with the morphologic manifestations. As the pathologist kept looking for newer ways to define "disease" microscopically, the clinician kept looking for better para-clinical techniques to diagnose the pathologist's "diseases". During this common search for "disease", the concept of prognostic correlation for clinical manifestations was lost.

At about the same time that Virchow was clarifying the microscopy and "causes" of disease, another group of "pathologic physiologists", containing many German investigators and led in France by Bernard, concentrated on function. Frequently rejecting both the bedside and the morgue, these investigators began using the laboratory for active experiments, exploring functional mechanisms of disease induced in animals and establishing the domain of physiology as an independent discipline devoted not to disease alone, but also to normal biologic function. These investigators were also relatively unconcerned with prognosis and treatment of human ailments. Their enduring contributions to medical science included the idea of performing laboratory experiments, the search for functional mechanisms, the concept of animal "models" of disease, and the principles of reductionist biology.

These two new activities, *histopathology* and *physiology,* were the earliest specialties in medical research that became established as clinically remote domains of the laboratory. After their common origins in "clinico-pathology", these two domains then separated from each other and, in turn, gave rise to two additional laboratory specialties. Toward the end of the 19th century, with further advances in technology, the pathologist's investigations of cause were rewarded by the laboratory discovery of bacterial agents in disease, and by the subsequent separation and development of the laboratory science that is now called *microbiology*. As the advancing knowledge of chemistry was applied by physiologists, *biochemistry* was separated from physiology to become another branch of "basic" medical science.

From all these contributions of the "basic" medical sciences that were developed away from the bedside, clinical nosology acquired the names of many additional morphologic "diseases" and all the etiologic and "functional" constituents of the modern pathologic diagnostic taxonomy. Such "diseases" as *thyroiditis, streptococcal infection, porphyria, atrial fibrillation, hypogammaglobulinemia, plasma cell myeloma, pulmonary alveolar proteinosis,* and many others cited earlier were "discovered" by the new methods of investigation. Many of the new names, however, represented "diseases" identified by laboratory workers, not by clinicians, and the "diseases" had been, if correlated at all, associated with isolated clinical states, not with prognosis. The laboratory workers, producing the observations and data of the new medical science, did not always have time for intensively studying the clinical courses of the "diseases" they were identifying. Even if the laboratory workers wanted to attempt such correlations, however, the necessary clinical data were often lacking. Clinicians were too busy learning the laboratory data and diagnostic techniques of the new science to give adequate attention to getting and correlating the appropriate clinical information.

During the 20th century in histopathology, ingenious staining techniques and powerful new microscopy have led to many additional expansions and refinements of morphologic knowledge. The 20th century successors of Bichat and Virchow, however, have pursued a taxonomic course analogous to that of Sydenham's successors in 18th century nosology. Histopathologists have classified, subclassified, and further subclassified elements of morbid anatomy, but have often failed to make satisfactory clinical and prognostic correlations for the morphologic categories of "disease". The "diseases" noted by physiologists, microbiologists, and biochemists have also often been defined and established without appropriate prognostic correlations.

Many clinicians of a century ago were markedly distressed by the histopathologic and chemical revolutions that were introducing so many "new" diseases and "alien" laboratory concepts into medicine. Referring to the new sciences being developed away from the bedside, the master French clinician Trousseau denounced the

... exaggeration of their importance, their pretentiousness, their being mixed up with our art in an inappropriate and impertinent manner.... Among ... all the compositions and decompositions, all the molecular movements ... there [may] be some which are governed by laws which govern dead matter, [but] ... others ... obey quite different laws—laws which perhaps chemistry may some day discover, but which for the present remain autonomous, special, unexplained, [and] inexplicable.... I wish [the laboratory scientists] to be modest.... I am quite willing to confess my ignorance as a chemist, but only on condition that chemists confess their ignorance as ... physicians.[99]

As for the new anatomic and etiologic names of disease, Trousseau preferred the older terms of clinical observation "because it imposes on me no doctrine nor opinion".[100] Said Charcot, another French clinical master, "Disease is very old, and nothing about it has changed. It is we who change as we learn to recognize what was formerly imperceptible." [101]

However the contemporary reader may view the comments of Trousseau, thoughtful clinicians will have little disagreement with Charcot. The "new diseases" of the 19th century and of our own often represent an identification of morphologic, microbial, biochemical, immunologic, chromosomal, molecular, and other abnormalities that have probably always been present in sick people but that could not be detected until suitable technology became available. Clinicians and pathologists today may talk of "new diseases" and "changing natural history" without recognizing that we see many of the same ailments treated by our ancestors, but that we apply new names and new etiologic concepts of "disease". The changes in prevalence of many "diseases" may merely reflect our new ability to diagnose them, rather than a true change in the interaction of man and nature.

Trousseau was also disturbed by the new nosology's lack of concern for the different "species" of clinical course that could be distinguished only from studying the natural history of a disease:

> How is it possible to estimate the value of a method of treatment ... if the operations of nature ... are ignored, operations which are different in the different species of diseases? By not discriminating between these different species, do we not incur the risk of attributing great virtues to medicines which have in reality no remedial power...? [102]

The differences among the clinical "species" of a "disease" are even more important today than in the time of Trousseau, because 20th century "diseases" are diagnosed in different ways and in different stages from those found in the wards of 19th century hospitals. A 19th century patient often entered the hospital expecting to die; when he died, his clinical and anatomic findings could be promptly correlated. A 20th century patient enters the hospital to live; his diagnosis and treatment occur in clinical circumstances utterly different from those that could so quickly attain pathologic correlation 100 years ago.

Although the concept of "ontology" in disease was rejected a century ago, many of its principles have since been proved.* We now know about specific "causes" and specific treatments for many "diseases" that can be specifically diagnosed. What clinicians continue to lack, however, is well-correlated data about natural history that can give us a knowledge of specific *courses* of "disease". Despite the many changes of the past half century, the pathologist's examination of tissue today is still an exercise mainly in diagnostic morphology; he has not adequately correlated his findings with our new knowledge of diverse clinical patterns in disease. He can tell us that the dead patient had a pulmonary embolus, a myocardial infarction, or a duodenal ulcer, but not why this particular embolus, infarction, or ulcer was painless. The pathologist can tell us that a surgical biopsy specimen is a cancer or an inflammation, but the morbid anatomy is not correlated well enough to predict accurately whether the cancer can be cured or the inflammation healed. The pathologist can tell us that a cancer is an epidermoid carcinoma, but he cannot consistently predict whether this particular epidermoid carcinoma grows rapidly or slowly; and whether it will spread to other sites, or remain localized.

Today's clinical pathologist can tell us that a diabetic patient has hyperglycemia and hypercholesterolemia, but not whether, when, or where vascular complications will occur. He can tell us that a cirrhotic patient has abnormal tests of liver function, but not whether ascites will develop or esophageal varices will bleed. The clinical pathologist can tell us that a patient with staphylococcal pneumonia has an organism that is "sensitive" or "resistant" to certain drugs; but not whether or when the patient will lose his fever, regain his appetite, and return to work.

In all of these, and in myriads of other prognostic distinctions, the

* The eventual vindication of "ontology" is particularly interesting in view of its initial rejection in favor of etiologic theories that have now come into question. The dictionary⁴⁴ defines *ontology* as "the science of being or reality".

pathologist provides a detailed nosology of disease that is excellent for precise diagnosis, but that lacks the clinical correlations necessary for science in modern therapy. Estranged for almost a century from correlation with direct clinical and epidemiologic observations, the pathologist's nomenclature of laboratory and morgue is no longer alone adequate for the operating room and bed.

*   *   *

The citation of these problems is by no means intended to denigrate pathologists, or to detract from the fundamental importance of morbid anatomy and laboratory work in medicine. Like the clinician, the pathologist has difficulties with observational criteria because he is human. Like the clinician, the pathologist has difficulties in how far he can draw conclusions from what he observes. Like the clinician, the pathologist has often been intellectually debauched by the guiles of technology. And like the clinician, the histopathologist, in particular, has new challenges for his role in 20th century diagnostic and therapeutic medicine.

The scientific problems of morbid anatomy and of clinico-pathologic correlation are no more solved today than are the problems of medical taxonomy and clinical therapy. Clinicians who still believe that the main goal of clinical medicine is to prevent illness and to care for sick people, and pathologists who still believe that the main goal of pathology is to study human disease, can advance medical science now, more than ever before, by collaborative research. The primary observations of the two specialties are too complex for both types of observation to be made often enough or consistently enough by single investigators. With the clinician and the pathologist bringing the precision of carefully organized scientific data to both ends of the clinico-pathologic (or pathologico-clinical) correlations, the present obscurity of natural history, prognosis, treatment, and many other features of human ailments can be clarified. If the latter half of the 19th century in pathology was the era of great discovery in "disease", the latter half of the 20th century can be an era of discovering what the former discoveries really mean in human illness.

This citation of problems in pathology is intended only to emphasize the simple and obvious point that pathology is not clinical medicine. The two domains are completely different in their sites, material, methods of observation and interpretation, and immediate goals. Nevertheless, although the pathologist works *his* way and uses concepts and vocabulary suitable for his work, the clinician, in working *his* way, often replaces his own concepts and vocabulary by those of the pathologist. In particular, the clinician continues to use the diagnostic taxonomy of pathology as an almost exclusive base for his therapeutic activities. If pathologists have failed to correlate their morphologic observations with clinical data, it is because clinicians have not made the data respectable and available. After carefully observing the personal distinctions of a host, and the symptoms and signs that are the clinical distinctions of an illness, the clinician then obliterates all these distinctions by converting them into the diagnostic name of a "disease".

Regardless of what type of diagnostic name is given to the "disease" —morphologic, microbiologic, chemical, biophysical, molecular, eponymic, "clinical", or combinations of these designations—a clinician's first step in treatment is to choose such a diagnosis from which to proceed. After diagnosing the "disease", however, the clinician has not finished all the diagnostic classification he must still do for the reasoning of prognosis and therapy. Within the "universe" of each "disease", there is still a diverse spectrum of illnesses and hosts to be classified, and the clinician cannot be a therapeutic scientist until he has reproducibly identified these other elements that characterize the material he treats.

Many aspects of the personal data of a host (such as age, race, sex, and occupation) already can be categorized in a reasonably good taxonomy, and these data are regularly cited in many classifications of treated patients. Such data can often be obtained, however, by observers with minimal or no clinical skill. The *sine qua non* of a clinician's skill is his ability to obtain the data of clinical manifestations— the symptoms and signs of the host's illness. The clinician is the unique apparatus that examines the sick host for obtaining the data of symptoms and signs, that reasons with these data, that draws conclusions from the reasoning, that executes therapeutic acts on the basis of these conclusions, and that appraises the consequences of the therapeutic acts. The quality of a clinician's clinical judgment depends on the way he has stored and evaluated these data; they are his "clinical experience".

Yet clinical data have no taxonomy at all. There currently exists no standard method, logic, order, system, structure, or rational procedure for classifying the clinical data of human illness. The clinician can do nothing specific with his clinical data except convert them, by an obliterating translation, into the diagnostic categories of the nomenclature of pathology. After deciding, for example, that the patient has had a myocardial infarction, the clinician has no way of diagnostically preserving the presence or absence of intractable chest pain, sweating, shock, dyspnea, cyanosis, arrhythmias, or other clinical manifestations from which the pathologic diagnosis was made. The patient's diagnosis is cited thereafter as *myocardial infarction,* and all of the original clinical distinctions are lost.

Pathologic diagnosis, however, is not the sole basis of therapeutic decisions. Every clinician knows very well that his choices of treatment are constantly influenced not just by a diagnostic label, but by the nuances of his distinctly clinical observations. Every clinician constantly classifies and applies those clinical nuances not just in the inferences of diagnostic reasoning, but specifically in the choices and evaluation of therapy. The clinician seldom recognizes his clinical classification and application of those distinctions, however, because he makes them informally, diversely, or subconsciously—with all the overt or subtle shades of variation of a *nuance.* Believing that the distinctions are unidentifiable nuances, and unable to designate the way he uses them, the clinician regards his therapeutic reasoning as a non-reproducible procedure, and gives it the name of *clinical judgment.* Yet, if the clinician looks closely at the nuances, and begins to think about them specifically, he can discern the clear distinctions of their contour.

He knows the many clinical distinctions that tell him when death is imminent or hope abundant; when to treat and when to wait; when to sedate with drugs and when to sedate with words; when to stop treatment, or change, or add; when to treat aggressively for cure, palliatively for relief, or consolingly for comfort. The clinician knows that these therapeutic decisions may depend on such distinctly bedside observations as the strength of a patient's hands, the posture of his body, the noise in his chest, the smell of his breath, the sweat on his brow, the grimace on his face, the quaver in his voice, and the anguish of his family. The clinician knows that the therapeutic decisions may depend on such distinctly clinical nuances as a particular combination of symptoms and signs, whether the patient complains of certain symptoms or tolerates them quietly, whether the disease was found before or after symptoms developed, whether the symptoms were of short duration or long, and whether one symptom had preceded another or followed.

The clinician knows all these and many more distinctly clinical features that are his harbingers of prognosis and determinants of therapy.
But he cannot express them specifically or consistently. Medical taxonomy has given him classifications for the host and for the disease,
but not for the illness of the patient who is the diseased host. Lacking
any formal means of classifying clinical observations, the clinician has
no place to put the information when he communicates with himself
or with his colleagues. He seldom finds the clinical information suitably
cited in the literature he reads, or in the conferences he attends, because
the clinical data are seldom deliberately arranged and deliberately correlated in the analyzed results of treatment for disease. He cannot speak
his clinical distinctions well, or think about them clearly, or read about
them specifically, or write about them formally, because he cannot
stipulate them—he has no ordered taxonomic vocabulary for them.

He has a taxonomic vocabulary for classifying the many personal
features of a host:

> age, race, sex, occupation, birthplace, religion, dietary intake, politi-
> cal beliefs, economic status, housing, familial kindred, geographic
> location, domestic pets, smoking habits, drinking habits, sexual habits,
> and many other demographic aspects of human life.

He has a taxonomic vocabulary for classifying the many features of
disease:

> organs, tissues, cells, cellular contents, molecules, atoms, electrons,
> chromosomes, antibodies, antigens, microbial organisms, electro-
> physiologic tracings, roentgenographic silhouettes, and the diverse
> ingredients of body fluids and excreta.

He even has a taxonomic vocabulary for classifying the agents of treatment: drugs, operations, and all the physical, chemical, and other procedures of contemporary therapy. But he cannot classify symptoms and
signs except by losing their distinctions with an inferred translation into
the diagnostic vocabulary of pathologic taxonomy. In the midst of the
articulate science that surrounds him, the clinician is left scientifically
aphasic, cacophonous, or mute. The diagnostic taxonomy of pathology
allows him no syntax for a language in which to express his own clinical
knowledge.

Lacking a taxonomy of his own, the clinician *must* grope for words
and concepts to describe scientific ideas that he often knows and practices full well. Lacking a taxonomy of his own, he *must* be "irrational"

in the intellectual storage of his strictly clinical observations and experiences; the "rational" spaces are all occupied by data of "disease" and of other modalities of classification, so he has to squeeze his clinical data into diverse interstices of his mind. Lacking a taxonomy of his own, he *must* be uncertain of where and how he got, put, or retrieved the data stored in those interstices. When asked how he does it, he cannot identify the process because it *had* to be done without a conscious order, so he regards it as an unscientific intuition, hunch, or mystique, and he calls it *clinical judgment.*

Human taxonomy provides a classification for designating a host who has a disease. Pathologic taxonomy provides a classification for designating (or diagnosing) the host's disease. There is no organized medical system, however, for classifying the illness that is the clinical interaction of host and disease. The illness of patients—an entity of nature constantly observed by clinicians, constantly analyzed by clinicians, and constantly treated by clinicians—has no taxonomy.

The construction of such a *clinical* taxonomy will be the first procedure of the "therapy" suggested in the remainder of this book. The foregoing discussion concludes the reasoning used to establish a "diagnosis" for the intellectual maladies that beset contemporary clinical science. It is now time to think about treatment.

PART II

Principles of Clinical Taxonomy

Chapter 8. Types, Uses, and Attributes of Clinical Data

Definitions
Clinical Data as Scientific Variables in Clinical Reasoning
The Preliminary Appraisal of Symptoms and Signs
The Clinical Attributes of Symptoms and Signs
    Iatrotropy; Toponymy; Chronometry

Chapter 9. Classification of Clinical Behavior of a Disease

Mode of Detection and General Clinical State
Cluster of Individual Clinical Manifestations
The Sequence of Clinical Manifestations
The Timing of Clinical Sequences
The Co-morbidity of Associated Illness

Chapter 10. A Clinical Primer of the "New" Mathematics

Definitions and Elementary Properties of Sets
The Operations of Boolean Algebra
Venn Diagrams and Relations of Sets
    Disjoint; Overlapping; Subordinate; Identical

Chapter 11. Spectrums of Disease and other "Mathemedical" Constructions

The General Spectrum of a Human Disease
Clusters and Spectrums in Specific Clinical Situations
    Acute Rheumatic Fever
        Spectrum of Sore Throats, Streptococcal Infections, and Sources of Rheumatic Fever
        Spectrum of Acute Rheumatic Fever
        Spectrum of Acute Rheumatic Carditis
        Prognosis of Acute Rheumatic Fever
    Spectrum of Cancer
        General Clinical Spectrum
        Prognostic Clinical Spectrum
        Prognosis in Cancer of the Lung
        Prognosis in Cancer of the Rectum
    Spectrum of Pain in Coronary Artery Disease
    Other Applications of Venn Diagrams
        The Etiologic, Prognostic, and Morphologic Spectrum of Fractures
        Clinico-Pathologic Correlation in Lung Disease
        Spectrum of Antibody Responses in Streptococcal Infections
        Spectrums of Observer Variability
Patterns of Sequence in Clinical Manifestations
    General Pattern of Possible Sequential Changes
    Recurrences of Acute Rheumatic Fever

Chapter 12. Biologic and Statistical Implications of Clinical Taxonomy

Biology of Human Illness
    The Evolution of a Disease; The Chronometry of Discovery; Concepts of Pathogenesis
Statistics in Human Disease
    Incidence and Prevalence of Disease
    "Random Sampling" and "Collected Cases"
    Identification and Enumeration
    Selection of Categories

8. Types, Uses, and Attributes
of Clinical Data

The performance of history-taking and physical examination provides clinicians with the personal (or demographic) data that describe the patient as a host, and with the clinical data that describe the patient's illness. The clinical data consist of different types of evidence, used for different purposes in clinical reasoning, and classified according to those purposes both before and after a diagnosis has been established.

DEFINITIONS

There are two main types of clinical data: symptoms and signs. A *symptom* is the name given to a subjective sensation or other observation that a patient reports about his body or its products. For example, the sensation of a pressing or pulsating discomfort behind the eyes may be designated as the symptom of *retro-orbital headache;* a substernal discomfort provoked by exertion and relieved by rest may be called the symptom of *angina pectoris;* an excessive amount of lower abdominal cramps or other extraordinary distress during menstruation may be called *dysmenorrhea.*

A *sign* is the name given to an entity objectively observed by the clinician during physical examination of the patient. For example, a *palpable liver* is the name of a sign manifested by a certain tactile sensation in the abdomen; *rhonchi* and *murmurs* are designations of certain noises heard during auscultation of the chest; *retinal exudate*

131

denotes a sign observed during ophthalmoscopic inspection of the ocular fundus.

Certain entities, such as jaundice, can be observed both by the clinician and by the patient, or by some other person who has no clinical training. Such entities may be called *subjective signs* or *objective symptoms*. They may be distinguished from *iatric signs*—such as retinal exudate, prostatic nodules, and most cardiac murmurs— which are discerned only with specific clinical techniques of examination. Objective symptoms (or subjective signs) can be *corporeal,* occurring in the patient's body, or *effluent,* occurring in various visible products that emerge from the patient's body. For example, a patient can report the presence of such corporeal objective symptoms as jaundice, a skin rash, a palpable superficial lump, and certain thoracic or articular noises that are loud enough to be overtly audible. The patient can also report the description of such effluent objective symptoms as bloody sputum, green vomitus, brown urine, and tarry stools.

Some of the clinical findings reported as symptoms and signs are thus noted exclusively by the patient, some are noted exclusively by the clinician, and others are noted by both. These distinctions are important for several reasons: a patient's complaint may often be directly verified, by the clinician or by non-clinical observers, if it is an objective rather than subjective symptom, since it is actually a sign; and the patient's own observation of these subjective signs may often be valuable in timing their duration and noting their variations before the patient comes to the clinician's attention.

For convenience of nomenclature in the rest of this book, the term symptom *will refer to either subjective or objective symptoms that are reported by patients. The term* sign *will refer to either iatric signs or the subjective signs (objective symptoms) observed by clinicians. The term* finding *will refer to either a symptom or a sign.*

CLINICAL DATA AS SCIENTIFIC VARIABLES IN CLINICAL REASONING

In the rational performance of diagnosis, prognosis, and therapy, clinicians reason with clinical data in three entirely different ways.

For diagnosis, clinical data are used to suggest a *group of possible causative or associated diseases* that account for the findings. From this group of diseases, clinicians choose the ones that are most likely to be present, and the unlikely ones that must be excluded. The appropriate laboratory tests and other diagnostic procedures are then selected and performed. The total data are then interpreted to establish diagnosis.

For prognosis and general therapeutic strategy, clinical data are used to suggest not a group of diseases, but a *group of patients with the same disease*. Prognosis and therapy, which are contemplated after diagnosis is established, require a review of the clinician's knowledge of all previous patients with the same disease. In this review, the clinician must identify those patients whose clinical (and other) properties most closely resembled the particular patient at hand. After determining what happened to the similar previous patients, the clinician assumes that the disease will evolve similarly in the current situation. He then recalls the treatment used in the previous situations and decides which treatment gave the best results. If the disease evolved in a satisfactory way without treatment, or if no mode of therapy offers any advantages over the anticipated natural course of the disease, the clinician's therapeutic decision may be to give no specific treatment.

For subsidiary aspects of therapy, clinical data are often used to suggest neither a group of diseases nor a group of patients, but a *group of findings distressing to the individual patient*. Although general therapeutic strategy is planned according to the established diagnosis and prognosis, clinicians choose many ancillary therapeutic procedures according to the patient's specific complaints. These complaints, which are not necessarily explained by the established diagnoses or affected by the general therapeutic plan, often indicate what the patient wants done for treatment to be successful.

To illustrate these procedures, consider the management of a patient who enters the hospital with acute substernal chest pain and severe respiratory distress. After reviewing the various pathologic disorders that can produce these clinical features, the physician decides tentatively that the patient's diagnosis (or pathologic state) is myocardial infarction, and that the clinical state of heart failure is also present. To confirm the pathologic diagnosis, the physician orders an electrocardiogram and other laboratory tests. He tells the family that the patient is gravely ill, and possibly moribund, not just because of the pathologic diagnosis, but because the patient's heart has also acutely decompensated. The physician may order anticoagulants if he believes they are helpful in the treatment of acute myocardial infarction. Almost all his other drugs, however, are intended to treat the clinical findings, not the pathologic diagnosis. Hypnotics and cardiotonic agents are given not for the pathologic diagnosis, but for the chest pain and cardiac decompensation. These drugs are maintained, altered, or stopped, not according to the pathologic diagnosis, but according to the duration and severity of the clinical manifestations.

The physician may also order additional measures—such as air-conditioning, cathartics, or sedatives—for the treatment of associated clinical or even atmospheric features that may or may not be related to the pathologic lesion of myocardial infarction. If the patient survives, and if the diagnosis is confirmed, the physician may then consider long-term management of the pathologic lesion with anticoagulants and lipid-altering procedures. In deciding about physical or occupational activities for the recovered patient, however, the clinician will base his judgment not merely on the pathologic diagnosis, but on the specific prognosis expected from observation of other patients whose heart attacks had similar manifestations.

Thus, clinical data have three separate roles in clinical reasoning. In diagnosis, they suggest causative diseases; in prognosis and in general therapeutic strategy, they indicate comparable patients; in subsidiary therapy, they indicate specific targets of treatment. The reasoning used for each of those different roles of clinical data involves different intellectual constructions and, consequently, different systems of classification.

To classify the same data in several different ways may seem unusual, but such taxonomic distinctions are common in everyday life. English words, for example, are arranged one way in a conventional dictionary,[44] another way in Roget's Thesaurus,[103] and yet a third way in Fowler's manual of usage.[104] Each of these three taxonomies of words is organized differently because it has a different purpose. A dictionary conveys the meaning of words, a thesaurus gives their synonyms and associations, and a manual of usage deals with the application of words in composition and in literary style. Similarly, the different rational roles of clinical data will require different types of classification procedures for diagnosis, for general therapeutic strategy, and for specific therapeutic evaluation.

THE PRELIMINARY APPRAISAL OF SYMPTOMS AND SIGNS

Before clinical reasoning can begin, the clinician must first decide which symptoms and signs he is going to think about. No symptom or sign exists as a distinctive entity. These clinical data exist only as the names given to certain sensations that must be perceived, communicated, and labeled with the appropriate designations. The acquisition of these data is the fundamental procedure of clinical examination: the observation and classification of the basic sensations reported by the patient and noted by the clinician. The methods of acquiring clinical data will be discussed later (Part IV) in greater detail, but their general principles are conveniently cited here. To decide that a particular symptom or sign exists, the clinician goes through a process of contemplating *sensation,* adding *specification,* and selecting *designation.* For a symptom, *sensation* describes the actual phenomenon perceived by the patient, such as a discomfort in the chest; *specification* adds such further description as substernal location, provocation by exertion, and prompt relief with rest; *designation* gives a name to the specified sensation—in this instance, *angina pectoris.* For a sign, the *sensation* may be a feeling of resistance palpated by the clinician in the right upper quadrant of the patient's abdomen; *specification* adds the further description of an outlined edge that moves with respiration; *designation* provides the specified sensation with a name—in this instance, *palpable liver.*

The designation of a finding often includes the concept of *deviance*—the abnormality of the finding. For example, the abdominal sensation just described may sometimes be called *enlarged liver* or *hepatomegaly,* rather than *palpable liver.* Many signs and symptoms have no significant deviance, and occur as normal phenomena. Exertional dyspnea, for example, is a normal symptom in a young man who has just raced 100 yards, but would be abnormal after a walk of the same distance. Many other minor discomforts of daily life—such as occasional headaches, sporadic insomnia, and minor menstrual cramps—are symptoms that fall within the range of normal for the experiences of human existence. Cutaneous freckles, gray hair in the aged, and slight asymmetry in the pendency of breasts or testes are physical signs that have no pathologic deviance.

After the examining process has established the existence of normal and abnormal findings, the clinical *pertinence* of each finding is evaluated. The pertinence of a finding refers to the importance assigned to it, by patient or by clinician, in that patient's illness. Any finding—normal or abnormal—becomes pertinent if the patient complains about it. For example, many noses and breasts that were anatomically and functionally normal have received plastic surgery because of a patient's esthetic complaints about their appearance. Conversely, many abnormal findings may be disregarded in the clinician's management of the most cogent features of the illness. For example, after examining a patient with an acute onset of crushing substernal pain, the clinician may give little or no immediate attention to such abnormal findings as menstrual irregularities, myopia, dental caries, and an ingrown toe-nail.

By identifying the existing symptoms and signs, and by classifying their deviance and pertinence, the clinician thus assembles a list of the significant findings to which he will give his principal diagnostic and therapeutic attention. With these preliminary evaluations completed, he is now ready for the main clinical reasoning.

His first main decisional act is to select diagnostic attribution for the pertinent findings. Each of the findings must be accounted for, and must receive a diagnosis that attributes the finding to a particular disease or combination of disease processes. A discussion of the deductive reasoning and other rational procedures used for diagnosis of disease is beyond the scope of this book, and will not be further considered here. Let us assume that the clinician has performed these procedures, has selected a diagnostic attribution for each of the findings, and has concluded that the patient has one or more individual diseases. Let us further assume that the clinician has selected a particular disease to be treated. The therapeutic reasoning can now begin.

THE CLINICAL ATTRIBUTES OF
SYMPTOMS AND SIGNS

In the diagnostic reasoning that was just completed, the clinician regarded symptoms and signs as evidence of disease(s), and used the clinical findings either as direct indications of diagnosis, as clues from which diagnostic deductions could be made, or as guides to the selection of appropriate ancillary tests.

With diagnosis of a disease established, the clinician now regards each clinical finding as an index for distinguishing patients who, although having the same diagnosed disease, have different forms of illness. Examples of such indexes for different forms of illness are the adjectives modifying the names of disease in phrases like *asymptomatic* lung cancer, *bleeding* peptic ulcer, and *acute* myocardial infarction. Each of these adjectives describes a different attribute of an illness. These general attributes of clinical findings—iatrotropy, toponymy, and chronometry—are briefly noted here, and will be discussed in greater detail in the next chapter.

IATROTROPY

When a disease produces a symptom in a host, the host may either ignore the symptom or complain about it. If he complains about it, he may mention it only to relatives and friends, or he may be sufficiently provoked by it to go to a doctor, thereby receiving medical attention and becoming a patient. The doctor gives the name of *chief complaint* to the patient's citation of the particular symptom or group of symptoms that bother him the most. Although the chief complaint is usually discerned by listening to the patient's first few statements, the doctor, in taking a complete history, may discover that the patient also has many other symptoms that were not cited as complaints.

The patient's total array of symptoms will therefore contain some that were *iatrotropic*, i.e., the complaints that made him seek medical attention. Other symptoms may have existed as complaints that were bothersome but not provocative enough to make the patient seek medical help. Still other symptoms may have been present as incidental findings that did not particularly concern the patient or motivate his decision to go to a doctor. In the usual written structure of a conventional medical history, the iatrotropic symptom is cited among the *chief complaints;* other symptoms noted as complaints are listed in the section called *present illness;* and symptoms that are not complaints are often recorded in the *review of systems.*

TOPONYMY

Every significant clinical finding not only can be diagnostically attributed to a disease, but also can be regarded as the toponymic consequence of a particular lesion, complication, or other effect of the disease. Certain findings are *primary* clinical effects: the direct consequence of the main pathologic lesion of that disease. Other findings are *secondary*, arising indirectly, remotely, or as a complication of the main lesion. Angina pectoris, for example, is a primary clinical feature in coronary artery disease, while dyspnea and edema (due to congestive heart failure) are secondary manifestations. Hepatic enlargement is a primary clinical sign in cirrhosis of the liver, while ascites and cutaneous "spider" angiomas are secondary.

The designation of a finding as either a primary or a secondary clinical feature will depend upon the particular finding and upon the particular disease of which the finding is a toponymic consequence. The same symptom may be a primary feature for one disease, but a secondary feature for some other disease. Dysphagia, for example, is a primary symptom of esophageal cancer (a direct effect of the main tumor) but is a secondary feature in bronchogenic cancer (the consequence of metastatic dissemination to the mediastinum). Hepatomegaly is a primary sign in cirrhosis but (when due to congestive heart failure) is a secondary feature of coronary artery disease.

The many clinical features attributable to a disease cannot always be simply classified as primary or secondary; the toponymic distinctions will often require many arbitrary decisions—as in any system of classification. So long as the distinctions are reasonable, clearly indicated, and consistently applied, however, the classification will be valid and reproducible. The decision about classifying clinical features as primary or secondary is relatively easy when the "disease" is a morphologic lesion localized to a specific site. For example, in coronary artery disease, infectious hepatitis, and benign prostatic hypertrophy, the pathologic lesion anatomically occupies a single region.

These decisions are somewhat more difficult when the lesions of the disease are present in several different sites that are anatomically separated (as sometimes happens in carcinomas, cerebral arteriosclerosis, rheumatic fever, and multiple sclerosis); or when the lesion is cellular rather than histologic (as in leukemia); or when the main lesion is chemical (as in diabetes mellitus or porphyria); or in the many disorders (such as lupus erythematosus and psychiatric ailments) for which no specific basic lesion has yet been identified. Nevertheless, no matter how the disease or the basic lesion is defined, its primary, secondary, and other toponymic clinical features can be appropriately designated. If the definition of the basic lesion should later change, of course, the corresponding categories of clinical features would need suitable revision.

T A B L E 1. Arbitrary Illustrations of Primary and Secondary Features in Various Diseases

Name of Disease	Basic Lesion	Examples of Primary Features	Examples of Secondary Features
Infectious hepatitis	Inflammation of liver	Anorexia; tender liver; jaundice	Cutaneous and abdominal manifestations of portal hypertension or cirrhosis (spiders, ascites, gastrointestinal bleeding)
Coronary artery disease	Narrowed lumen of coronary arteries	Chest pain of at least three different types: angina pectoris; "coronary insufficiency"; "myocardial infarction"	Congestive heart failure; atrial fibrillation; ventricular aneurysm; mural thrombus
Carcinoma of lung	Carcinoma of lung	Hemoptysis; wheeze; recent cough	Anorexia; weight loss; hoarseness; superior vena cava syndrome; bone pain; neurologic manifestations
Regional ileitis	Inflammation of parts of ileum	Fever; abdominal pain; diarrhea	Weight loss; anemia; fistulas
Diabetes mellitus	Abnormal glucose metabolism	Nutritional (polyuria, polydipsia, polyphagia, weight loss); metabolic (acidosis, ketosis); susceptibility to infection (furuncles, etc.)	Peripheral vascular disease; nonperipheral vascular disease (retina, heart); nephropathy; neuropathy
Rheumatic fever	Post-streptococcal inflammation of selected tissues	Articular manifestations; erythema marginatum; subcutaneous nodules; chorea; murmurs of vulvulitis	Cardiac enlargement; congestive heart failure
Myelogenous leukemia	Immature leukocytes	Fever; anemia; splenomegaly	Weakness; infections; purpura
Multiple sclerosis	Degenerative lesions in nervous tissue	Optic neuritis; nystagmus; speech difficulties; ataxia	Locomotor incompetence; speech incompetence; decubiti; infections
Lupus erythematosus	Uncertain	Skin lesions; arthritis; nephritis	Hypertension; renal failure; anemia; psychosis

139

A series of examples is shown in Table 1 to illustrate an arbitrary classification of primary and secondary clinical features in several different diseases.

CHRONOMETRY

Symptoms have many temporal characteristics. They may begin abruptly or insidiously; they may slowly or rapidly rise to a peak intensity; they may wax and wane, or persist at a continuous level, or disappear at various rates of speed. When the patient's disease is medically detected, each symptom will have been present for different lengths of time; moreover, certain pertinent symptoms that appeared early in the illness may have disappeared before the patient sought medical attention. Finally, when a patient has had two or more symptoms, the symptoms will have had a succession, or order of appearance. Symptom *A,* for example, may have occurred at the same time as symptom *B,* or may have preceded or followed it. Symptom *C* may have occurred contemporaneously, or before or after symptoms *A* and *B*.

The chronometric classification of a symptom, therefore, will indicate the length of time it has been present, its order in the succession of symptoms, and perhaps other temporal attributes as well.

*   *   *

Using these clinical attributes of the appropriate symptoms and signs, a clinician can classify the different types of illness that occur in patients who have the same disease.

9. Classification of Clinical Behavior of a Disease

In a psychologic or social sense, the word *behavior* refers to a person's deportment in various situations of daily life. In a more general sense, the concept of behavior applies to the interaction of an entity with its environment. With that concept, we can contemplate the behavior of a disease during its interaction with the human host who provides the environment in which the disease conducts its "life". The disease can behave morphologically, to alter structures in the host's body; or biochemically and biophysically, to affect functions of the body; or clinically, to produce the signs and symptoms of the host's illness.

Until the host receives medical attention, he is unaware of effects inside the body that are not clinically perceptible. He may, however, observe external or other overt features of illness that constitute the clinical behavior of the disease. Encountering these clinical features of illness, the host will respond with psychic, social, and other reactions determined by his own personal patterns of behavior. He may become anxious and frightened by the symptoms, or may remain calm and serene; he may tolerate the symptoms stoically or exaggerate them dramatically; he may perceive many subjective signs that are barely detectable objectively, or he may fail to note others that are grossly evident; he may seek medical attention promptly after the symptoms appear, or he may procrastinate, postpone, or otherwise delay his visit to a doctor; he may choose his doctor to be a family physician, or may go directly to a highly specialized consultant.

Thus, as an evolving disease produces illness in a host, the host's response to the illness will affect both the time at which the disease first comes to be medically detected, and the particular medical setting at which the detection occurs. No matter how these events take place, however, the detected disease will have produced a describable and classifiable set of phenomena in its clinical behavior as an illness. The classification of those clinical phenomena helps to distinguish different patients with the same disease—and is a fundamental ingredient of clinical judgment.

In observing the illness of sick people, in formulating principles of therapeutic management, and in evaluating the subsequent results, clinicians constantly classify the clinical behavior of disease. These observations, formulations, and evaluations constitute a clinician's *clinical experience*. The appraised events of the past are the background for the judgment with which he designs, executes, and appraises his future activities in the bedside experiments of clinical care. (The procedures of "experience" and "experiment" are so closely related that the same word is used in some languages, such as French, to represent both activities.) A clinician achieves his "experience" by observing the illness of his patients, by categorizing the observations, by analyzing the contents of the categories, by storing the information in his memory, and by later retrieving the data selectively when he engages in the reasoning processes of judgment. The information stored in this rational background includes many types of classified data, but the particular distinction of a clinician's experience is an intellectual collection of data in which disease is classified according to its clinical behavior.

Because every clinician classifies his experience differently and because no specific taxonomy exists for an organized arrangement of the information, contemporary classifications of clinical data are unstandardized, inconsistent, and sometimes chaotic. Although the same events may often be contained in the clinical experiences of different clinicians, the clinicians may use many different categories for rationally collecting and sorting the events.

Nevertheless, no matter how each clinician gets and arranges the data, the possession of an organized background of clinical experience is the main knowledge that distinguishes a clinician from all his other medical colleagues. Of the many participants in the panorama of contemporary medical science, a clinician is the only doctor who constantly observes the illness of patients, who constantly classifies the clinical data to make therapeutic decisions, and who constantly analyzes the data to evaluate the accomplishments of therapy. Pathologists classify disease by pathologic behavior; radiologists, by radiologic behavior; biochemists, by biochemical behavior; immunologists, by immunologic behavior. Clinicians classify disease by clinical behavior.

The purpose of this chapter, and of several that follow it, is to demonstrate a formal, systematic construction for this classification—to develop a specific taxonomy for the clinical manifestations of human illness. This chapter is concerned with the rational methods of arranging pre-therapeutic clinical data for classifying patients in "design" of the experiments with which prognosis is estimated and treatment selected. The *post*-therapeutic rational arrangements—for evaluating the subsequent accomplishments of treatment—require separate analytic classifications, and will be discussed later in Part III.

*   *   *

Once the existence of a particular disease has been established (or diagnosed), the patient's clinical properties at that moment can be further classified according to five main features:

1) The manner in which the disease was detected in that patient and his general clinical state at the time of detection.

2) The cluster of individual clinical manifestations that constitute the general clinical state.

3) The sequence in which those manifestations appeared.

4) The timing, or duration, of each sequence.

5) The co-existence of illness due to other diseases.

Each of these five aspects of clinical behavior in a human disease has its own kind of variations. Although multiple and complex, the variations are finite and classifiable.

MODE OF DETECTION AND GENERAL CLINICAL STATE

Although patients usually seek medical aid for complaints of specific symptoms, a patient may go to a doctor for many other reasons. The examination may be a routine check-up, scheduled periodically regardless of the patient's state of health, or it may be solicited because of anxiety engendered in the patient (or in his family) by the illness of an acquaintance, the publicity of a health campaign, or other non-clinical reasons. Sometimes the examination is imposed upon the patient by external circumstances such as employment, insurance, or military service. On other occasions, the doctor comes to the patient, as in the investigations of an epidemiologic survey.

The symptoms or other conditions that bring a patient to medical attention, together with the information obtained during the clinical examination, will generally suggest certain specific diseases and diagnostic procedures. In addition, however, the clinician may order many other tests, either as part of the "routine" investigation or because additional clinical findings, suggestive of other diseases, were noted in the general examination. From all these procedures, the clinician may thus discover the presence of an additional disease (or diseases) whose existence was not implied by the chief complaint, or by any of the clinical findings.

To describe the many possible modes of detection of a diseased patient, the traditional term *chief complaint* is semantically and clinically inadequate: some patients may have no complaints and no symptoms; the symptoms stated as chief complaints in many patients may not be attributable to the main condition established as diagnosis; and a complaint of long duration may have undergone changes that introduce many other important symptoms. A more inclusive term is needed to refer to the reason why the patient came to see the physician. For the rest of this discussion, the phrase *iatrotropic stimulus* will be used for this purpose. The *chief complaint* is the patient's answer to the question, "What bothers you the most?", but the *iatrotropic stimulus* is his answer to the question, "Why did you decide to go to the doctor at this particular time?".

Although the iatrotropic stimulus and the chief complaint will often be the same, they will differ in some of the circumstances just cited, and even when they appear to be the same, they may still have subtle but distinct differences. For example, in a patient whose chief complaint is "chest pain on exertion for 8 months", the iatrotropic stimulus for the current examination may have not been the chest pain itself, but the patient's concern over the unexpected recent death of an acquaintance. As another example, the iatrotropic stimulus may have been a recent bout of chest pain that lasted longer or was more severe than the episodes of the previous 8 months. As a third possibility, the chest pain might have been unchanged for the past 8 months, but the iatrotropic stimulus may have been a transient recent episode of distressful but painless palpitation. Finally, the patient himself may have been unconcerned about the chest pain, and may have sought medical attention only in response to the prodding of an anxious wife.

Because of variations in iatrotropic stimuli, the medical diagnostic discovery of a particular disease in an individual patient can occur either deliberately or by accident. In a deliberate discovery, the patient comes to the doctor because of complaints due to that disease. In an accidental discovery, the patient's iatrotropic stimulus is something other than a complaint due to the particular disease: the stimulus may have been some type of para-medical purpose, as cited earlier, or a complaint due to some other disease.

To describe these different clinical properties among patients with the same disease, several additional terms become necessary. In the spectrum of patients with a particular disease, a *complainant* patient is one in whom the disease is discovered deliberately because of specific clinical complaints arising from it. A *lanthanic** (or non-complainant) patient is one whose disease is discovered "accidentally"; his iatrotropic stimulus contains no complaints referable to that disease. He may be wholly asymptomatic, or asymptomatic for that disease while symptomatic for another, or symptomatic for that disease with complaints arising from another.

For example, in the spectrum of coronary artery disease, a patient who seeks medical attention for angina pectoris is complainant. If the patient came to the doctor complaining of blindness (due to ocular cataracts), and if the symptom of angina pectoris is noted during the routine "review of the systems", the patient is lanthanic. Another example of a lanthanic patient with coronary artery disease is an asymptomatic man who, during a "routine check-up", is noted to have pathognomonic abnormalities in his electrocardiogram.

It is important to note that *lanthanic* and *complainant* refer only to the patient's state in regard to one particular disease. The same patient can be lanthanic for one disease and complainant for another disease. In the case of co-existent ocular cataracts and coronary disease, cited in the foregoing example, the patient was complainant for his cataracts and lanthanic for his coronary disease.

Thus, in the population of patients with a particular disease, the lanthanic ones may have "clinical" or "subclinical" features of that disease, and may be symptomatic or asymptomatic. The property that

* From the Greek λανθάνω, to escape attention. Chemists have applied this same root to name the lanthanide (rare earth) elements. The use of the word in this sense was suggested to me by Dr. Katerina Haka.

characterizes a patient as *lanthanic* is the absence of iatrotropic complaints due to that disease. (The more conventional words *latent, occult,* and *subclinical* are not satisfactory for this purpose, since they refer to disease that is not clinically evident. The lanthanic patient's disease may be clinically evident, but he does not complain to a doctor about it.) If a lanthanic patient's disease is medically detected, the detection comes as a clinical "accident" in the course of an examination performed in response to some other stimulus.

With these considerations, the clinical spectrum of a particular disease can be broadly divided into two groups of patients who are either complainant or lanthanic. In complainant patients, the disease can usually be diagnosed or suspected while the patient is alive, because the patient has come to a doctor complaining of it. In lanthanic patients, the disease may be detected either during life, after death, or not at all. The disease in a lanthanic patient can be discovered during life in the accidental circumstances described earlier, when a general examination is performed for some other purpose or complaint. At that examination, the physician obtains a routine laboratory test that discloses evidence of the disease, or he encounters the clinical evidence that arouses suspicion and further testing. The lanthanic patient's disease is discovered after death if necropsy is performed and reveals a previously unsuspected pathologic lesion. A lanthanic patient's disease remains undiscovered if he is examined during life but the correct diagnosis is not established, or if he dies without necropsy, or if the necropsy fails to show a lesion. In the last situation, a lesion may not be found at necropsy if the pathologic examination is inadequate, if the disease produces no visible lesion (e.g., porphyria or hypothyroidism), or if the lesion is in a site not routinely examined at necropsy (e.g., calf veins or temporal bone).

In addition to these features of mode of detection, the detected disease has a distinctive clinical state that depends on the presence or absence of the primary and secondary clinical features described earlier (Chapter 8). At the time of detection, the patient may have no clinical findings attributable to the disease, or primary clinical features only, or secondary features only, or a combination of primary and secondary features. The different possibilities of deliberate or accidental detection and of different types of clinical features create seven different subgroups of patients. These subgroups form clinical stages of the disease, delineated by the presence or absence, alone or in

T A B L E 2. **The Subgroups or Clinical Stages of a Disease: Mode of Detection and General Clinical Features of the Patients**

Subgroup Number	Code Name of Subgroup	Mode of Detection: Iatrotropic Stimulus Was a Complaint Arising from the Disease	General Clinical Features	
			Primary	Secondary
1	Lanthanic asymptomatic	0*	0	0
2	Lanthanic primary	0	+	0
3	Lanthanic combined	0	+	+
4	Lanthanic secondary	0	0	+
5	Complainant primary	+	+	0
6	Complainant combined	+	+	+
7	Complainant secondary	+	0	+

* Legend: + = present; 0 = absent.

combination, of specific complaints, primary features, and secondary features. The contents of these different stages are listed in Table 2, which also gives identifying clinical code names for the different subgroups of patients.

It should be noted that the term *clinical stage* is often applied incorrectly, in studies of cancer, to categorize the anatomic or pathologic states of the neoplasm as localized, or disseminated regionally or distantly. Such distinctions are morphologic, not clinical. The term *clinical stage,* as used here, refers to particular combinations of symptoms, signs, and iatrotropic stimuli.

To illustrate the application of these classifications, seven general clinical stages of a population of patients with coronary artery disease (or ischemic heart disease) are described in Table 3. For the purpose of this particular classification, chest pain is regarded as a primary clinical feature of the disease, and such manifestations as arrhythmias and congestive heart failure are considered to be secondary features. The symptom of dyspnea was arbitrarily chosen to represent a secondary clinical feature. Swollen legs, irregular heartbeat, or various other symptoms could have served equally well. The specific examples given in Table 3 do not cover all possible manifestations and circumstances of coronary disease, and serve only to indicate how the particular situations described here might be classified. It should be noted that some lanthanic patients listed in Table 3 are wholly asymptomatic and that others, with symptoms of coronary disease, have complaints due to symptoms of the other cited diseases.

T A B L E 3. **Illustration of Iatrotropic Stimuli and Clinical Features in Subgroups of Patients with Coronary Artery Disease**

Subgroup Number	Code Name of Subgroup	Iatrotropic Stimulus	Clinical Features of Coronary Artery Disease
1	Lanthanic asymptomatic	Routine check-up or painful inguinal hernia*	None†
2	Lanthanic primary	Urinary frequency due to benign prostatic hypertrophy*	Mild angina pectoris
3	Lanthanic combined	Decreased vision due to ocular cataracts*	Mild angina pectoris; symptomatic atrial fibrillation
4	Lanthanic secondary	Loss of hearing due to otosclerosis*	Mild peripheral edema due to early congestive heart failure‡
5	Complainant primary	Chest pain	Angina pectoris, or more severe chest pain
6	Complainant combined	Chest pain or dyspnea or both	Chest pain and congestive heart failure
7	Complainant secondary	Dyspnea	No chest pain; congestive heart failure‡

* These particular conditions are *arbitrarily chosen* to represent various iatrotropic stimuli. The same one could have been used for each subgroup here.

† Diagnosis of coronary artery disease made from electrocardiographic evidence only.

‡ Diagnosis of coronary artery disease made by exclusion of other forms of heart disease; electrocardiographic evidence may also be present.

CLUSTER OF INDIVIDUAL CLINICAL MANIFESTATIONS

The concepts just cited are applicable to any disease. The clinical spectrum of a disease comprises the seven stages cited in Table 2, and every patient—according to his disease, his iatrotropic stimulus, and his clinical findings—can be classified into one of those general stages (or subgroups) of the disease.

For this general classification, many different signs and symptoms were arbitrarily combined, or clustered, into the categories designated as *primary* and *secondary clinical features*. In infectious hepatitis, for example, a patient would be regarded as having primary features if he had any one of the appropriate entities cited in Table 1 as a primary feature of infectious hepatitis. Many citations of entities regarded as primary or secondary features also represent a categorical cluster. The term *neuropathy,* for example, as a secondary feature of diabetes mellitus, might be applied to a patient with any one of such clinical findings as numbness in the foot, loss of peripheral vibratory sense, or sphincteric incontinence.

Any one of the seven main clinical stages of disease can thus contain many subordinate stages, forming a more complex spectrum of clinical subgroups. The contents of the accessory spectrum will depend on the particular manifestations that form the primary and secondary features of the disease. Since these features are distinctive for each disease, the specific composition of the clinical subdivisions cannot be described in general terms, and will vary according to each particular disease. A patient with primary features of infectious hepatitis, for example, may have a tender liver but not jaundice, or jaundice but not a tender liver; or jaundice *and* a tender liver. A patient with neither jaundice nor a tender liver may still be in the primary features stage of hepatitis if he has anorexia. Similarly, in the secondary features (or cirrhotic) stage of hepatitis, patients may have cutaneous spiders alone, ascites alone, both, or neither.

The existence of so many different classes of patients, having diverse combinations of individual primary and secondary features, creates a major obstacle in clinical taxonomy. If patients are to be identified with scientific exactness, then each of these different combinations would need a separate classification. The number of categories required for this purpose would be enormous, exceeding the scope and complexity of even the most elaborate clinical taxonomies proposed in the 18th century. Such complexity would be necessary, however, only if contemporary clinical taxonomy had classification as its sole purpose—if it were to be a taxonomy *qua* taxonomy.

In contemporary medicine, fortunately, the purpose of clinical taxonomy is not merely to classify. The classifications have a purposeful significance in prognosis and therapy. Prognostic and therapeutic analyses of disease provide a correlation for the clinical categories— and a method of selecting appropriate categories. By studying the evolution of the various clinical forms of a disease, clinicians can select those clinical entities that are distinctive enough to warrant separate categorical designations and those that may be clustered together into a combined category. Entities that are of no prognostic or therapeutic significance can often be ignored; entities that are clinically important can be specifically noted and labeled.

Consider, for example, some of the major clinical manifestations[5] and the subsequent course of patients with the acute post-streptococcal inflammatory disease that is called *rheumatic fever*. Among the primary clinical features of this disease are the diverse articular symptoms and signs of arthritis, the musculokinetic evidence of chorea, the dermatologic manifestations of subcutaneous nodules and erythema marginatum, and certain auscultatory noises that clinically represent carditis. The secondary features of rheumatic fever would include physical or radiographic signs of cardiac enlargement, and clinical evidence of cardiac decompensation. From studies of the natural course of rheumatic fever,[11, 17] it may be noted that 1) arthritis, chorea, subcutaneous nodules, and erythema marginatum all subside without leaving any specific residual damage, whereas carditis often leaves permanent deformities; 2) arthritis, chorea, and carditis can often occur alone, rather than in combination, whereas subcutaneous nodules and erythema marginatum rarely appear alone and almost always occur in conjunction with one or more of the other major manifestations; 3) chorea has a longer acute course than arthritis, and often begins as or after arthritis (or other evidence of acute inflammation) has subsided; and 4) patients with the secondary features of carditis are much more likely to have residual heart disease than those patients whose cardiac manifestations are confined to primary features only.

From these observations, we can select the categories to be cited in a prognostic classification of the specific clinical spectrum of rheumatic fever. The categories should include arthritis, chorea, and carditis; and the carditis should be separated into mild (primary) and severe (secondary) divisions. The acute cutaneous manifestations, having no particular prognostic or therapeutic importance, do not require specific categorical demarcations in the spectrum. (The composition of this clinical spectrum will be further described and illustrated in Chapter 11.)

As another example, consider the secondary clinical features of patients with cancer. Some of these features, such as weight loss, do not *per se* denote anatomic dissemination of the tumor; other features, such as bone pain (in a non-osseous cancer), indicate anatomic spread of the tumor beyond the primary site. From observation of the clinical course of patients with cancer, it can be noted that these different secondary features are associated with distinct differences in survival rates.[25] Consequently, in preparing prognostic categories for the clinical spectrum of a cancer, the secondary clinical features might be divided into one group, called *systemic,* and another, called *metastatic.* (The composition of this spectrum will also be illustrated later in greater detail in Chapter 11.)

To make the types of taxonomic decisions described in these two examples requires close clinical observation and follow-up data on large numbers of patients with each disease under surveillance. Such decisions regarding categories of clinical classification cannot be made for many of the diseases whose surveys are described in the existing reports and tabulations of clinical literature. The data of existing publications have three major defects:

1) The population surveyed in older studies of many diseases does not have its diagnostic "purity" assured by the precision of modern technologic adjuncts. Consequently, the existing studies often contain data from many erroneously diagnosed patients who would have been excluded from a modern survey. Since the magnitude of the diagnostic errors is unknown, the data are unreliable for citing incidence of manifestations and for documenting concepts and correlations of clinical behavior in the "universe" of that disease. Such diagnostic "impurities" are particularly common in older surveys of populations of patients with syphilis, tuberculosis, coronary artery disease, rheumatic fever, renal disease, cancers, and many other diseases.

2) In most existing surveys, the clinical features of patients have usually been tabulated without regard to the manner in which the disease was detected. Although lanthanic, complainant, and other varieties of symptomatic patients need not always be separated in the prognostic and therapeutic correlations of every disease population, the distinction is critical in certain chronic illnesses, such as diabetes mellitus, coronary artery disease, rheumatic heart disease, and neoplasia.

3) Existing survey data often list the total number of individual clinical properties present in a population, but seldom cite the co-existence and inter-relationship of *combinations of properties.* Older surveys of acute rheumatic fever, for example, indicate the number of patients with arthritis, carditis, or congestive heart failure but not how many patients with arthritis also had carditis, or how many arthritic carditic patients also had congestive heart failure.

For these reasons, the construction of effective prognostic categories of classifications for each disease will require new studies, specifically intended for that purpose, and performed from direct appraisal of patients or of patients' medical records.

THE SEQUENCE OF CLINICAL MANIFESTATIONS

The two aspects of classification that have just been described deal with the iatric detection and cluster of manifestations in the clinical stages of a disease. A separate feature of clinical classification is the sequence, or order, in which the manifestations occurred. As a disease evolves, it may proceed from one manifestation to the next, or from one general clinical stage to another.

The classification of the sequential pattern of events may be necessary to indicate differences that still exist among patients having the same clinical stage and the same individual manifestations. Two patients with coronary artery disease, for example, may each have angina and congestive heart failure. Yet the one who had angina *before* he developed congestive heart failure is clinically different from the one whose angina did not begin until *after* the congestive heart failure. In diabetes mellitus, a patient who develops renal failure after the onset of visual difficulty is different from one in whom the order of these events was reversed.

For many investigative or prognostic purposes, the classification of clinical sequence may not be necessary, but the refinements and distinctions provided by different orders of sequence in a disease must always be considered before this property is dismissed as a factor of negligible importance in evaluating treatment. When sequence is deemed important enough to warrant its classification, appropriate terms or symbols can be introduced. The indexing nomenclature can ordinarily be attained by verbal designations of the changes, but can be given a formal structure, when necessary. (An illustration of such a structure will be demonstrated later in Chapter 11.)

THE TIMING OF CLINICAL SEQUENCES

As the clinical sequence of events unfolds in a patient's disease, each clinical manifestation (or stage) lasts for a certain amount of time. These different durations can be measured as they occur naturally, or as the sequence is interrupted or altered by therapeutic intervention. The *intervals* of a sequence are the periods of time that elapse, for example, in the transition from lanthanic to complainant stages of disease, or from the onset of one individual manifestation to another. The measurement of these durations is easy when they are marked by symptoms or overt events, but is difficult when the major events begin insidiously or undetectably. For almost all intervals, however, an upper time limit can usually be approximated or demarcated by means of the careful history-taking and data-seeking techniques to be described later (Chapter 11 and Part IV). Intervals can then be classified according to their actual durations or upper time limits.

The formal classification of time intervals, like that of sequence, may not be necessary in many clinical circumstances, but also cannot be ignored or dismissed until the significance of interval in each disease's clinical taxonomy is carefully appraised. Patients who seek treatment "late" in a disease may be different from those with apparently similar manifestations and sequences who seek treatment "early". The differences may sometimes arise not because the "late" group is stoic or phlegmatic, but because of profound subtle distinctions in the severity and clinical behavior of the disease. In cancers of the lung or rectum, for example, patients with a long duration of only primary clinical features (i.e., no systemic or metastatic features) had significantly higher survival rates than patients with a short duration of the same features.[25] (These distinctions will also be illustrated later in greater detail in Chapter 11.)

THE CO-MORBIDITY OF ASSOCIATED ILLNESS

Of the many clinical elements that compose a patient's illness, some may be attributable to the particular disease for which his clinical state is being classified. Many other elements of illness, however, may be due to some other disease or diseases. The associated illness arising from these other diseases produces a *co-morbidity* that may affect the patient's prognosis and therapeutic responses in the particular disease under consideration.

For example, a patient with peripheral arteriosclerosis may have intermittent claudication while walking. His claudication may vanish, however, if he develops coronary artery disease with angina pectoris so severe that the chest pain keeps him from walking fast enough or far enough to develop leg pain. In a patient with an asymptomatic localized cancer of the lung, prognosis may be poor not because of the cancer, but because of severe co-existing congestive heart failure due to rheumatic heart disease. A patient's response to treatment of acute pneumococcal pneumonia may be affected by the simultaneous presence of poorly controlled diabetes mellitus or of underlying chronic bronchitis.

Thus, patients with the same disease, having similar properties in the four previously cited types of associated clinical characteristics, may nevertheless have striking differences in the co-existing illness arising from other disease(s). The additional aspects of co-morbidity will therefore require separate classification.

*   *   *

These five categories of clinical variation within the spectrum of a single disease—iatric detection, clinical stage and clusters, sequence, duration, and co-morbidity—are features of human illness constantly observed by clinicians. Although these features generally receive an informal classification during the reasoning of clinical judgment, they have not hitherto been designated with specific names and categories. Some of the terms that have been cited—such as *iatrotropic stimulus, complainant, lanthanic,* and *co-morbidity*—had to be newly devised for this discussion, although they represent concepts well known to every observant clinician.

Why have these clinical entities not previously received a distinct nomenclature and classification? Perhaps the main reason has been that the diagnosis and pathogenesis of disease, rather than treatment, have received most of the intellectual attention of clinical science during the past half century. Since the study of diagnosis and pathogenesis does not ordinarily require the types of additional clinical taxonomy discussed here, clinical scientists have not perceived a need for the classification. As the treatment of patients becomes recognized as a major intellectual challenge in contemporary clinical science, the additional taxonomy will be discerned as a scientific necessity for identifying the sick people who are the "material" of therapeutic experiments.

Another significant reason, however, for the previous absence of clinical taxonomy has been its complexity. The classification of a disease can usually be stated in a single diagnostic phrase, but the classification of a patient's clinical distinctions requires many different designations. Each of the five types of clinical properties just cited can have many variations, and all five types often must be contemplated simultaneously. The many different possibilities create a staggering taxonomic problem for which no previously existing techniques of classification have been adequate. Previous methods of taxonomic procedure could not cope with the multiple, co-existing variables that had to be identified, and—even if methods were available—no human memory would be equal to the task of properly storing and recalling all the necessary details in different patients.

Thus, the classification of these many clinical variations of human illness previously seemed neither necessary nor possible. Today, as clinicians recognize a therapeutic purpose and necessity for the classification, they can also discover the existence of effective new intellectual procedures that enable formation of the classifications and management of the complex data. To form the classifications, clinicians can use the "new mathematics"—symbolic logic, set theory, and Boolean algebra. To aid their imperfect human memories in storing and retrieving the multiplicity of data, clinicians can use a technologic device whose factual capacity is vast and whose mnemonic recall is total—the digital computer. An ironic, awesome paradox of contemporary scientific technology is that so apparently esoteric a discipline as abstract mathematics and so apparently dehumanized a device as a digital computer can be used to help clinicians improve the practical humanistic art of patient care.

Since a digital computer's circuits are arranged according to the new mathematical concepts, an elementary understanding of these concepts is basic to both forming and using a systematic clinical taxonomy. The necessary mathematical concepts, simple and few, are presented in the next chapter.

10. A Clinical Primer of the "New" Mathematics

Like the character in Molière's *Le Bourgeois Gentilhomme*, who was astonished to learn that he spoke in prose, clinicians may be startled to discover that they *think* in mathematical sets. The thinking occurs during every act of diagnosis, prognostic estimation, therapeutic decision, and correlation of clinical and laboratory data. As exercises in deductive and inductive reasoning, these acts can be described in mathematical terms.

The branches of mathematics (or philosophy) used for these rational activities are called set theory, and symbolic logic; they are about a century old. As relatively new developments in mathematics, they were not included in the pre-medical training of most contemporary clinicians. These new subjects, however, are now being taught in many curriculums of undergraduate or even elementary education. Clinicians who have never heard of set theory or symbolic logic may find that their children are learning the new mathematics in school.

The new mathematical procedures can be used to catalog the background information and to demonstrate the procedures of logical reasoning. With these techniques, a precise identification can be given to many hitherto unspecified elements of the data and deliberation used in clinical judgment.

In applying clinical experience as a background for clinical judgment, the clinician classifies the previous observations he has stored in his memory, selects those that pertain to the situation at hand, draws tentative conclusions, acts on the basis of those conclusions, observes what happens thereafter, and lets the results confirm or refute his initial decisions. He then relates all these events back to the original observations, and uses the total outcome to integrate and augment his existing store of knowledge. He performs some of these processes by conscious discipline, using specific data, overt classifications, and delineated, conscious reasoning. He does others so quickly and almost reflexly that the rational process may become subconscious or intuitive, leaving him unaware of exactly what he did during the thinking. Often unable to identify the stored elements that were used initially or those that were added and altered subsequently, the clinician may begin to regard his reasoning as a type of mystique—an exercise in intellectual artistry that can often be neither documented nor delineated.

Human beings organize their thoughts for logical reasoning in a way that resembles their organization of words for grammatical speaking. The very word *logic* comes from the Greek word *logos*, which refers to either reason or speech. Occasionally, people think or talk deliberately, aware of their rational processes and of their grammar. At other times, they think rapidly in flowing ideas, without pauses for rational analysis; or they talk instinctively in fluent phrases, without pauses to select the grammar. The laws of rational thought, like the laws of grammar, have been studied and established. The rational laws are a part of the new mathematics, which provides a system of logical constructions and visual illustrations for describing the ingredients of human reasoning. The use of these procedures gives clinicians an opportunity to convert many mystical aspects of clinical judgment into the rational precision of science.

The application of new mathematical concepts in clinical medicine may seem strange, unnecessary, or artificial. A clinician who has already established his own good system of reasoning may suspect that formal mathematical analysis will bring only confusion to what he now does well, subconsciously and sometimes intuitively. Similarly, a native of a country often finds no need to study the grammar of its language; from years of continuous experience, he may speak and write the language well, without any conscious attention to rules of style or syntax. Nevertheless, in trying to explain subtle uses of the language to a foreigner, the native is forced to analyze his grammatical constructions.

The "foreigner" that has come to clinical medicine today is the digital computer. It brings with it the capacities for facilitating diagnosis, for making multiple analytic correlations rapidly and accurately, and for processing the myriads of data used in scientific decisions about prognosis and therapy. The computer comes to the clinician at a time when he desperately needs rational technologic aid in managing the other consequences of modern technology. The new therapeutic technology—in pharmaceuticals, surgical operations, and radiotherapy—enables the clinician to perform the extraordinary experiments of modern treatment. The new observational technology —in roentgenography, electrophysiology, chemistry, and other laboratory techniques—has given the clinician vast hordes of new data to be correlated with bedside observations in the evaluation of those experiments.

The total amount of information for even a single patient is often difficult to remember. For the large numbers of patients whose descriptional details must be recalled to plan and evaluate clinical treatment, the accumulation of data is generally beyond the capacity of any human memory. The mind of man is unsurpassed in the ability to perceive, think, analyze, imagine, and create—but is greatly limited in the ability to store large numbers of facts permanently and to recall the data precisely.

To supplement the fallibility of human memory, clinicians use various types of written or printed records. Although excellent for storing data, the records must be individually collected, classified, and enumerated for any analysis of their content. The manual procedures for sorting and counting large amounts of written data are cumbersome and often inaccurate. To store and retrieve the massive amount of information obtained in the experiments of modern clinical therapy, a clinician cannot rely on the limited capacities of human memory or on awkward compilations of conventional medical records. The digital computer is the instrument that offers clinicians a new mnemonic technology for mastering the operation of the new observational and therapeutic technologies.

Like a foreigner learning a new language, the computer can easily be taught a simple vocabulary and the construction of elementary sentences. But also like the foreigner, the computer must be taught nuances of grammar if the language produced is to have either elegance or poetry. Even if computers did not exist, however, and even without the incentive of "educating" the computer, clinicians have much to gain by studying their own clinical "grammar". Despite excellent instructions in the use of a language, a foreigner may never learn its idioms perfectly and may always speak with an alien accent. The native, however, in performing the grammatical analysis needed to instruct the foreigner, will emerge with an increased power and precision in the command of his own language. The native may thereby learn much more from studying grammar than the foreigner who incited the study.

The logic and symbols of the new mathematics offer clinicians a sublime intellectual mechanism for describing the procedures of clinical reasoning. Before those clinical procedures can be illustrated, however, an elementary understanding of the new mathematics is necessary. The rest of this chapter is devoted to a brief outline of the basic ideas that are pertinent and adequate for a clinician's needs in using the techniques. This outline has been deliberately condensed and simplified, and is not intended to be a complete presentation of the new mathematics. The object here is to describe the few concepts that are most useful for clinical activities. A more comprehensive account of the mathematical procedures can be found in appropriate textbooks.[105]

DEFINITIONS AND ELEMENTARY PROPERTIES OF SETS

Students of conventional algebra learn to use such letters as a, b, x, or y to represent individual objects, and to maneuver the letters in such operations as addition, subtraction, multiplication, and division. Set theory deals with collections (or classes) of objects, rather than with single objects; its maneuvers deal with the operations (or relations) that occur among the various collections or classes.

A *set* is a collection of objects or elements all having some common defined property. We can speak of the set of all human beings, the set of all patients, the set of all men, the set of all people who have diabetes mellitus, the set of all diseases that can produce hemoptysis, or the set of all disorders found only in newborn infants. Every object contained in a set must have the characteristic property of that set, but can have many other properties as well. A single object can therefore be a member of many sets. Thus, a particular man can belong to the set of all human beings, the set of all patients, the set of all men, and the set of all people who have diabetes mellitus.

A set may contain many divisions, called *subsets*. Every subset is itself a set, having its own characteristic properties as well as the characteristic property of the parent set. Thus, the set of adult human beings can be divided into three subsets: the set of women, the set of men, and the set of adult hermaphrodites.* The set of men contains many subsets, among which are the set of brown-haired men, the set of old men, the set of rich men, and the set of men with blood glucose levels higher than 105 mg. per 100 ml. The set of old men may contain, as a subset, the set of old rich men.

A single object may belong to one, many, or none of the sets under discussion. Thus, a particular man may be a member of the set of old men but not of the set of rich men; he may be in the set of brown-haired men but not in the set of men with blood glucose levels higher than 105 mg. per 100 ml. If he is young, poor, blond-haired, and normoglycemic, he belongs to none of the four sets just cited.

Sets are always considered within a framework of reference called a *universe*. Thus, sets of different patients would be contained in the parent universe of human beings, or in the universe of·people who have had medical attention. The universe of human diabetes mellitus contains sets of patients who have polydipsia, sets of patients with acidosis, sets of patients with vascular lesions, and many other sets. The set of patients with diabetic acidosis contains a subset with ketosis, a subset with hyperventilation, and a subset with coma. The set of patients with diabetic retinopathy contains a subset with retinal hemorrhages and a subset with retinal exudate. The set with exudate contains a subset with exudate in the macular area, and so on.

In any particular universe, the *complement* of a set consists of all objects in the universe that do *not* belong to that set. Thus, in a universe composed of all adult human beings, the complement of the set of all men is the set of all women (and the set of hermaphrodites). In the universe of diabetes mellitus, the complement of the set of patients with vascular lesions is the set of all diabetic patients who do not have vascular lesions. In the universe of human disease, the complement of the diabetes mellitus set consists of all diseases other than diabetes mellitus.

Symbolic logic provides a means of formulating some of the features just described. If x indicates a particular object, and A a particular set, the symbol ϵ is used to indicate membership in a set. Thus,

$$x \in A$$

means that the object x is a member of (or belongs to) set A. The symbol $\subset$ is applied exclusively to sets, and means "is contained in".

* For this discussion, a hermaphrodite is regarded as neither man nor woman.

Thus,

$$A \subset B$$

means that set A is contained in set B, or A is a subset of set B. With the symbol reversed, this statement could be alternatively written as

$$B \supset A$$

or, set B contains set A as a subset. The symbol $^-$ above the letter of a set indicates the complement of that set. Thus

$$\overline{A}$$

refers to the set containing all objects, in the parent universe of set A, that do not belong to A.

THE OPERATIONS OF BOOLEAN ALGEBRA

Since sets are not individual objects, they cannot be maneuvered in the same arithmetical operations—addition, subtraction, multiplication, and division—that are used in conventional algebra. The operations performed upon sets are considered in a branch of mathematics called Boolean algebra.* Three main operations can occur in Boolean algebra: *union* (depicted by the symbol $\cup$), *intersection* (depicted by $\cap$), and *complementation* or *negation* (depicted by $^-$).

The operation of *union* ($\cup$) forms a new set that joins the contents of the two sets. Thus, in the expression

$$C = A \cup B,$$

C is a set that contains all the elements in set A, and all the elements in set B. An element that belongs to both set A and set B will obviously be included in set C. Thus, when we state that $x \in A \cup B$, we mean that the element x belongs to the set formed by the union of A and B. A verbal logical equivalent of the union symbol $\cup$ is the expression "and/or", because the element x, in this statement, can belong to A alone, to B alone, or to both A and B.

The operation of *intersection* ($\cap$) forms a new set that contains

---

* Devised by George Boole (1815–1864), an English mathematical logician who later worked in Ireland. His pioneering contribution to this field has recently been reprinted in paperback form.[106]

only those elements that belong both to set A and to set B. Thus, in the expression

$$C = A \cap B,$$

C is a set that contains whatever elements A and B have in common. Thus, when we state that $x \in A \cap B$, we mean that the element x belongs to the set formed by the intersection of A and B. A verbal logical equivalent of the intersection symbol $\cap$ is the expression "both . . . and . . .", because the element x, in this statement, belongs to both A and B. If A and B have no elements in common, then the set formed by their intersection is empty. Any set that contains no elements is called the *null set*.

The operation of negation ($^-$) forms a new set that contains, in that particular universe, all the elements that do not belong to the original set. Thus, in the expression

$$C = \overline{A},$$

set C is the complement of set A. Thus, when we state that $x \in \overline{A}$, we mean that the element x does not belong to A; it is a member of the complement of A. The verbal logical equivalent of the symbol $^-$ is the expression "not". (For any universe U, containing any set A, $U = A + \overline{A}$.)

Parentheses are used in Boolean algebra in much the same way they are used in ordinary algebra: to avoid ambiguity in indicating the order of operations. Thus, in ordinary algebra, the expression $a \times b + c$ might represent $(a \times b) + c$ or $a \times (b + c)$. Similarly, in the algebra of sets, the expression $A \cup B \cap C$ must be clarified to indicate whether it is $(A \cup B) \cap C$ or $A \cup (B \cap C)$. Just as no parentheses are necessary in ordinary algebra when all the operations are the same, such as $a + b + c$ or $a \times b \times c$, no parentheses are needed in Boolean algebra when the operations are all union or all intersection. Thus, $A \cup B \cup C$ is an unambiguous expression, representing the set formed by the union of the three sets, and $A \cap B \cap C$ is also unambiguous, representing the set formed by their common intersection.

When the operation of negation is applied to a single set, no parentheses are necessary. When the union or intersection of sets is negated, however, parentheses should be used. Thus $(\overline{A \cup B})$ means the complement of the set formed by the union of A and B; and $(\overline{A \cap \overline{B} \cap C})$

means the complement of the set formed by the mutual intersection of three sets: A, the complement of B, and C.

For convenience and review, the various symbols of Boolean algebra are listed, together with illustrative explanations, in Table 4. With these operational procedures, we can characterize the many properties (or attributes) that an individual object may possess. Each of the properties can be cited as the name of a set, and the object's membership in that set will indicate that it possesses that particular property.

To illustrate these activities, consider the subgroups of diseased patients listed earlier in Table 2 (Chapter 9). In the universe of this disease, let L represent the set of lanthanic patients, P the set of patients with primary clinical features, and S the set with secondary clinical features. Let x represent any patient under consideration. Then $x \in L$ means that the patient is a member of the lanthanic set, or is lanthanic; $x \in \overline{L}$ means that the patient belongs to the complement of the lanthanic set; i.e., he is complainant.

The expression $x \in P \cup S$ means that the patient belongs to the set that is the union of the primary and secondary features sets. Thus, this particular patient may have either primary clinical features, or secondary features, or both. It should be noted that the union of these two sets will comprise three subsets: patients with primary features only (written as $P \cap \overline{S}$), patients with secondary features only (written as $\overline{P} \cap S$), and patients with both primary and secondary features (written as $P \cap S$). The expression $x \in P \cup S$ denotes only that the

T A B L E 4. **The Symbols of Bloolean Agebra**

Expression	Meaning
$x \in A$	Object x belongs to set A
$A \subset B$	Set A is contained in set B
$B \supset A$	Set B contains set A
$\overline{A}$	The complement of set A
$A \cup B$	The set formed by the union of sets A and B
$A \cap B$	The set formed by the intersection (or overlap) of sets A and B
$x \in \overline{(A \cup B)} \cap C$	Object x is a member of the set formed by the intersection of set C with the complement of the set formed by the union of sets A and B

patient belongs to one of these three subsets, but the expression does not specify which one.

The expression $x \in P \cap S$ would mean that the patient belongs to the intersection of the primary and secondary features sets; i.e., he has both primary and secondary features. A patient in the complainant primary set (subgroup 5 of Table 2) would be indicated as $x \in \overline{L} \cap P \cap \overline{S}$; i.e., he is non-lanthanic, and has primary features but no secondary features. A patient in the lanthanic secondary set (subgroup 4 of Table 2) would be indicated as $x \in L \cap \overline{P} \cap S$.

The $\cap$ symbol is a particularly useful clinical tool because a series of intersections can be extended indefinitely to indicate a patient's possession or non-possession of many different properties (i.e., membership in sets with those properties). For example, if N is the set of nurses, R the set of rich people, Y the set of young people, B the set of brown-haired people, and G the set of patients with blood glucose levels higher than 105 mg. per 100 ml., then

$$x \in N \cap \overline{R} \cap \overline{Y} \cap B \cap G$$

would indicate a patient who is a poor, old, brown-haired, hyperglycemic nurse.

This type of Boolean notation is convenient for demonstrating the co-existence of many different properties in patients. By indicating the presence or absence of each property, the notation can immediately label the particular combination of properties found in that patient. Such notational concepts are also used in planning the programs for processing the data used in digital computers, whose circuits are organized according to the operational principles of Boolean algebra.

VENN DIAGRAMS AND RELATIONS OF SETS

For most practical purposes, a clinician needs no knowledge of Boolean algebra beyond what has just been cited. Moreover, the rather abstract notation of the Boolean symbols can often be replaced by a graphic illustration of the concepts. These graphic illustrations will be the focus of discussion for the remainder of this chapter and will be used to depict all of the clinical examples presented later in Chapter 11.

The graphic illustrations of sets are provided by Venn diagrams,*

* John Venn, 1834–1923, was a British logician who introduced[107] this technique of illustration for sets.

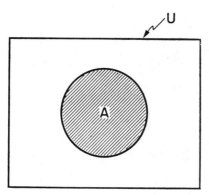

FIGURE 1
   A set, *A,* in a universe, *U.*

which portray a set as the contents of a circle (or some other enclosed space, such as an oval or rectangle). In such diagrams, the size of the space is arbitrary and has no relation to the number of members in the set. The object is to portray *qualities* rather than *quantities.* Figure 1, for example, shows a universe, *U,* containing a particular set *A.* We have no idea of the number of objects in set *A* or the size of the universe *U.* The diagram demonstrates only that set *A* has the qualitative property of being contained in that universe. It may also be noted that $\overline{A}$, the complement set of *A* is everything in *U* that is not *A*; thus, $\overline{A}$ is the unshaded area of U.

In the inter-relationship of two sets, four possible situations can occur: *a)* the two sets may be *disjoint,* or *mutually exclusive,* having no members in common; *b)* the sets may be *overlapping,* having some members in common but other members that are distinctive to each set; *c)* one set may be *subordinate* to the other, being contained as a subset; or *d)* the two sets may be *identical* in that every member of one is also a member of the other. These relations are clinically described below, and illustrated in Figure 2.

DISJOINT (FIG. 2*a*)

The set of patients (*A*) who complain of sore throats and the set of patients (*B*) without complaint of sore throats are entirely disjoint

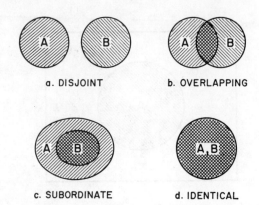

FIGURE 2
The four possible relationships of two sets, *A* and *B*.

in that no patient simultaneously belongs to both. If the disjoint sets are complements of each other, as in this example, they need not be specifically portrayed as separate circles. Thus, in Figure 1, if *U* were the universe of patients, and *A* the set of patients with complaint of sore throats, then the patients without complaint of sore throats would simply be the entire unshaded area outside *A*. A second circle would be unnecessary. Two sets, however, may be disjoint without being exact complements of each other. Thus, in the universe of adult human beings, the set of men and the set of women are disjoint, but not exact complements. Although the two sets have no members in common, because no person can simultaneously be "man" and "woman", the complement of the set of men includes more than just the set of women, and vice versa. A true hermaphrodite, being neither man nor woman, would be included as part of the complement of the set of men. A hermaphrodite would also be part of the complement of the set of women.

OVERLAPPING (FIG. 2*b*)

The set of patients (*A*) with clinical evidence of myocardial infarction and the set of patients (*B*) with electrocardiographic abnormalities are overlapping sets. Some patients belong to A but not B; some belong to B but not A; and some belong to both.

SUBORDINATE (FIG. 2c)

The set of patients (B) with acute infectious hepatitis is entirely contained within the set of patients (A) who have abnormal sulfobromophthalein retention. Not all of the patients in A, however, have infectious hepatitis. Since B is a subset of A in this illustration, all patients in B are also in A, but not conversely. Further examples of this subset relationship can be provided by considering A as the set of all human males, and B the set of boys; A as the set of patients with any type of chest pain, and B the set of patients with angina pectoris; A as the set of patients with acute rheumatic carditis, and B the set of patients with severe carditis.

IDENTICAL (FIG. 2d)

Identical set relations are rare in clinical medicine, but can be artificially created. For example, if bacteriuria is made a prerequisite to the diagnosis of urinary tract infection, and if urinary tract infection is arbitrarily diagnosed whenever bacteriuria is found, then the set of patients with bacteriuria will be identical to the set with urinary infection. Every member of one set will be a member of the other.

One additional definition will be useful in future discussion: two sets are called *independent* if each set contains members that are not present in the other set. Thus, disjoint or overlapping sets are independent, but subordinate or identical sets are not.

The size of the circles (or other shapes) used to portray the relationships of two or more sets has no quantitative connotations. Thus, the situations portrayed in Figure 3, a to c, all have exactly the same meaning as that shown in Figure 2b. The situations portrayed in Figure 3, d to f, all have the same meaning as that of Figure 2c. To indicate quantitative distinctions in the membership of sets and subsets, numbers are added to the drawings, as shown later in Chapter 11.

Venn diagrams can also be used to illustrate the results of the operations of Boolean algebra. The shaded areas in the four parts of Figure 4 show, respectively, a) a set A in a universe; b) the complement of set A; c) the set that is the union of two intersecting sets,

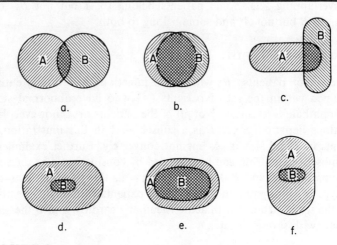

FIGURE 3

Alternative ways of portraying the relationships shown in Figure 2*b* (*a, b, c*), and in Figure 2*c* (*d, e, f*).

A and *B*; and *d*) the set that is the overlap (or intersection) of two intersecting sets, *A* and *B*.

It should be noted that the Boolean algebra of sets provides a type of addition in which 2 plus 2 does not necessarily equal 4. If we want to determine the sum of the number of members of two sets, the usual results of conventional addition can be used only if the two sets are disjoint. For any other relationship of two sets—overlapping, subordinate, or identical—the total number of members in the two sets will be *less* than the sum of their individual members. Suppose, for example, that set *A* contains 100 patients and set *B* contains 100 patients. In conventional addition, we would expect the sum of the two sets to contain 200 patients. If the two sets overlap, however, as in Figure 2*b*, some of the patients counted in *A* are also members of *B*. Thus, the 100 patients of each set do not exist disjointly; the total number of patients contained in the two sets may be 150, 175, or some other number less than 200, depending on the quantity of patients present in the common intersection of the two sets, *A* ∩ *B*. If the two sets are subordinate, as in Figure 2*c*, the total number of patients present in the two sets, *A* and *B*, is simply the total number

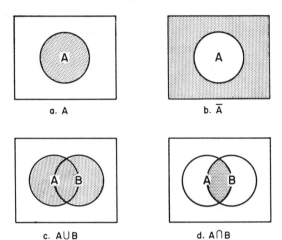

FIGURE 4

The sets produced by Boolean operations of complementation (*b*); union (*c*); and intersection (*d*).

present in *A* alone. If the sets are identical, as in Figure 2*d*, the total number of patients is simply the number present in either *A* or *B*.

Venn diagrams can also directly illustrate a type of reasoning called syllogisms. For example, Figure 2*c* can depict the famous syllogism: *All men are mortal; Socrates is a man; therefore Socrates is mortal.* For this illustration, let set *A* in Figure 2*c* be the set of all mortals; let set *B* be the set of all men. Let *x* = Socrates. Then *x* ϵ *B*, and *B* $\subset$ *A*. Therefore *x* ϵ *A*. The diagram of Figure 2*c* can also be used to illustrate a common error in logical reasoning. Thus, an incorrect phrasing of the foregoing syllogism would be: *All men are mortal; Socrates is mortal; therefore Socrates is a man.* It is clear from the diagram of Figure 2*c* that *B* $\subset$ *A*, but the new second part of the statement just made here is *x* ϵ *A*, not *x* ϵ *B*. In this circumstance, we cannot be certain that *x* ϵ *B*, because of the possibility that *x* ϵ *A* $\cap$ $\bar{B}$, thus being a member of the non-human subset of mortals. For example, "Socrates" might be the name of a dog.

Syllogisms are not the only type of logic that can be illustrated by Venn diagrams. For example, the set arrangements already described in Figure 2*b* are a demonstration of the statement: *some patients with* *myocardial infarction do not have electrocardiographic abnormalities.* Since *A* (in Fig. 2*b*) is the set of patients with myocardial infarction, and *B* is the set with electrocardiographic abnormalities, the subset *A* that does not overlap *B* represents the group of patients cited in the statement. Figure 2*c* could be used to illustrate the old aphorism: *all that glitters is not gold.* In this case, *A* would represent the set of objects that glitter, and *B* would represent the subset of glittering objects that are made of gold. The subset $A \cap \overline{B}$ would represent non-golden glittering objects. If we were given the additional statement, *all that is gold does not glitter,* we could use a Venn diagram of intersecting (rather than subordinate) sets to illustrate the combination of two statements.

The discussion thus far has been confined to the four patterns of relationship in two sets. For three sets, the number of possible patterns increases markedly. The third set can be disjoint, overlapping, subordinate, encompassing, or identical to any of the previous two sets or subsets depicted in the four patterns of Figure 2. Some of the many possible patterns of relationship for three sets have been illustrated elsewhere (Fig. 2 in Ref. 22), and will not be repeated here. For practical clinical purposes, the most useful three-set pattern is that formed by the "full intersection" of three independent sets. In this circumstance, each set intersects with every other set and with the subset of every dual intersection. A total of seven distinct subsets are formed. The different distinct subsets, together with other combinations that are possible within the full intersection of three independent sets, are shown in Figure 5. The associated labels indicate the Boolean specification of each of the shaded sets and subsets.

*   *   *

Because of the unique ability to identify *overlapping* collections of objects, set theory and Venn diagrams are powerful tools for the classification of clinical types of human illness. In other forms of taxonomy, the different categories are cleanly separated according to morphologic or dimensional specifications; there is no overlap of categories and no need to classify various combinations of properties. In every taxonomy used in contemporary natural science, the object of classification is to separate, to dissect, or to analyze—not to synthesize.

When we classify the phylums of living organisms, for example, we

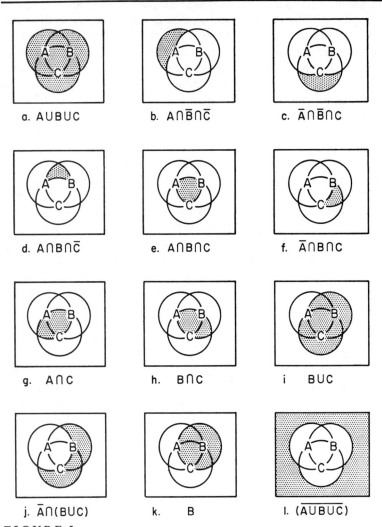

FIGURE 5

The identification, by Venn diagram or by Boolean notation, of various sets and subsets contained in three intersecting "independent" sets. The label under each diagram indicates the particular set that is shaded in the diagram.

divide them into such categories as arthropods, mollusks, or chordates. Except for certain rare organisms that do not conform to the rigorously separated categories, there is no overlap of phyla, and no need for classifications to manage the overlap. When we classify height, we use a discretely separated range of measured increments or categories. A particular person then belongs to one, and only one, of these dimensional categories. His height may be in the range of 67 to 69 inches, but it cannot be also in the range of 72 to 74 inches. He may be either short, average, or tall, but he cannot have two of these attributes or all three.

In classification of clinical manifestations of a disease, however, the overlap is a critical, distinctive feature of the population. In rheumatic fever, for example, a patient may have arthritis alone, chorea alone, carditis alone, or arthritis and chorea, arthritis and carditis, chorea and carditis, or all three of these properties. The seven subgroups just described have different features that distinguish patients of one group from those of another. For precise classification, the patients cannot be separated merely according to the isolated properties of either arthritis, or chorea, or carditis; the overlap of properties must be considered for appropriate delineation of subgroups.

The classification procedures of clinical taxonomy must be able to deal not only with these aspects of clinical cluster, but also with the co-existing *combinations* of different types of iatric detection, sequence, duration, or co-morbidity in patients with the same disease. Moreover, the comprehensive study of biologic structures or of disease populations requires more than just a division of the material into component parts. The constituent parts must also be synthesized into the whole of an intact organism or into the total spectrum of a human disease. The synthesis of a whole demands an overlapping of components that creates additional variations far more complex than a mere sum of the parts.

A successful clinical taxonomy must therefore be able to demonstrate the overlapping combinations or syntheses of the many different properties that make clinical phenomena so intricate and difficult to classify. The main value of set theory, Boolean algebra, and Venn diagrams in modern medicine—their unique contribution to the mental technology of the contemporary clinician—is that they provide the means of constructing such a taxonomy. They offer methods for indicating the analysis and performing the synthesis simultaneously.

11. Spectrums of Disease and Other "Mathemedical" Constructions

Venn diagrams can be used to illustrate the systems of classification described in Chapter 9, and to portray many other situations of clinical (or para-clinical) taxonomy. Some of the methods and results are demonstrated in this chapter.

THE GENERAL SPECTRUM OF A HUMAN DISEASE

At the time a particular disease has been diagnosed, the patient may be lanthanic or complainant for that disease, and may have primary clinical features, secondary features, both, or neither. The full intersection of these three independent sets of properties—lanthanic, primary features, and secondary features—is shown in Figure 6, producing a Venn diagram that is the *clinical* spectrum of a human disease. Each of the subsets created by the intersections of these three over lapping circles contains subgroups of patients with different properties. The numbers of the subsets and properties of the patients in this figure coincide with those of the subgroups listed earlier (page 147) in Table 2.

The clinical spectrum of Figure 6 contains and classifies those patients whose disease is detected while the patients are alive. Not all people in the universe of a particular disease, however, receive a diagnosis during life. The lanthanic set also contains a subset of patients in whom the disease is first found after death. During life, such patients may have had primary features, secondary features, both, or

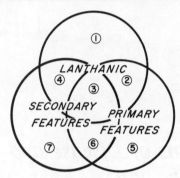

FIGURE 6
The clinical spectrum of a human disease.

neither. The details of the clinical history can often be obtained, if necessary, from the patient's medical record or from surviving relatives and friends. In addition to these "necropsy discoveries", the universe of a disease contains other patients whose disease has not been medically diagnosed. When these other features of detection of disease are added to Figure 6, the result is Figure 7, which shows the medical spectrum of a human disease.

Another way of portraying the spectrum of Figure 7 is to regard the "undiscovered" group of patients as a subset of the lanthanic set. Thus, the lanthanic set would contain three subsets that are disjoint because the disease in a particular patient can first be found (or not found) in only one of the three ways: during life, after death, or not at all. These subsets of the lanthanic set are illustrated in two alternative arrangements—both demonstrating the same properties—in Figure 8, *a* and *b*. In Figure 8*b,* the arrangement is eccentric rather than concentric because the three sets are all subsets of the lanthanic set, but are not subsets of each other.

Adding the distinctions of Figure 8*b* to those of Figure 6 produces the analytic synthesis of the total spectrum of a human disease. This spectrum, shown in Figure 9, is similar to that of Figure 7, except that the surrounding "universe" has been removed and its "undiscovered" patients have been placed within the lanthanic set.

By a slight logical distortion that provides diagrammatic symmetry and simplicity without affecting the consistency of subset classification,

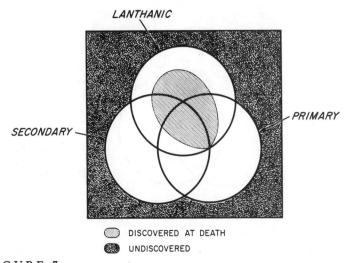

FIGURE 7
The total spectrum of a human disease.

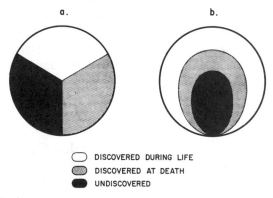

FIGURE 8
The time of discovery of disease in the lanthanic set.

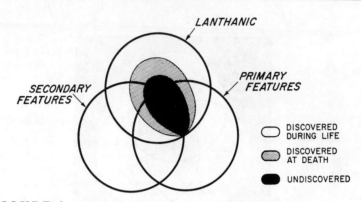

FIGURE 9
    The total spectrum of a human disease. (An alternative arrangement
    of Figure 7.)

the additional subsets of the lanthanic set can be shown concentrically
as subsets of each other. This arrangement is depicted in Figure 10,
which is esthetically preferable to Figure 9 as an analytic synthesis of
the total spectrum of a human disease. Figure 10 contains the seven
clinical subsets of disease discovered in life (shown in Fig. 6), and adds
four more subsets discovered at death. The central subset of the
lanthanic set of Figure 10 is not further divided according to clinical
features, and represents the "core" of wholly undetected disease.

By using these subset numbers, or the code names cited earlier in
Table 2 (Chapter 9), the mode of detection and general clinical stage
of a diseased patient can be described, classified, and indexed.

CLUSTERS AND SPECTRUMS IN SPECIFIC CLINICAL SITUATIONS

Venn diagrams are particularly useful for depicting the *cluster* of
manifestations that form the clinical spectrum of specific diseases
and other situations. Such clusters of multiple, overlapping properties
can also be classified, in the traditional manner, with verbal designations
that avoid the new mathematical techniques. The mathematical procedures, however, offer the following advantages:

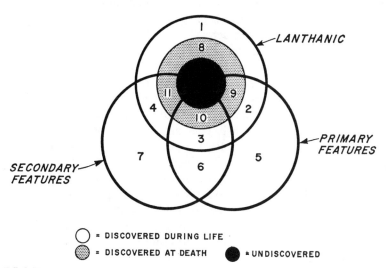

FIGURE 10

The total spectrum of a human disease. (An alternative arrangement of Figure 9.)

1) The diagrams and symbols can identify subgroups for which existing nomenclature is difficult, inadequate, or absent. Proper use of the mathematical maneuvers will demand the formation of specific definitions for the groups (or properties) to be cited as major sets. Such definitions will increase the precision with which patients are counted and analyzed in clinical reasoning or in statistical procedures performed by computational devices.

2) Although clinical relationships, like those of other data, can be expressed in tabular form, the Venn diagrams are a method of depicting these relationships visually as patterns; the diagrams (or patterns) of overlapping independent variables are thus analogous to the linear or curvilinear graphs drawn for data of dependent variables.

3) The concepts of union, intersection, and complementation of sets enable a recognition of overlap, or different combinations of properties, that might escape attention in a classification system formed verbally without formal logical rigor.

The principles of designing Venn diagrams for clinical spectrums are much more easily demonstrated by practical example than by theoretical discussion. Nevertheless, certain general methodologic principles can be summarized here:

1) For each disease or clinical situation to be classified, large numbers of patients are surveyed, and all the pertinent clinical (and other) properties are noted as present or absent for each patient. When a particular clinical property has shades of gradation—such as mild, moderate, or severe dyspnea—each shade of gradation can be considered a separate property, to be cited as present or absent.

2) From the tabulated results, the properties are analyzed for frequency of appearance, alone or in combination.

3) From these analyses, a series of individual properties, or aggregates of properties, is chosen to represent the independent sets whose overlap will cover the total spectrum of the situation (or disease) under consideration. To provide a complete spectrum, the particular properties or aggregates that are chosen to represent major sets should be independent rather than subordinate. For example, in classifying the spectrum of diabetes mellitus, we could represent an aggregate of clinical properties by a set labeled *vascular abnormalities*. This set, and the *polyuria* set, are good choices for major sets, because they are independent and overlap. The property of *polydipsia,* however, would not be a good choice as an additional major set, because the *polydipsia* set is usually subordinate (as a subset) to that with *polyuria*.

4) After the major sets of the main diagram have been arranged, subsets can be added when they are clearly discerned and useful. In coronary artery disease, for example, a complete clinical spectrum can be obtained as the intersection of three sets marked *chest pain, congestive heart failure,* and *other cardiovascular abnormalities.* A *dyspnea* set can be shown, if desired, on the main diagram as a subset of the *congestive failure* set. After the main diagram has been constructed, specific parts of the spectrum can be selected for "magnification" in separate sub-spectral diagrams of the components not cited in the main spectrum. Thus, a separate subdivisional pattern or sub-spectrum could be constructed for the different clinical features of *chest pain,* of *congestive heart failure,* and of *other cardiovascular abnormalities.* The congestive heart failure spectrum could then be "magnified" and shown as the intersection of three sets marked *respiratory abnormalities, right-sided abnormalities,* and *arrhythmias.* The *respiratory abnormalities* spectrum could be further "magnified" and shown as the intersection of sets marked *dyspnea, basilar râles,* and *other pulmonary abnor-*

malities (such as pleural effusion). The *right-sided abnormalities* spectrum could also be further portrayed as the intersection of sets marked *hepatomegaly, peripheral edema,* and *venous distention.* An appropriate sub-spectrum could also be designed for the *arrhythmias* set.

5) The subtle choice of appropriate properties and sets for these patterns must be individualized for each situation. The choices will always vary with the purpose and application of the classification. A spectrum constructed for correlations with prognosis and therapy may have different ingredients from one constructed only to show the range of clinical manifestations in a particular disease. In some of the illustrations to be shown later, the Venn diagram was constructed to depict the results in different laboratory tests or in the diagnoses of different clinical observers, rather than to demonstrate the prognostic or clinical features of patients. After the major sets are selected in most clinical situations, their patterns of overlap in the Venn diagrams will identify specific subgroups of patients who can be counted and compared for correlation with other properties determined either by laboratory tests or by subsequent clinical observations. The results of these correlations may often suggest alternative choices and arrangements for the main sets or diagrams.

6) The actual construction of the Venn diagrams involves artistic decisions about size, shape, positional rotation, margination, and shading. Each of these decisions is arbitrary—a matter of esthetic taste, subservient to clarity and to maintenance of correct logical implications. Since the size of the circle has no quantified meaning, it can be made as large or small as necessary. The shape of a set need not be circular; ovals, ellipses, rectangles, or any other enclosed form can be used. The different sets can be rotated clockwise, counterclockwise, or in other positional relations to each other, as long as the appropriate logic is preserved. (For example, Figure 11 illustrates four alternative ways—varying in size, shape, and position of the sets—for portraying exactly the same spectrum shown in Figure 6. In Figure 8, *a* and *b,* the same situation was illustrated in two different ways.) For margination, one may follow the convention of keeping an equal thickness for the lines that are boundaries of major sets, and using somewhat thinner lines for subordinate sets. The interior of the sets may be shaded, if shading contributes to clarity. Thus, the three sets of Figure 6 were left unshaded, but the subordinate sets added in Figures 9 and 10 were shaded. In the later Figure 14*a,* the initial three sets were shaded to distinguish them from the additions made in Figures 14*b* and 15.

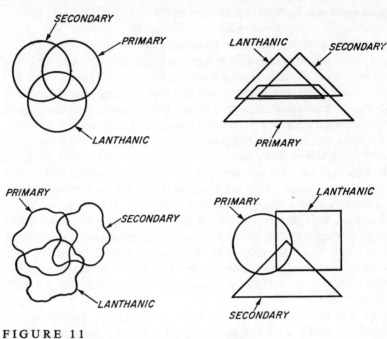

FIGURE 11
Four alternative arrangements of Figure 6.

7) Other artistic decisions deal with labeling and insertion of numbers. The verbal label of a set can be placed inside the contents, or outside the perimeter, connected with a line or arrow. An interior label should preferably extend into, or touch, all the subsets to which it refers. When shading is used, clarity can be achieved without the need for "trans-subset" labels. The insertion of numbers in the interior of the diagrams can be done for two purposes. One purpose—shown in Figures 6, 9, and 10—is for identification only, to label the subsets. (Such "label" numbers can often themselves be encircled, as in the figures just cited and in the later Figures 21 and 28.) A more important use of numbers is to represent the count of objects in that subset. Such counted numbers may be left "free", as in the later Figures 17, 20, and 24 through 30, or the numbers can be enclosed in a small rectangle, as in the later Figure 33. The sum of counted objects within subsets of

a single set can be shown adjacent to the main verbal label, as in the later Figures 26 and 29.

The techniques just described for forming the Venn diagrams of clinical patterns have now been applied extensively in acute rheumatic fever, and have been used more recently to illustrate cancer of the lung, and several other taxonomic situations. These illustrations will be presented here to exemplify the procedures, and some of their value.

ACUTE RHEUMATIC FEVER

Spectrum of Sore Throats, Streptococcal Infections, and Sources of Rheumatic Fever

Figure 12 shows the overlapping complex relationships in the "universe" that contains patients with sore throats and patients with streptococcal infections. In this universe, streptococcal infections are identified by a positive laboratory test either in throat culture, or in serologic rise of antibody titer, or in both. Sore throats are identified as a symptom reported by the patient. The inter-relationships of the Venn diagram of Figure 12 show the many possible situations that can occur; streptococcal infections need not produce sore throats, and sore throats need not be streptococcal. Clinical and epidemiologic study[12, 108-110] of large numbers of patients in these different situations, however, has demonstrated that rheumatic complications emerge from only a portion

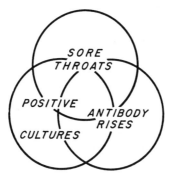

FIGURE 12

The universe of sore throats and of streptococcal infections.

of this total spectrum. The epidemiologic data of those studies have shown that rheumatic fever can develop in patients with or without a sore throat, and with or without a positive throat culture. The critical feature that makes a streptococcal infection potentially rheumatogenic is a rise in antibody titer.

Thus, rheumatic fever is a "subset" of antibody-rise streptococcal infections. The subset can be portrayed by adding it to Figure 12 in several alternative ways, two of which are shown in Figure 13, *a* and *b*. The shaded area in Figure 13, *a* or *b*, indicates the rheumatic fever subset of the universe of sore throats and streptococcal infections. The location of this subset helps to explain several pertinent clinical features of the occurrence of rheumatic fever. "Typical" pharyngitis, with a sore throat, often fails to appear in many patients who have a serologically positive streptococcal infection. In such patients, the infection can produce rheumatic fever insidiously, without a previous symptomatic warning. Conversely, when adequate serologic evidence is available to exclude a significant effect on antibodies, a positive throat culture in a patient with sore throat denotes that the event is streptococcal intrusion, or the "carrier state", but not potentially rheumatogenic infection.

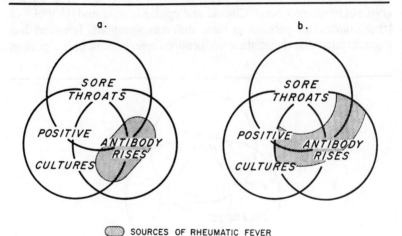

SOURCES OF RHEUMATIC FEVER

FIGURE 13
    Sources of rheumatic fever in the universe of sore throats and of streptococcal infections.

Spectrum of Acute Rheumatic Fever

As a subset of the universe of streptococcal infections, rheumatic fever is a clinical entity whose contents are arbitrarily defined by the Jones criteria.[5] The universe of rheumatic fever contains a series of sets whose relationships were described in Chapter 9, pages 149–150. The intersection of the sets of patients with arthritis, chorea, and carditis is portrayed in Figure 14*a*. A subset of patients who have severe carditis is added in Figure 14*b*. As already noted (page 150), two other "major" features of rheumatic fever—erythema marginatum and subcutaneous nodules—seldom occur alone, and have no prognostic or therapeutic significance. Hence they have been omitted from the main diagram.

A "minor" manifestation of post-streptococcal inflammation is *arthralgia*—the complaint of aching joints, without overt manifestations of arthritis. The arthralgia set, defined in this way, is not part of the arthritis set. Patients with arthralgia may also have carditis or chorea (or both), but patients with arthralgia alone do not have rheumatic fever, as arbitrarily defined by the Jones criteria. Thus, the arthralgia set may be suitably added to the diagram of Figure 14*b* to produce Figure 15, the clinical spectrum of acute rheumatic fever. In this spectrum, the arthralgia and arthritis sets were defined to be disjoint, and a

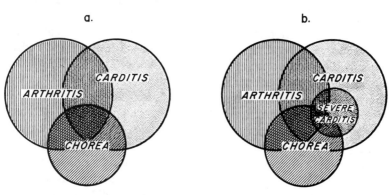

FIGURE 14
Sets included in the clinical spectrum of acute rheumatic fever.

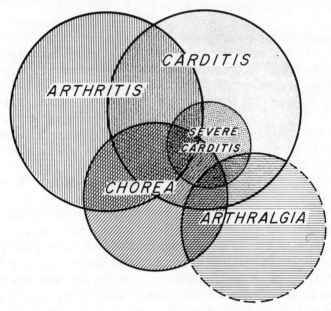

FIGURE 15
The clinical spectrum of acute rheumatic fever.

dashed border has been used for the outer perimeter of the subset with arthralgia only.

The common denominator in the sets and subsets of clinical events portrayed in Figure 15 is not "rheumatic fever", but the antecedent symptomatic or asymptomatic streptococcal infection. The subsequent inflammatory complications triggered by the infection need not appear with the arthropathic or febrile manifestations implicit in the name "rheumatic fever". Thus, when chorea occurs alone, it is not an aberrant variety or *forme fruste* of "rheumatic fever", but a distinct entity in the post-streptococcal spectrum. When carditis occurs alone, the patient has no chorea or joint pains, and may also lack fever or congestive heart failure. With none of these symptoms to act as an iatrotropic stimulus, the patient may not seek medical aid during acute carditis. Because he is lanthanic, his acute rheumatic fever may remain medically unrecognized and unidentified. When the acute carditis subsides in such patients, leaving residual scars found at some later date, rheumatic heart disease is said to have developed "without a history of rheumatic fever". The heart disease found in these circumstances is often called "insidious". To some clinicians, the implication of the word "insidious" is that *acute* cardiac inflammation continually persisted over a period of many years. Actually, the period of acute inflammation may have been no more than a few months, and the truly "insidious" aspect of the disease was the absence of symptoms that would have enabled the patient to be complainant and medically detected during the *acute* phase of the carditis.

Spectrum of Acute Rheumatic Carditis

Within the parent universe of post-streptococcal inflammation, acute rheumatic fever has the spectrum of sets and subsets just shown in Figure 15. Within the parent universe of rheumatic fever, acute rheumatic carditis also has constituent sets and subsets that form its spectral pattern, shown in Figure 16. In a large population with acute rheumatic carditis,[17] all patients were observed to have either mitral

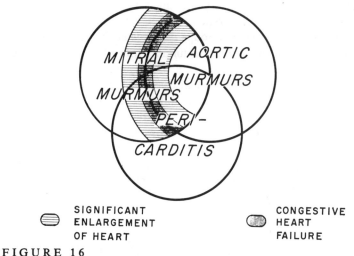

SIGNIFICANT ENLARGEMENT OF HEART

CONGESTIVE HEART FAILURE

FIGURE 16
The clinical spectrum of acute rheumatic carditis.

valve murmurs, aortic valve murmurs, or pericardial rubs, occurring singly or in combination. Within these sets of carditic patients, there was a subset with severe carditis, manifested by cardiac enlargement and/or congestive heart failure. All patients with significant cardiac enlargement were observed to have mitral murmurs (of pathologic or organically functional origin) during the acute attack, and some such patients also had aortic murmurs, pericarditis, or both. Cardiac enlargement is thus shown in Figure 16 as a subset of the mitral murmur set, located in a zone that contains mitral murmurs alone, as well as in a zone where mitral murmurs overlap with aortic murmurs and pericardial rubs. Congestive heart failure was found to occur only in patients with cardiomegaly, and is therefore depicted on the diagram as a subset of the cardiac enlargement set.

The clinical relationships demonstrated in the patterns of Figures 12 through 16 have been discussed with regard to the concepts they illustrate in etiology, pathogenesis, and epidemiology of rheumatic fever. Another important function of these patterns is their delineation of the patients whose properties are to be correlated with other data and subsequent observations. The subsets in the Venn diagrams contain groups of patients who are homogeneous in the properties cited, and who are reproducibly identified as members of distinct portions of the spectrum of streptococcal infections, or of rheumatic fever. With specific clinical subgroups demarcated by these classifications, the other data obtained concomitantly or subsequently can be correlated with a meaningful precision that is unattainable when the diverse "species" of a "phylum" of disease are left unrecognized and undefined. In rheumatic fever, such different clinical "species", or combinations thereof, form the basic subgroups of patients for correlation of other data in the investigations of such phenomena as occurrence of post-therapeutic rebounds,[10] experimental provocation of rebounds,[19] effects of temporal delays in therapy,[18] rates of rheumatic recurrence per subsequent streptococcal infection,[12, 109, 110] and cardiac effects of rheumatic recurrences.[12, 13]

Prognosis of Acute Rheumatic Fever

If the outcome of rheumatic fever is correlated with its acute clinical events, the Venn diagram of Figure 15 can be used to demonstrate prognostic distinctions. These distinctions are provided in Figure 17,

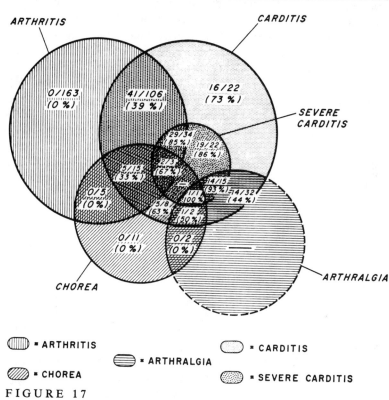

ARTHRITIS   CARDITIS

0/163
(0 %)

41/106
(39 %)

16/22
(73 %)

SEVERE
CARDITIS

29/34
(85 %)

19/22
(86 %)

5/15
(33 %)

2/3
(67 %)

14/15
(93 %)

14/32
(44 %)

0/5
(0 %)

1/1
(100 %)

5/8
(63 %)

1/2
(50 %)

0/11
(0 %)

0/2
(0 %)

ARTHRALGIA

CHOREA

▨ = ARTHRITIS   ▨ = CARDITIS

▨ = ARTHRALGIA

▨ = CHOREA   ▨ = SEVERE CARDITIS

FIGURE 17

The prognosis of acute rheumatic fever. (Denominators = number of patients in each subset; numerators = number of patients with clinical evidence of rheumatic heart disease 8 years later.)

whose contents enumerate the occurrence of residual heart disease for patients in each of the different acute clinical stages. The data represent the observed sequelae of attacks of acute rheumatic fever in a population of 441 patients,[7, 11] and show the striking distinctions in prognosis among different subsets of patients who all had the same disease: *acute rheumatic fever.*

Patients without carditis remained free of residual heart disease, regardless of the associated clinical findings. Patients with severe carditis had much worse results than the non-severe carditic groups.

Among patients with non-severe (or mild) carditis, the subsets with concomitant arthritis or arthralgia (with or without chorea) had a better prognosis than the subsets that had no joint symptoms. The percentages of residual heart disease were 39%, 33%, 50%, and 44% in the mildly carditic subsets with joint symptoms, versus 73% and 63% in those with no articular abnormalities. The combined data show that residual heart disease occurred in 61 (39%) of 155 patients in the four subsets with mild carditis *and* joint symptoms. By contrast, residual heart disease was found in 21 (70%) of 30 patients with the same degree of acute cardiac damage but no joint symptoms. The difference is statistically significant at $p < 0.01$ ($x^2 = 8.4$) and suggests, in this cardiac group, that the presence of joint symptoms has a more favorable prognostic import than their absence.

SPECTRUM OF CANCER

General Clinical Spectrum

The spectral pattern of rheumatic fever shown in Figure 15 was originally planned only after direct empiric clinical observations of the patients.[17] An approximate spectrum could have been constructed *a priori,* however, from general clinical knowledge of the disease. Similarly, from logical consideration of ordinary clinical experience, a spectrum can be formulated for the mode of detection and general *clinical* stage of patients with a cancer. One satisfactory spectrum could be the Venn diagram depicted earlier in Figure 6. If Figure 6 were used for cancer, the *primary features* set would refer to patients with symptoms or other clinical findings attributable to the tumor at its primary site. The *secondary features* set would refer to patients with findings that arise remote from the primary site of the tumor. Such a diagram would adequately encompass the clinical spectrum of cancer, but would omit certain important details. In particular, the *secondary features* set has too much diversity, and is preferably divided (as discussed on page 151 of Chapter 9) into a *systemic* set and a *metastatic* set. With these additional divisions, the Venn diagram of the general clinical spectrum of a cancer should theoretically contain four independent sets with the properties of (*A*) lanthanic, (*B*) primary, (*C*) systemic, and (*D*) metastatic clinical features.

The full intersection of four independent sets (*A, B, C, D*) in a Venn diagram would produce 15 subsets, having the properties of *A, B, C,*

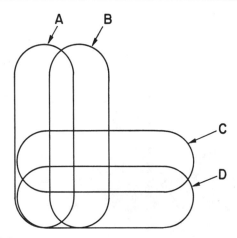

FIGURE 18
Venn's original diagram of the full intersection of four independent sets, A, B, C, and D.

D, AB, AC, AD, BC, BD, CD, ABC, ABD, ACD, BCD, and $ABCD$.* Such a four-set diagram cannot be drawn in two dimensions if the sets are portrayed as circles. In the original description of the diagrams that now bear his name,[107] Venn achieved a satisfactory four-set arrangement by using ovals, as shown in Figure 18. Although Venn's diagram is a satisfactory portrayal of the full intersection of four sets, the shape of the subsets is not convenient for the insertion of numbers. A modification of Venn's diagram, with rectangles instead of ovals, would produce a four-set pattern more suited for the subsequent enumeration of patients. Such a modification† is shown in Figure 19.

* If there are n independent sets fully intersecting in a Venn diagram, the number of anticipated subsets is $2^n - 1$. Since each of the n properties can be present or absent in a particular subset, the number of possibilities is $2 \times 2 \times 2 \times \ldots$. From this total, one subset is subtracted because it will contain none of the n properties, and will hence be omitted from the interior contents of the diagram. Thus, 3 subsets are produced by the full intersection of 2 independent sets, 7 subsets by 3, 15 by 4, 31 by 5, and so on.

† The idea of replacing curved shapes by rectilinear ones was given to me by Miss Judith Seligson. At the time she made the suggestion, she was 12 years old, and neither of us had yet seen Venn's solution to the four-set drawing.

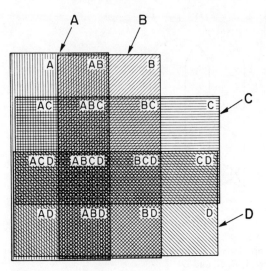

FIGURE 19
A modification of Venn's four-set diagram, indicating the properties present in each subset.

The type of four-set pattern shown in Figure 19 can be used to illustrate the intersection of lanthanic, primary, systemic, and metastatic sets that form the clinical spectrum of a cancer. The diagram is shown in Figure 20, together with its clinical enumeration for 596 patients with histologically demonstrated lung cancer. At the time of clinical detection, 34 of these patients were lanthanic asymptomatic discoveries. An additional 43 patients (25 + 3 + 11 + 1 + 2 + 1) were lanthanic but symptomatic in regard to the lung cancer. The remaining 519 patients came to a doctor complaining of symptoms attributable to their lung cancer.[111]

When the subsequent course of these 596 patients was observed, the 34 asymptomatic patients had significantly higher survival rates than the rest of the population. Among the 562 symptomatic patients, however, there was no prognostic difference (in comparable groups) among the 43 who were lanthanic and the 519 who were complaint. Therefore, the complainant-lanthanic distinction might be ignored

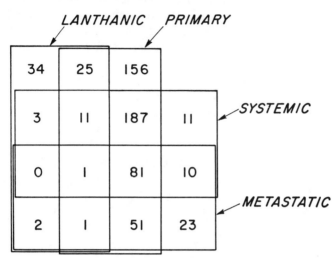

FIGURE 20
The clinical spectrum of lung cancer: distribution in a series of 596 patients.[25]

among symptomatic patients, and the clinical spectrum of symptomatic cancer could be portrayed as a standard three-set diagram of primary, systemic, and metastatic sets. To make the clinical spectrum complete, an extra section would have to be appended to indicate asymptomatic patients. Figure 21 shows such a three-set symptomatic spectrum, together with an extra crescent denoting the asymptomatic set. The result is an eight-subset diagram, simpler than the 15 subsets of Figure 20, but showing significant symptomatic distinctions in the clinical spectrum of a cancer.

Prognostic Clinical Spectrum

On the basis of clinical experience and ordinary clinical logic, the spectrum of Figure 21 can be re-arranged to demonstrate prognostic anticipations in patients with cancer. Of the eight subsets of patients demonstrated in Figure 21, the four with metastatic symptoms (subsets 5 through 8) have a manifestly poor prognosis because the symptoms *per se* indicate the functional effects of spread of tumor beyond the primary site. These four subsets are demarcated in Figure 22*A*. In the remaining four subsets—in which the patients have no metastatic symptoms—the presence of systemic symptoms in subsets *3*

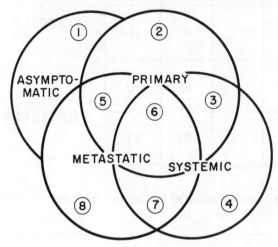

FIGURE 21
Simplified clinical spectrum of a cancer.

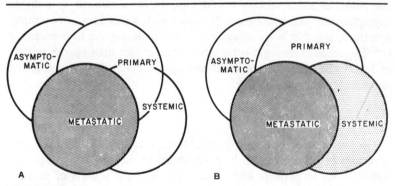

FIGURE 22
Prognostic demarcations in the clinical spectrum of a cancer.

and *4* suggests a prognosis less favorable than in the patients of subsets *1* and *2*, who have neither metastatic nor systemic symptoms. The two systemic subsets are demarcated in Figure 22*B*.

In the patients of subsets *1* and *2*, whose symptoms *per se* have no unfavorable morphologic or functional connotations, an additional feature of clinical taxonomy—the duration of symptoms—can next be considered. For patients with primary symptoms only (subset *2* of Fig. 21), the duration of symptoms indicates a minimal time for the duration of the tumor, since the tumor has been present at least as long as its symptoms. If the symptoms are of short duration, no conclusion may be drawn about the rate of growth of the tumor. The symptoms may be short because the tumor has grown rapidly; or the tumor might have grown slowly, remaining silent and iceberg-like in the undetected core of the spectrum, so that symptoms did not appear until quite late in the tumor's development. If the symptoms are of long duration, however, the tumor is likely to be slow-growing. The only way a patient could continue to have primary symptoms only, for a long time, without developing systemic or metastatic symptoms, would be to have a slow-growing tumor.

In the asymptomatic patients of subset *1*, whose disease is discovered by accident during an examination performed for an iatrotropic stimulus not due to the cancer, the duration of the cancer's symptoms cannot be assessed, since no symptoms exist. In such patients, the tumor has been present for an unknown length of time and, without the accidental discovery, might have remained symptomatically silent even longer.

With these considerations, subset *2* can be partitioned into two parts, as shown in Figure 23, to form a spectrum with five main symptomatic groups or "clinical stages". In the arrangement shown in Figure 23, subset *1* of Figure 21 remains intact as the asymptomatic group (stage I). Subset *2* of Figure 21 has been divided into two parts, according to whether the duration of symptoms was short or long. If 6 months is used as the boundary of "short" and "long", the "long primary" group (stage II) contains patients who have primary symptoms only, with at least one of the symptoms being older than 6 months. The "short primary" group (stage III) contains patients with only primary symptoms, none of which is older than 6 months. Subsets *3* and *4* of Figure 21 have been combined to form the "systemic" group (stage IV), and subsets *5, 6, 7,* and *8* have been joined to form the "metastatic" group (stage V).

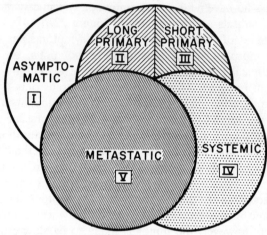

FIGURE 23
Clinical stages in the prognostic clinical spectrum of a cancer.

From the foregoing discussion and from MacDonald's hypothesis of "biologic pre-determinism",[23] a prognostic gradient can be anticipated among these five symptomatic stages. The survival rates should be highest in stages I and II, declining through stages III and IV to the lowest rates in stage V. Such a gradient, if present, would identify critical aspects of the biologic behavior of cancer. Yet the gradient, particularly in stages I through IV, would not be discernible from the conventional morphologic data of cancer, and could be detected only from the taxonomic analysis of symptoms.

Prognosis in Cancer of the Lung

Figure 24 shows the 5-year survival rates, regardless of therapy, in 596 patients with cancer of the lung,[25] classified according to the five clinical stages cited in Figure 23.

For these classifications, the clinical manifestations of lung cancer were designated as follows: primary symptoms were a recent cough; hemoptysis; chills, fever, or sweats of an associated pneumonia; subjective wheezing; recent dyspnea; or appropriate types of chest pain. Systemic symptoms were significant anorexia; significant weight loss;

CANCER OF LUNG
5 YR. SURVIVAL

ALL CASES: 56/596 (9%)

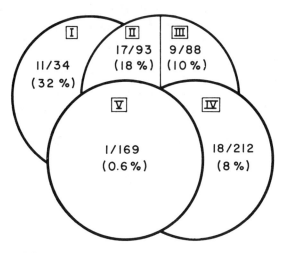

FIGURE 24
Prognosis of cancer of the lung: 5-year survival rates in 596 patients.[25] (Denominators = number of patients in each clinical stage, as specified in the text and in Figure 23. Numerators = number of patients who survived 5 years or more.)

fatigue; or the clubbing or joint pains of hypertrophic pulmonary osteo-arthropathy. Metastatic symptoms were such mediastinal manifestations as hoarseness (with a non-moving vocal cord), dysphagia, or the swelling of the upper torso indicative of the superior vena cava syndrome; and such extra-thoracic manifestations as cutaneous nodules, neurologic findings, bone pain, and abdominal masses.

The results of Figure 24 demonstrate that the anticipated prognostic gradient is indeed present among the five clinical stages. Although the total 5-year survival was 9% for the entire population of 596 patients, the rates ranged from 32% in stage I, to 18% in II, 10% in III, 8% in IV, and 0.6% in V. The prognostic gradient in these clinical stages persisted when the patients were further subdivided into subgroups that had the same morphologic features and the same modes of therapy.[25]

Prognosis in Cancer of the Rectum

Figure 25 shows the 5-year survival rates, regardless of therapy, in an analogous recent study[25] of 201 patients with cancer of the rectum, classified according to the concepts of Figure 23. For these classifications, primary symptoms were rectal bleeding; a significant recent change in stool appearance or in bowel habits; ano-rectal discomfort; or appropriate types of abdominal pain. Systemic symptoms were anorexia, significant weight loss, or fatigue. Metastatic mani-

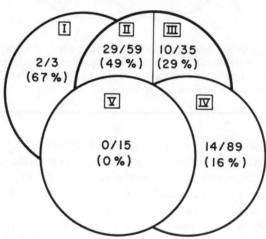

CANCER OF RECTUM
5 YR. SURVIVAL

ALL CASES: 55/201 (27%)

Ⅰ 2/3 (67%)

Ⅱ 29/59 (49%)

Ⅲ 10/35 (29%)

Ⅴ 0/15 (0%)

Ⅳ 14/89 (16%)

FIGURE 25

Prognosis of cancer of the rectum: 5-year survival rates in 201 patients.[25] (Denominators = number of patients in each clinical stage, as specified in the text and in Figure 23. Numerators = number of patients who survived 5 years or more.)

festations included ascites, jaundice, bone pain, and an unequivocally enlarged, nodular hard liver.

The results show the same type of prognostic gradient noted for lung cancer. The over-all 5-year survival was 27% but, in the individual symptomatic stages, the rates went from 67% in the three patients of Stage I, to 49% in II, 29% in III, 16% in IV, and 0% in V. This prognostic gradient persisted when the patients were further subdivided into subgroups that were morphologically similar.

These data demonstrate that the symptoms of cancer indicate functional effects and rates of growth that cannot be discerned morphologically. The distinction, although often suspected, has not been previously specified and quantified. In the absence of a clinical taxonomy the biologic implications of symptoms were often not analyzed. Without a classification for specific symptomatic subgroups, the significance of temporal distinction is lost if duration is calculated as an average for *all* types of symptoms, instead of being restricted to patients with primary symptoms only. In many investigations of cancer, the survival data have demonstrated a paradoxically good prognosis for patients discovered "late" rather than "early". The data were often dismissed, however, as isolated peculiarities of the behavior of cancer and man, and the biologic significance of the data was not further considered.

A patient's iatrotropic stimulus is the result of many different features of man or of disease. Different people, developing the same types of symptoms, will respond in diverse ways. Some people will seek medical attention promptly; others may wait. Nevertheless, few people will long ignore symptoms that are rapidly progressive, frightening, severe, or incapacitating. On the other hand, many patients may not rapidly seek medical help when the early symptoms of the tumor are neither inconveniencing, dramatic, nor debilitating. Such patients are often not motivated to visit a doctor until much later in the illness when more significant symptoms have developed. In this way, many "favorable" tumors are not detected until a long duration of symptoms has elapsed.

The implications of these aspects of clinical taxonomy in cancer have been discussed elsewhere,[25] and are particularly important in estimating prognosis for individual patients, in planning and evaluating therapeutic trials, and in correlating the results of laboratory research. The morphology of the tumor is an important index of its biology, but so is the clinical history of the patient. Slow-growing tumors produce symptoms slowly.

THE SPECTRUM OF PAIN IN CORONARY ARTERY DISEASE

During a survey of patients who received coronary arteriography, Proudfit, Shirey, and Sones[112] analyzed and correlated the various types of chest pain found in 475 patients with coronary artery disease. Using appropriate criteria, the authors described five types of pain, designated as:

> Angina pectoris, classes I through III
> Coronary failure
> Angina pectoris, class IV
> Rest pain (without any of the preceding three
>   manifestations)
> Myocardial infarction

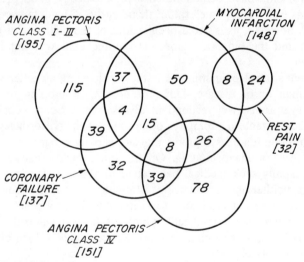

FIGURE 26

Spectrum and epidemiologic distribution of chest pain in 475 patients with coronary artery disease. (Adapted from the Venn diagram of Figure 2 of Ref. 112, by Proudfit, Shirey, and Sones.)

The overlapping spectrum of these different types of pain, and the number of patients who had each type, is shown in Figure 26. The largest single set was angina pectoris, classes I through III, with 185 patients, and the same property, occurring alone, provided the largest single subset, 115 patients. Although this spectrum of pain was not constructed for prognostic purposes, the seven different subsets of the myocardial infarction set demonstrate some of the clinical complexity that must be considered when survival rates or various modes of therapy for this disease are evaluated.

OTHER APPLICATIONS OF VENN DIAGRAMS

THE ETIOLOGIC, PROGNOSTIC, AND MORPHOLOGIC SPECTRUM OF FRACTURES

The group of orthopedic surgeons led by G. H. C. Bauer have applied Venn diagrams for characterizing different aspects of fractures, and for later evaluations of prognosis and treatment.

Alffram[113] has analyzed the "etiologic" and prognostic spectrum of 1109 cases of fracture of the proximal end of the femur, portrayed as shown in Figure 27. In his definitions of the major sets, *disease* referred to a known abnormality other than old age; *trauma* referred to a definite accident, however trivial; and *old age* referred to patients older than 70 years. The largest single subset, comprising almost half his population, contained 462 traumatized healthy old people. The 243 traumatized old people with disease had the highest 3-month mortality rate, 25%.

Edwards[114] has analyzed the morphologic spectrum of fractures of the tibial shaft in a series of 492 patients, portrayed in Figure 28. The three major sets were characterized according to easily observable anatomic features: displacement, skin injury, and type of bone injury. Of the 492 fractures, 439 (89%) occurred in a combination of three (subsets *1, 4,* and *5*) of the eight subsets in this universe. Nine of the fractures, which were neither open, displaced, nor transverse, are shown outside the immediate spectrum. Edwards noted a direct correlation between the cause of the fractures and their morphologic manifestations, and he found that the additional procedures of classification were helpful in planning rational treatment.

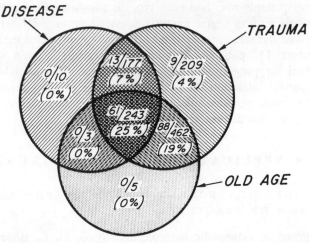

FIGURE 27

Etiology and 3-month mortality rates in fractures of the proximal end of the femur. (Denominators = number of patients in each category; numerators = number of patients who were dead 3 months later.) (Adapted from the Venn diagram of Figure 19 and from data in Table 43 of Ref. 113, by Alffram.)

CLINICO-PATHOLOGIC CORRELATION IN LUNG DISEASE

After establishing appropriate criteria for the clinical and morphologic designations, Mitchell, Ryan, Petty, and Filley[115] performed a clinico-pathologic correlation cf lung disease in 175 patients subjected to necropsy. Morphologic evidence of either emphysema (EMPH), mucous gland hyperplasia (MGH), or both, was found in 72 patients. Among these 72 patients, 47 had had clinical evidence of severe airway obstruction. The extremes of the clinical spectrum were "pink and puffing" (PP), which occurred in 14 of those 47 patients, and "blue and bloated" (BB), which occurred in 17. The clinical manifestations of the remaining 16 patients were somewhere between these two functional extremes, and were categorized as "neither PP nor BB".

The Venn diagram drawn by Mitchell and his co-workers to dem-

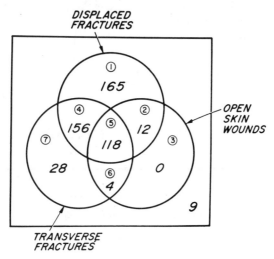

FIGURE 28

Distribution of cases in the anatomic spectrum of fractures of the tibial shaft. (Adapted from the Venn diagram of Figure 2 and from data in Table 3 of Ref. 114, by Edwards.)

onstrate the enumerated clinico-pathologic correlations is shown in Figure 29A. The diagram is unusual in that the size of each subset has been made proportional to the number of members it contains. Such constructions are technically difficult because of the requirement for using graph paper, or some other method of measuring area, in order to calculate the relative size of each constituent subset. Although such a "proportional" Venn diagram has the advantage of demonstrating quantitative relations, its qualitative aspects may be less clear in this form than when depicted in a more conventional "non-proportional" Venn diagram. The latter type of diagram, demonstrating exactly the same data as Figure 29A, is presented for esthetic comparison in Figure 29B.

The pulmonary investigation cited here is particularly noteworthy for its demonstration of the frequent dissociations, discussed earlier on pages 66–70, between morphologic form and clinical function in a human disease. No significant clinical evidence of airway obstruction had appeared in 25 of the 72 patients in this series of cases with

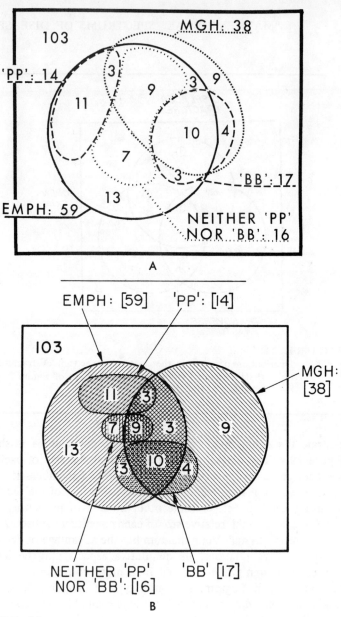

FIGURE 29

Distribution of cases in a clinico-pathologic correlation of lung disease. Abbreviations are explained in the text. *A* is the original Venn diagram, kindly loaned by Dr. Roger S. Mitchell, of Figure 4 in Ref. 115 by Mitchell, Ryan, Petty, and Filley. *B* is an alternative construction of a Venn diagram showing the same principles and data.

morphologic evidence of severe lung disease. The 47 patients with severe clinical symptoms showed a trend toward distinct correlation, in that the PP group had mainly emphysema alone, with a few patients also having mucous gland hyperplasia, whereas the BB group had mainly MGH, with or without EMPH. Nevertheless, the distribution of clinical and morphologic findings was so diverse and so often dissociated that no consistent correlation can be assumed for the clinical and morphologic aspects of this type of lung disease. Such dissociations between form and function have also been frequently noted in other recent studies of lung disease,[116, 117] and also in studies of cirrhosis,[118] gastritis,[119] hemiplegia,[120] osteo-arthrosis,[121] and "rheumatic activity".[122]

SPECTRUM OF ANTIBODY RESPONSES IN STREPTOCOCCAL INFECTIONS

Several different antibodies can be found in human serum as a result of infection with group A β-hemolytic streptococci. Among the antibodies that have been most thoroughly tested are anti-streptolysin O (ASO), anti-hyaluronidase (AH), and anti-streptokinase (ASK). Not all of these antibodies will show a rise in titer in response to a streptococcal infection. The rise may occur sometimes in only one of the antibodies, sometimes in two, and sometimes in all three. The antibody rises found in 226 infections detected during a large epidemiologic study[123] are shown in the Venn diagram of Figure 30. All three antibodies showed a rise in titer in 54 infections; two of the three rose in 88 (55 + 22 + 11) infections; and only one antibody rose in 84 (51 + 25 + 8) infections.

The diagram demonstrates that the ASO titer was the most "effective" of these three antibodies for identifying streptococcal infections. The ASO titer rose in 182 cases, as compared with a total of 145 for AH and 95 for ASK. It should be noted, however, that 19% of streptococcal infections would not have been identified if ASO were the sole titer examined in serologic testing, because the ASO titer rose in only 81% of the 226 infections. Thus, although a rise in ASO titer can indicate a streptococcal infection, the absence of a rise does not exclude infection. If AH testing were added to the routine ASO procedure, 96% of the infections (218/226) in this series would have been detected.

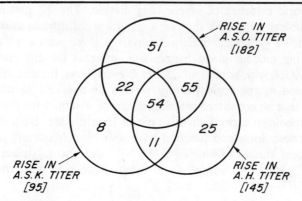

FIGURE 30

Distribution of antibody responses in 226 group A streptococcal infections. (Constructed from data presented in Table 10, page 38, of Ref. 123, by Wood, Feinstein, Taranta, Epstein, and Simpson.)

SPECTRUMS OF OBSERVER VARIABILITY

Venn diagrams can also be used to demonstrate the agreements or disagreements in diagnostic opinions reached by different means of observation. Figure 31 shows the diagnosis of esophageal varices in 39 patients examined by two different endoscopists and by barium-contrast radiography. In this series, which was reported by Conn, Smith, and Brodoff,[124] complete agreement of all three observers was reached in 20 instances, 8 with varices and 12 without. Spagnuolo, Taranta, et al.[125] have also used Venn diagrams to illustrate observer variability in cardiac auscultation.

PATTERNS OF SEQUENCE IN CLINICAL MANIFESTATIONS

The types of Venn diagram formulated in the first three sections of this chapter have dealt with the constituents of a clinical or other situation at a single point in time. The diagrams can also be used to illustrate such temporal changes as the sequence of manifestations in a disease.

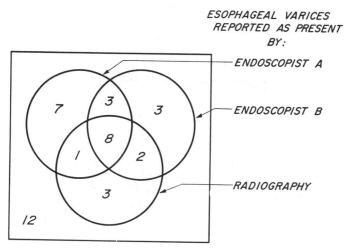

ESOPHAGEAL VARICES
REPORTED AS PRESENT
BY:

ENDOSCOPIST A

ENDOSCOPIST B

RADIOGRAPHY

FIGURE 31

Observer variability in the endoscopic and radiographic diagnosis of esophageal varices in 39 patients. Numbers in each subset represent the number of patients in whom a positive diagnosis was made by each "mode" of observation. In 12 patients, no varices were noted by any observer. (Adapted from the Venn diagram of Figure 1 of Ref. 124, by Conn, Smith, and Brodoff.)

GENERAL PATTERNS OF POSSIBLE
SEQUENTIAL CHANGES

In Figure 32, a series of arrows have been added to the general clinical spectrum of disease first shown in Figure 6. The arrows indicate different transitions that can occur from one clinical stage of disease to another. The diagram shows 42 arrows, demonstrating the movement from any one of the seven main clinical stages into any one of the other six. For indexing the transitions, the arrows themselves could be marked from 1 to 42 and each transition then numbered; alternatively, a change from stage 5 to stage 6, for example, could be designated as "$5 \rightarrow 6$".

Although the diagram of Figure 32 contains 42 arrows, the total number of possible transitions in clinical stages is actually 56, not 42.

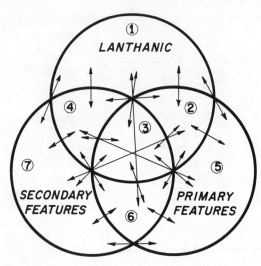

FIGURE 32
Possible clinical transitions in the clinical stages of a disease.

From each of the seven clinical stages, the disease can move into two other alternatives not cited in the diagram: death, and health (or disappearance of the disease). Since each of the seven clinical stages of disease can move into any of the six other stages, into death, or into health, the total number of possible transitions is $7 \times 8 = 56$.

For changes of *individual* clinical manifestations, instead of changes in the *general* clinical stages noted in Figure 32, the number of sequential possibilities is enormous, and their classification must be individualized for each disease.

RECURRENCES OF ACUTE RHEUMATIC FEVER

Patients with recurrent attacks of acute rheumatic fever provide an opportunity for arrow-marked Venn diagrams to show the sequence of change in clinical manifestations of a disease. Figure 33 correlates the clinical features of an antecedent attack of acute rheumatic fever with the manifestations that appeared in the same patient during a recurrent attack.[13] The basic spectrum of Figure 33 is the same spec-

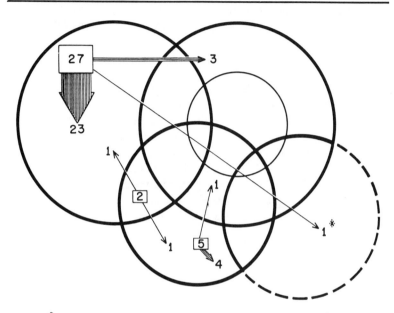

* GLOMERULONEPHRITIS

FIGURE 33

    Sequence of manifestations in antecedent and recurrent attacks of rheumatic fever, for 34 patients without carditis in the antecedent attack.[13] (For further details, see text and also Fig. 15, page 184.)

trum of acute rheumatic fever shown earlier in Figure 15. The numbers inside the rectangles denote the number of patients in each initial subset who had the cited clinical manifestations during the antecedent attack. The point of each arrow indicates the manifestations present in the recurrent attack; the number next to the arrow's point indicates how many patients had that manifestation; the shaft of the arrow has a thickness proportional to the number of patients.

    This particular diagram shows the fate, in rheumatic recurrences, of 34 children and adolescents who had no carditis in the antecedent attacks. In 27 cases, the recurrences were mimetic: 23 patients had only arthritis, and 4 patients had only chorea, in both attacks. Only 4 patients developed carditis in the new attacks, and the evidence of carditis later disappeared in all 4 instances.[13] This type of diagram visually portrays data that would otherwise require a long tabular listing for individual patients.

*   *   *

The many "mathemedical" applications of Venn diagrams should now be apparent. The diagrams can help improve the state of science in clinical reasoning, while simultaneously offering a new outlet for clinical "artistry". To construct the diagrams, a clinician must fulfill the scientific demands of logical and biological stipulation; but he can also exercise free artistic taste in esthetic choices of configuration for the drawings. Although the ingredients of clinical judgment can still be an "art", Venn diagrams will enable the art-work to be designed and communicated in the form of a precise, reproducible clinical portrait.

12. Biologic and Statistical Implications of Clinical Taxonomy

The patterns of classification just cited are not necessarily the only or the best ways of managing each particular situation. Future thought and research will probably bring other patterns or other classifications that are preferable to those just described. To "design" a new project in clinical research, an investigator can use existing clinical classifications when they seem applicable and effective; he can establish new clinical patterns from surveys of appropriate patients or medical records; he can use his existing knowledge to form approximate patterns as transient hypotheses to be confirmed; or he can create special *ad hoc* classifications for studies that involve several diseases or that include clinical situations not previously classified. What is most important about clinical taxonomy is not so much the particular categories chosen for the distinctions, as the realization that such clinical distinctions are a necessity of medical science.

Classification of patients according to the clinical behavior of disease is imperative for understanding the biology and statistics of human ailments. Without such classification, diverse mixtures of patients cannot be separated into subgroups that are clinically similar enough for precision in epidemiologic delineations, prognostic estimations, therapeutic selections and evaluations, correlations of clinical and laboratory data, and appraisal of subsequent clinical or other events in studies of natural and post-therapeutic history. Unless patients with a particular disease are divided into groups that are comparable, with suitable homogeneity in clinical properties, the precision of science is lost. The experimental "design" is non-reproducible.

The implications of these clinical distinctions affect every aspect of conceptual thinking and scientific comprehension in human disease. Some of the many implications are discussed in the sections that follow.

BIOLOGY OF HUMAN ILLNESS

THE EVOLUTION OF A DISEASE

The Venn diagram of Fig. 10 (p. 177) can illustrate the evolution of a disease in its host. A disease always begins in the (black) central undiscovered core of the spectrum. As the disease develops in a particular host, it moves outward to stages (subsets 8 through 11) where it is medically detectable although not yet clinically discovered. The disease can then advance either to subset 1, where it is discovered while subclinical, or to the clinical manifestations of subsets 2 through 7. In those subsets, the disease may be discovered by accident before the patient complains of symptoms (subsets 2 through 4), or the symptoms may provoke the patient to seek medical aid (subsets 5 through 7).

THE CHRONOMETRY OF DISCOVERY

The time that elapses in the transition from undiscovered core to a clinical stage, and from inception of clinical stage to actual clinical detection, is critically important for determining the total duration of a patient's disease and how "early" it is found. The chronometry of a disease in a particular patient can be assessed in two ways: 1) from retrospective comparison of results found in routine examinations (such as physical findings, roentgenograms, and urinalyses) that were performed before the onset of symptoms, and 2) from the duration of appropriate symptoms. The first of these assessments would help indicate the length of time that the disease was in its "undetected" core, and the symptomatic intervals would denote the durations of different clinical stages.

For example, despite the attention devoted to the concept of "early" discovery in diseases such as cancer, the "earliness" is seldom actually measured in units of time, and is usually deduced from the different anatomic stages of the tumor. A small, localized tumor is assumed to be "early"; a large or disseminated tumor is assumed to be "late". Most discussions of "early" treatment in cancer are thus completely speculative—being based on anatomy, rather than chronometry. Nevertheless, as indicated in Figures 24 and 25, and in the associated discussion on pages 191–198, slow-growing tumors produce symptoms slowly, and the symptoms are an important index of biologic behavior of the disease. When time is actually measured, an "early" tumor may be already metastasized; a "late" tumor may still be resectable for cure.

Rheumatic fever provides another illlustration of the importance of clinical details in chronometric analysis of disease. For many years, clinicians had noted that rheumatic patients treated promptly after onset of symptoms had less residual heart disease than those treated late. The therapeutic conclusion was that early treatment had effectively prevented residual heart disease. Nevertheless, when patients with acute rheumatic fever were subclassified and compared in suitable clinical categories, promptness of therapy did not appear to influence the occurrence of residual heart disease.[11, 18] The biologic behavior of rheumatic fever produces an inverse clinical phenomenon: when the disease "licks at the joints", it often "bites at the heart", but when it "bites" at the joints, it often licks at or spares the heart.[17] Thus, patients with the most severe arthritis often have no carditis, while those with carditis often have no articular symptoms. Joint pains, however, are a cogent iatrotropic stimulus, whereas carditis *per se* is asymptomatic. Consequently, the patients with arthritis sought treatment early because of their joint pains but often had no cardiac involvement; the patients with cardiac involvement often had no articular or other symptoms that would evoke early treatment. Regardless of whether treatment began soon or late after onset of symptoms, residual heart disease occurred in none of the patients without carditis, and in almost all the patients with severe carditis. The erroneous old belief that prompt treatment regularly prevented heart disease had arisen because the "early" population consisted mainly of patients whose painful joints made them seek aid promptly. Such patients often had no heart disease to be "prevented".

CONCEPTS OF PATHOGENESIS

Several apparently "peculiar" aspects of pathogenesis in disease are explained by the existence of subsets *4* and *7*—clinical stages in which patients have had the secondary features (or complications) of a disease but none of the primary features. These subsets account for the occurrence of patients who have rheumatic heart disease without a history of rheumatic fever, or hepatic cirrhosis without a history of acute hepatitis, or chronic nephritis without a history of acute pyelonephritis or of acute glomerulonephritis. In each of these instances, the patient did not develop the symptomatic primary clinical features regarded as "typical" of the acute disease. Lacking arthritis or chorea, a patient may not be recognized as having acute rheumatic fever. In the absence of jaundice, acute anicteric hepatitis may escape diagnosis. Without red urine or edema as an iatrotropic stimulus, acute glomerulonephritis may be medically undetected.

Similarly, the spectrum of every disease that is a morphologic or chemical entity will contain subset *1*—the patients who are asymptomatic. Thus, clinicians should not be surprised to encounter patients who have streptococcal infections without sore throats, myocardial infarctions without chest pain, diabetes mellitus without polyuria, and duodenal ulcer without peptic symptoms.

When the diagnosis of a disease is established in patients of subsets *1, 4,* or *7,* the absence of a history of primary features often makes clinicians doubt the reliability of the patient's perception or reporting. Thus, a teetotaler who develops cirrhosis after anicteric hepatitis may be suspected of lying when he denies alcohol ingestion, because he has never had the jaundice that would usually be expected with acute hepatitis. All these "atypical" forms of disease are clinically uncommon rather than atypical; they are legitimate parts of the clinical spectrum of a disease, but they are generally found, in clinical settings, less frequently than the "typical" cases. Epidemiologic studies outside the medical center may find many more of the cases now regarded as uncommon or "atypical". The history given by patients in this uncommon part of the spectrum will not be "diagnostic" of the disease —but is a critical feature of classification in understanding pathogenesis and in comparing the results of treatment.

Of particular importance in therapy is the fact that clinicians, without better knowledge of natural history of each stage in the spectrum of a disease, cannot be sure that an instance of disease discovered in subset *1* would necessarily advance to other subsets if left untreated, or that subsets *2* and *5* (with primary features only) would necessarily undergo transitions into secondary clinical stages. Patients discovered with only primary features must be appraised differently

from those discovered with secondary features (subsets *3, 4, 6,* and *7*)
—particularly if therapy is intended to prevent complications. This
same stricture applies to the evaluation of treatment planned to prevent development of primary or secondary features in the lanthanic
asymptomatic patients of subset *1.*

These spectrums of illness also contain important implications
for investigators of etiology and pathogenesis. No matter what agent is
found or suspected as a cause of a disease, the pathogenetic mechanism is not fully explained until the susceptibility of the host is accounted for. Why did this particular host, among the general population of people, get this disease? And why did this particular patient,
among the hosts who became diseased, develop this particular form of
the disease? Most current investigations of etiology and pathogenesis
are confined to the alleged causative agent and to external environmental factors (such as poverty) in patients who are identified only as
having the disease. No further correlations are usually made for patients in different clinical stages of the disease.

For example, when pathogenesis is analyzed in patients with
tuberculosis or cancer, the patients are seldom divided into lanthanic
or complainant groups, or into those first detected with primary only,
secondary only, or combined clinical features. Thus, the heterogeneous
spectrum of each of these diseases is usually studied pathogenetically
as though all the sick patients had developed the same kind of disease.
Yet it is possible that a patient who develops only secondary features
is different in susceptibility and in mode of pathogenesis from a patient
whose disease is found while he is asymptomatic. Many important
laboratory data now being discarded as showing no significant correlation in cancer or tuberculosis might show meaningful importance if the
data were analyzed for homogeneous clinical subgroups of patients,
instead of being distributed throughout the diverse total mixture of a
disease population. The investigator who works fastidiously to achieve
precision in his laboratory data may compromise their value by correlating them with the diffuse *brei* of a "disease" that is not clinically
subclassified.

Rheumatic fever provides another example of inadequate pathogenetic correlation in contemporary laboratory research. The strepto-
coccus that triggers this disease has been the focus of major investigation for at least two decades, yet almost no research has been done
during that time to distinguish the susceptibility of hosts who get

arthritis but no carditis from hosts who get carditis but no arthritis. The post-streptococcal pathogenetic mechanisms may be entirely different in these two types of patients, although both groups have the same "disease". Nevertheless, despite the attention given to the "strepto-coccology" and immunology of rheumatic fever, there has been almost no investigation of the fundamental pathogenetic clues offered by these different clinical forms of illness in the susceptible host.

STATISTICS IN HUMAN DISEASE

INCIDENCE AND PREVALENCE OF DISEASE

It is readily apparent from Figure 7 or Figure 10 that almost all statistical data on the general incidence and prevalence of a disease are inaccurate. Statisticians can never determine the true frequency with which a disease occurs; the statistician tabulates *diagnoses,* not diseases. He never knows how many people in a general population really have a particular disease; all he knows (at best) is how many people have received the diagnosis of that disease. Any collection of data on general incidence or prevalence of disease must necessarily omit the hard "core" of undiscovered and undiagnosed disease, whose true magnitude can seldom be determined. Disease of this type occurs in patients who are inadequately diagnosed, and in lanthanic hosts who are omitted from epidemiologic surveys or who die without necropsy or without lesions demonstrable at necropsy.

The "vital statistics" data that represent facts of demography—age, sex, date of birth, place of birth, date of death, place of death—are indisputable, and are of extraordinary value in medicine. Birth rates, death rates, and incremental changes in the geography of populations provide important information for many medical activities. When the data of "vital statistics", however, represent clinical opinions—cause of death, incidence of "disease", prevalence of "disease"—the results must be appraised cautiously. Different "diseases" may be increasing or decreasing in frequency from one year to the next merely because of changes in diagnostic techniques, or variations in the fashions of diag-nostic opinion.

A simple example is the contemporary disappearance of the disease "dropsy". A reader who compares the vital statistics of a century ago with those of today would note that this "disease" was a common cause of death 100 years ago, but is almost never reported today. The reader might therefore conclude that one of modern medicine's greatest triumphs was the eradication of a scourge responsible for so much mortality in the past. The triumph, of course, belongs to changes in medical nomenclature. "Dropsy" is still with us in abundance, but we now call it something else: *congestive heart failure, cardiac decompensation, nephrotic syndrome,* etc. From the data of "vital statistics", it is difficult to decide how much of the old *consumption* and *tuberculosis* has been replaced by the modern *cancer of the lung;* and whether *rheumatic fever* has declined in frequency only because we can treat streptococcal infections to prevent it, or also because we now give the names of *lupus erythematosus, rheumatoid arthritis, viral arthralgia,* and *congenital heart disease* to what previously may have been called *rheumatic fever.* The recent unexplained decline in frequency of *gastric cancer* in the United States may also be due to changes in diagnostic techniques, rather than to a lesser prevalence of the disease in nature.

Despite obvious inaccuracies and uncertainties, the "vital statistics" data of incidence and prevalence of disease are often accepted too credulously, and are made the basis for major investigations of etiology. For example, when a disease has a low rate of occurrence in one geographic population and a high rate in another, investigators may accept the data as reliable and may begin to search the demographic characteristics of the two populations—in such features as ethnic groups; occupations; smoking, drinking, or nutritional customs—for factors that might be causing the difference in rates of the "disease". Yet these variations in the statistical freqency of a "disease" in different localities may often have nothing to do with its etiology or pathogenesis. The variations may arise solely from differences in techniques (or criteria) for diagnosis, or for detecting lanthanic hosts.

"RANDOM SAMPLING" AND "COLLECTED CASES"

A more subtle and equally important problem in statistics arises from the failure of most clinicians and of many statisticians to recognize that *no* clinical collection of patients can be a valid random sampling of the total population of a disease. The impossibility is demonstrated by the diagram in Figure 10. In any medical locality, the number of patients with a given disease who are undiscovered, or first found at necropsy, will vary greatly according to the standards and techniques of diagnosis and of medical care. More significantly, the type of locality at which discovered patients are collected will inevitably bias the contents of the collection. The reason for the bias is that the clinical and personal properties of the sick patients, and not the pathologic diagnosis and laboratory data, will determine the time, the provocative stimuli, and the type of doctor or hospital at which the patients seek medical care.

Consequently, no two hospitals or two doctors will see exactly the same type of clinical population. Although many fundamental concepts of contemporary biostatistics are based on theories about "random sampling", the biologic reality is that doctors don't choose patients; patients choose us. The place where the doctor works and the kind of work he does will often determine the particular type of patient that comes to him. Figure 34 shows how the doctor's location affects his view of the spectrum of disease shown in Figure 10. The view is inevitably distorted by where he stands when he looks.

Pathologists, at the morgue, see the dead. Epidemiologists, in a field

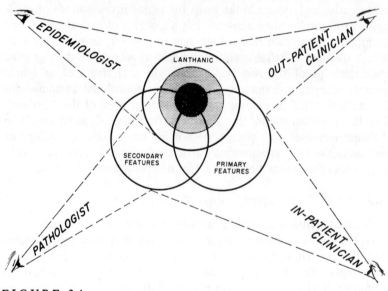

FIGURE 34
Site of the observer and view of the spectrum of a disease.

survey, see the asymptomatic. Clinicians see the hospitalized sick as in-patients and the ambulatory or mildly ill as out-patients. The contents of a population of patients with the same disease will also differ if collected on ward or private pavilion, in municipal or voluntary hospital, on surgical or medical service, in specialized referral units or in general treatment centers, in large or in small cities. Because observers at these different posts will inevitably see different parts of the spectrum of a disease, the proportional distribution of subsets in the observed collection of patients will always differ. The observers may all describe the same disease, but not the same percentages of different subsets of patients.

When doctors reach into the complex spectrum of a disease, select "random samplings" or "collected cases", and draw conclusions about the whole from the part they have observed, they are often placed in the position of the six blind men examining the elephant. (One of the blind men, feeling the tusk, thought the elephant was like a spear; another, feeling the trunk, thought it was like a snake; and so forth.) The observers may thereafter disagree violently about the whole that they have extrapolated from the examined part, while failing to recognize the source of the dissension. Many contemporary therapeutic controversies—such as anticoagulants in cardiovascular disease, steroids in rheumatic fever, and types of surgery or other therapy for cancer—are problems of this type. The "statistically significant" results of many therapeutic trials or surveys often reflect not the effects of therapy, but the effects of undetected important variations in base populations that seemed similar only because they were not adequately classified.

Suppose that a patient must meet certain requirements in order to receive a particular mode of therapy, but that the clinical severity of his illness keeps him from fulfilling the requirements. For example, he may be too sick to travel even a short distance to the hospital where the treatment is given, or he may not be well enough to travel a long distance to a research or referral center where a special new agent is being tested. If he reaches the appropriate hospital, his state of health may still be so bad that he is regarded as an unsuitable candidate for surgery, or for the diagnostic tests prerequisite to administration of the new treatment, or for withstanding some of the expected "complications" of the treatment. In all of these circumstances, the patients who are the most severely ill with a particular "disease" will have been excluded from the population who receive the treatment under study.

The population given the treatment will thus, in general, contain more people with a milder form of illness and a higher proportion of "good risks" in prognosis than the population to whom the treatment was denied. If the treated and non-treated groups are later compared only on the basis of having the same "disease", and if the severity of clinical illness is ignored, the treated groups will generally have better results—as they would have even if untreated. This type of problem constantly occurs in modern medicine, regardless of whether the investigations of therapy are "retrospective" or "prospective".

To receive surgical treatment for cancer, for example, a patient must be "operable"—which means that his tumor must be anatomically localized enough to be removed, *and* his clinical state must be healthy enough to enable him to tolerate both the operation and its consequences. A patient with an anatomically "operable" tumor may therefore be denied surgery because he is too old; because he may be unable to adjust to the new anatomic or functional situation that would be created by the surgery; because the functional clinical effects of the tumor have made him cachectic; or because a co-existing disease, such as cardiac decompensation, makes him a "poor operative risk". The clinical severity or co-morbidity of the illness in many such patients is often followed by early death. The "operable" and "inoperable" groups are thus clearly not comparable, although they may all have the same cancer and even same morphologic lesions. Nevertheless, the results of *surgery* and *no surgery* for cancer are often compared without regard to such distinctions.

Patients rejected from surgery for other reasons of severity of neoplastic disease, such as morphologic or clinical evidence of metastasis, are usually referred for radiotherapy or chemotherapy. Nevertheless, when the results of surgical treatment are compared with those of the other agents, consideration is seldom given to the surgeon's preselection of a relatively "healthier" population. The superiority of the post-surgical survival rates is often attributed only to the surgery.

The problem is even more subtle for many diseases that are usually treated by physicians rather than by surgeons. In rheumatic fever, for example, if a certain new drug is restricted only to patients treated "early" enough, the time limitation on the duration of symptoms will exclude many anarthritic patients with carditis. The patients who report for treatment promptly after onset of symptoms usually have joint pains, but in such patients, as demonstrated earlier (page 188), the carditis has a better prognosis than in the anarthritic group. If the investigator's "controls" are taken from previous medical records, and if no provision is made for the appropriate temporal and clinical distinctions of the compared patients, he may draw false conclusions about the effectiveness of his new drug.

In the universe of diabetes mellitus, patients who are "brittle" may refuse to continue treatment with a doctor who demands that his patients keep themselves normoglycemic. The "brittle" diabetic patient, who cannot maintain a normal blood sugar without the discomfort of frequent insulin shocks, may transfer to a different doctor whose therapeutic program is more easily maintained. Since "brittle" diabetics seem to be more likely to develop vascular complications than patients who are non-"brittle", the first doctor's therapeutic strictness may succeed only in limiting his population of patients to those who have disproportionately good results in avoiding vascular complications. The strict therapeutic regimen that drove the "bad risks" away may then be given credit for the success of the "good risks" who remained.

In acute myocardial infarction, many deaths occur almost immediately or within the first day after the infarction. Consequently, the patients who live long enough both to be admitted to the hospital and to begin oral anticoagulant therapy are often a relatively "mild" subset of the clinical spectrum of myocardial infarction. If the "controls" selected from medical records are compared with a treated population, and if no provision is made for the clinical severity of the infarction, the patients treated with anticoagulants may have better results mainly because they were "healthy" enough to be treated. Retrospective comparisons of this kind prompted the formulation of what might be called Rytand's law of *post hoc* cardiac statistics: "The prognosis for a patient with myocardial infarction is worse when anticoagulants are given to someone else".[126]

These problems in clinical classification are not solved merely by making the therapeutic investigation prospective and by getting a statistician to design it. In a large-scale, statistically designed, prospective study of anticoagulants for myocardial infarction, the participating doctors knew that anticoagulants would be given to patients admitted on certain days, but not on others. A patient whose heart infarcted on the wrong day could be kept at home long enough to be admitted the next day, if the doctor wanted him to get anticoagulants.

If the patient was able to survive the delay, however, he was thereby often "healthier" than a patient admitted immediately to the "control" group.

In the foregoing examples, the cited investigations were not given specific reference numbers because many alternative examples could have been chosen. All of these and many other unsolved problems in the design of therapeutic comparisons are to be expected in a science that is so relatively young. Although the "numerical method" was introduced[127] into clinical medicine more than a century ago by Pierre Ch. A. Louis (1787–1872), very few clinicians or statisticians today have been trained to appreciate the subtleties of applying statistics to the results of *therapy,* and the design of comparative prospective trials of treatment has received attention from statisticians only during the past 20 years.

As a pioneer in clinical statistics, Louis helped end the popularity of blood-letting by counting and comparing the results of patients treated in various ways. His general statistical techniques had many defects,[128] however, as might be expected of any new approach in science. After a brief period of influence and renown, his concepts were not firmly established and his work has been generally forgotten.

The fate of Louis should be a *caveat* for any clinician who questions an accepted therapy of his era and who urges his colleagues to make better use of their senses and of statistics in evaluating therapy. Louis concluded his treatise on blood-letting with these "radical" comments: "Let those, who engage hereafter in the study of therapeutics, pursue an opposite course to that of their predecessors. Let them not think that they have done any thing effectual, when they have only displayed their own theories, or stated what is done by the most celebrated physicians in such or such a case. But let them labor to demonstrate, rigorously, the influence and the degree of influence of any therapeutic agent, on the *duration, progress, and termination of a particular disease".*[129]

This type of strong intellectual medicine may be too distasteful to clinicians. At the time of Louis, the intellect of clinicians was being assaulted, from other sources, by conceptual revolutions taking place in the traditional nosologic and etiologic principles of medicine. The old "clinical" diagnoses of disease were being replaced by the nomenclature of pathologic anatomy, and the old Hippocratic theory of humoral causes for disease was being supplanted by Virchow's doctrine of cellular etiology.

Shaken by the destruction of the foundations of medical theory, clinicians must have been stunned and furious to have blood-letting, their old standby in therapy, also taken from them. Louis was attacked, sometimes vilified,[130] and defended, sometimes lauded. Although Jackson,[131] Bowditch,[132] Osler,[133] and other prominent American physicians who praised him had predicted that his name would endure among the greats in medicine, a century later he is almost unknown here.*

Louis's relative obscurity today is not surprising. Unlike his contemporary countrymen, Laënnec and Trousseau, who are known to medical students everywhere, Louis described no "new" diseases or physical signs to give his name an eponymic memorial. He was apparently[132] not an inspiring lecturer, so he earned no reputation as a great teacher. His prose style also seems uninspired, so he left no aphorisms to be collected in anthologies of medical writing. Since he did not actively practice and did most of his research from medical records, he gained no fame as a great clinician. And he produced no new systems of etiologic conjecture to take their place among the many other speculations immortalized in medical history.

Laënnec's memory is also perpetuated by the stethoscope he developed for aiding the clinician's auditory perception, but Louis's "numerical method" was a rational instrument for helping the mind. What he did was to initiate a science of clinical statistics that no one wanted. He had developed new methods, rather than new theories or tangible substances. He urged doctors to become better clinical observers and counters, but he failed to convince good clinical observers who felt no need to count, good counters who felt no need to clinically observe, and etiologic theorists who felt no need to do either.

Medicine today is also undergoing sieges that may lead to revolutionary change in our now-traditional nosologic and etiologic principles. The anatomic nosology of disease is being threatened by the nomenclature of biochemistry, and the Virchovian cellular theories

* I had never heard of Louis during my medical training, and, despite a good deal of subsequent reading about epidemiology, medical statistics, and numerical clinical trials, I had not encountered his name until about a year ago, when Dr. Lloyd G. Stevenson, Professor of the History of Medicine at Yale University School of Medicine, mentioned him to me. Louis might possibly also be remembered at Harvard, where his influence on Bowditch[132] was responsible for establishment of the "Clinical Conferences of the Medical School of Harvard College", and where his portrait hangs in the Bulfinch Staff Room of the Massachusetts General Hospital.

of etiology may be supplanted by molecular theories. Many clinicians today are perturbed about the possible overthrow of the basic principles of "disease" taught them in medical school. Let this historic parallel be warning to any contemporary clinician or statistician who dares be skeptical about an "established" procedure in modern therapy!

For the century that followed the work of Louis, the development of medical statistics gave almost no attention to problems in *treating* human illness. Medical statisticians were concerned mainly with getting "vital statistics" of the occurrence of disease, and with using such statistics and demographic data for studying the etiology of disease. As techniques became available to prevent infectious diseases, statisticians became more "clinically" oriented, but the information they dealt with was still either the demographic data that characterized the initially healthy host, or the para-clinical data and diagnostic names that characterized the "disease". With the advent of antibiotics to treat infectious disease, medical statistics finally reached the era of the therapeutic clinical trial. The first such trials were still relatively simple to design, however, because the critical data in the infectious diseases could be easily obtained bacteriologically. The patient either did or did not have laboratory evidence of the infectious disease, and the bacteria either did or did not go away after treatment. Hence, in planning and evaluating such therapeutic trials, there was relatively little need to consider the nuances of the patient's *clinical* state.

Only in the past two decades have statisticians become concerned with the design and appraisal of therapeutic trials in non-infectious or chronic diseases. To this problem, the statistician thus brings a long tradition of intellectual neglect of the significance and management of clinical data. He finds, as his collaborators, clinicians who have a long tradition of intellectual fear of statistics. The science of therapeutic trials is thus young and growing and has much to learn.

The clinician's problem as he enters the domain of "clinical biostatistics" is his ignorance or awe of the statistics. He usually knows nothing about it, or he has been taught too much. For most practical purposes, all he needs to know is some simple distinctions about different types of averages (such as means, medians, and modes), and a few simple tests of determining the numerical significance of different results (such as the *t test* and *chi-square*). Instead of learning when and how to use these convenient practical tests, however, his mind may have been inundated with multi-variate linear regression equations, complicated analyses of co-variance, stochastic processes, principles of bio-assay, rank order tests, and other numerologic procedures which, however useful in non-clinical activities, often have no value or pertinence in therapeutic trials. His intellect reeling with this clinical excess of statistical theories, the clinician may be reluctant to ask the statistician in a therapeutic trial to justify the choice and execution of needlessly complex statistical maneuvers.

The statistician's problem as he enters the domain of "clinical biostatistics" is that he usually knows a good deal about "statistics", a little about "bio", and almost nothing about "clinical". By neglect or by deliberate exclusion, for the reasons already cited, his statistical training did not include an appreciation of *clinical* activities and data. The pioneering work of Louis, for example, is not cited in most contemporary textbooks of epidemiology or biostatistics, and, with the exception of Mainland's detailed text,[134] almost none of the books on medical or biologic statistics discuss the effects of different stages of *clinical illness* in therapeutic trials and surveys of "disease".*

---

* It is tempting to speculate retrospectively about the etiology of Louis's failure to establish his "numerical method" for posterity. One possible reason is that after his successful clinical investigation of blood-letting, his later work became too "statistical". Instead of continuing to study the outcome of treatment, he began mainly to tabulate the occurrence of different manifestations in disease. These numerical accounts may have given his work the "dry" quality noted by both Faber[135] and Greenwood[28]—a quality still often present in contemporary statistical reports of such occurrence rates. Trousseau, a leader of French clinical medicine and an earlier collaborator[36] of Louis, perceived that these prognostically uncorrelated tables of frequency were of little help to clinicians in studying the outcome of treatment. For these clinical problems Trousseau recommended,[137] as an alternative to Louis's statistical occurrence rates, the use of Bacon's inductive approach to the observation of nature. Since the Baconian approach was based on multi-temporal correlations, rather than the uni-temporal numbers of occurrence rates, it was better suited then, as now, to evaluating prognosis and treatment—with or without statistical calculations.

Another contributing factor, of course, was the anti-therapeutic intellectual medical fashion of the era. In demolishing the Hippocratic humoral theories about etiology and in rejecting the ontologists' concept of specific courses for disease, Virchow's cellular doctrines of etiology also established a tradition of therapeutic nihilism among pathologists. "Since there are no specific disease entities", said Virchow, "there are no specific therapies." [138a] If treatment did not count in medical science, there was no apparent need for a counting medical science.

My own suspicion, however—unfettered, in the traditional etiologic manner, by any valid proof—is that Louis was ultimately done in neither by the "dryness" of his non-therapeutic statistics, nor by the nihilism of the pathologists. It was

There is a word clinicians constantly use for discussing the different stages of a patient's illness: the word is *sick*. We use the word judgmentally to describe distinctions in a patient's clinical state; we may say that he looks *sick,* or is not as *sick* as he was yesterday, or that he "is a *sick* myocardial infarction." We often do not define the word, but we know what it communicates: a sense of urgency in the need for treatment, or a poor prognosis, or a difference between two patients with the same diagnosed disease. The reasons for calling a patient *sick* are often such clinical distinctions as intractable pain; the severity of dyspnea; the height of fever; the presence of shock, oliguria, or congestive heart failure; and the co-morbidity of a disease that exists in addition to the one under treatment. But all of these clinical distinctions of sickness, which so profoundly affect the choice of treatment and the outcome of "disease", may be unfamiliar to a statistician. He has been trained primarily in the management of demographic and numerical data, and of categories in diagnostic nomenclature, and he may have little or no appreciation of the clinical data that demarcate prognosis and treatment for sick people.

These clinical distinctions, if not analyzed, will be major sources of unrecognized bias in any clinical survey or trial. Vaguely aware of the bias, the statistician may assume he can remove it by "random allocation" of therapy without attempting to "stratify" the patients into different clinical subgroups. The concept of "random" does not apply to the way patients choose doctors and doctors choose treatment. If these "decisional" distinctions are not considered, the entire principle of "random allocation" may have no validity in therapeutic trials.

Still reluctant to make and classify the clinical distinctions, however, the statistician may assume he can remove the non-random bias if the population sampled is large enough or sufficiently analyzed by various numerologic formulas. Increasing the size of the "sample" often serves only to increase the magnitude of the error if the bias is not removed, and no amount of statistical manipulation can possibly identify what was initially left unspecified.

The problem of statistical comparisons is a problem in comparison, not in statistics. If the clinical analyses of one doctor and

---

competition from another "numerical method": the dimensional measurements of laboratory technology. If clinicians could use all the new tests for measurements, they could get numbers easily and accurately without the laborious personal efforts needed to observe and count clinical numbers à la Louis. "Technology", Max Frisch[138b] has said, "is the knack of so arranging the world that we don't have to experience it." Technology had won another round.

another, of one medical center and another, or of patient groups within the same medical center are to be comparable, then the populations must be identified and divided according to their pertinent clinical properties. These properties delineate not only the components of the population, but also the clinical characteristics responsible for the different proportions of the disease seen by different observers. Without such identifications, subgroups of patients cannot validly be compared. Without the identifications, unreproducible clinical investigations are perpetuated and increased.

IDENTIFICATION AND ENUMERATION

The many different subgroups established by these distinctions may distress the statisticians working in clinical trials, and the clinicians working in actual practice. A single clinician may encounter patients of exactly the same subgroup too infrequently for his own previous observations to be useful or valid. Statisticians may find the numbers of patients in each category too small for application of the pertinent statistical formulas. The distress is inevitable and necessary, but can be assuaged as long as clinicians and statisticians will recall that the purpose of their analyses is medical, not merely statistical, significance. Small amounts of consistent, homogeneous, reproducible data will be clear and meaningful even if not "statistically significant". Large mixtures of unknown proportion and unidentified content may attain numerical differences that are statistically significant, but medically misleading or meaningless.

Confronted with a patient in an unfamiliar subgroup, clinicians can turn to information stored elsewhere (in a colleague's experience, in medical literature, or in a computer file) and find the data they need. When stored data are sparse, clinicians can contribute their own observations to the total knowledge. For accuracy in these procedures, the clinicians and the storage apparatus must be able to identify the same subgroup of patients. Such identifications are often impossible today, however, because neither the experience of many clinicians, the reports and surveys of the medical literature, nor the data now being enthusiastically stored in computer programs have been arranged with consistent, uniform classifications for differentiating precisely among clinical subgroups. Whether stored in clinician, literature, or computer, the data of one system or source often cannot be compared with those of another: physicians in one location may find they cannot rely on interpretations made elsewhere; statistical and computational analyses therefore yield precise but useless generalities, often inaccurate and often valueless in application to individual patients.

Beginning with the small enumerations of multiple but distinct subgroups, statisticians can increase the size of numbers by combining results of the same subgroups in different studies, or of different subgroups in the same study. The first type of combination is possible only when the basic clinical data of the investigations are obtained by standardized techniques and classified similarly. The second type of combination, within groups of the same study, is regularly feasible provided that the contents of the consolidation are identified and recognized. When dissimilar, unidentified groups are *inadvertently* consolidated, neither statistician nor clinician can determine the reason or source for subsequent differences observed in the population.

The separation and combination of objects for classification is sometimes referred to as "lumping" and "splitting", and taxonomists often choose their tactics arbitrarily. In clinical analyses, however, the initial "splitting" is mandatory. Without these initial divisions, the clinician "lumps" a melange of unknown entities. Having "split", he can always "lump" later, but he then has the major scientific advantage of knowing what he "lumps", and why.

SELECTION OF CATEGORIES

No matter how a statistical analysis is performed—with manual arithmetic, abacus, desk calculator, or digital computer—the basic first step in the procedure is to decide what data to analyze and how to classify the collected data. In a particular study, for example, is it worthwhile to test for differences in the age of patients? If so, what categories of age should be tested? Should patients be divided into two groups (*old* and *young*), or into decades (ages 0 to 9, 10 to 19, 20 to 29, 30 to 39, etc.), or in some other partition?

This crucial first step in the design of a statistical analysis may be fatally flawed if inappropriate properties and categories are chosen. In selecting results for analysis, statisticians often prefer to work with laboratory and demographic data, rather than clinical data. Compared with clinical data, laboratory and demographic information is usually more reliable, more dimensional (expressed in numbers rather than words), and more easily classified. Consequently, non-clinical data generally are more likely than clinical data to be chosen as variables for analysis in statistical procedures. The consequence of this "statistical bias" is often a right answer to the wrong question. For example, the prognosis of acute rheumatic fever has no significant relationship to such laboratory data as sedimentation rate and anti-streptolysin O titer, or to such demographic data as age, race, and sex. The important prognostic correlations are with such clinical data as cardiac murmurs and congestive heart failure. Yet these significant prognostic correlations would be completely missed if clinical data were not selected for analysis.

The choice of properties and categories in the analysis of data is an intellectual exercise requiring the highest order of clinical judgment. The initial choice cannot be made by a statistician who lacks a background of experienced clinical observation to tell him what is likely to be important and what is not. Nor can the choice be made by a computer, since the machine has no idea of what to do with the data until man decides what data to give it and what to tell it to do. Even if man decides to give the computer all the data, and then let it test for everything, many human decisions will still have to be made, in advance, about "all" the data to be given the computer as input.

For example, in coding cardiac murmurs as data for computer or other statistical analysis, is it sufficient to note the murmurs only as systolic or diastolic? Should we also code such information as the loudness and transmission of the murmur? Or its time of inception and time of cessation in relation to the associated heart sounds? Or its thoracic site of maximum loudness? Or its pitch and quality? In some studies, many of these distinctions in acoustic clinical data are superfluous. In other studies, the many distinctions just cited will not be enough. Yet the decisions about how to code the data of murmurs must be made *before* the computer gets the information and *before* the statistical analysis begins.

The choice of what to analyze and how to classify it is the fundamental aspect of a statistical analysis in clinical medicine, and the "basic science" that is the background for this crucial procedure is neither statistical theory nor any form of computational wisdom. The "basic science" is thoughtfully interpreted clinical experience.

*   *   *

Like any other system of taxonomy, the classification of patients according to the clinical behavior of a disease is a means of sorting or separating heterogeneous mixtures into homogeneous subgroups. The description of a series of patients with a particular disease could indicate, for example, that the population contained so many patients in clinical subset A, so many in subset B, and so on. The results of treatment (or of other investigations) could then be correlated and assessed for each of those subsets. As a separation or partition technique, clinical taxonomy offers the same scientific advantages—in reproducibility and precision of results—that have come in the past from better separation procedures for identifying the material of chemistry and physics.

In any scientific domain, progress has always been achieved by improvement of techniques for classifying the observed material. In clinical medicine, the techniques proposed here were not previously necessary, useful, or attainable. They have become necessary to achieve scientific validity in "design" of the constant therapeutic experiments made possible by modern pharmacology and surgery. They have become useful because modern technology has brought organized precision in management of laboratory and demographic data, so that clinical data are left as the major unclassified features of organic human illness. They have become attainable because modern mathematical systems provide the structural mechanism for managing a formal classification of overlapping, multiple, independent properties.

The types of taxonomy described here may improve the *design* of therapeutic experiments, but are not sufficient to answer questions about the accomplishments of therapy. No matter how well an experiment is designed, it must still be executed, its results must be observed, and its observations analyzed. The appraisal of therapeutic response poses separate issues in clinical taxonomy—issues that are often closely related to those already discussed, but that are different enough, in basic concepts and methods, to warrant their own discussion separately.

If we have now begun to think about treatment, the next step is to think about what treatment does.

PART III

Evaluation of Therapeutic Accomplishment

Chapter 13. The Objectives of Treatment

The Targets of Treatment
The Actions of Treatment
  Prevention
    In Healthy People
    In Sick People
  Alteration
    Of Diseases
    Of Clinical Manifestations

Chapter 14. Indexes and Criteria of Therapeutic Response

Verbal and Dimensional Precision in Scientific Data
Establishment of Indexes and Criteria
  Citation of Objectives
  Types of Criteria
    Existence Criteria
    Gradation Criteria
    Transition Criteria
    Aggregate Criteria
  Selection of Appropriate Targets and Indexes
  Description of Index Variables
  Problems in Choice of Clinical and Laboratory Criteria
  Pathognomonic versus Therapognomonic Indexes
  Statistical Collaboration

Chapter 15. Retrospection, Experience, and Medical Records

The Problems of Retrospection
Problems in Execution and Design of Doubly-Prospective Therapeutic Studies
The Use of Medical Records in Therapeutic Research
  Attempts To Compare Different Therapeutic Agents
  Choice of a "Zero Time"
  Classification at "Zero Time"
  Classification of the Severity of Illness
  Acquisition of Complete Data
  Management of Uncertain Data
  Choice of Appropriate Topics for Investigation
  Research Methods and Personnel
The Quality of Data in Medical Records

230

13. The Objectives of Treatment

By coming to a doctor, a patient asks to participate in the extraordinary experiment that constitutes clinical care. If asymptomatic, the patient hopes the experiment will prevent or suppress the future development of a disease; if symptomatic, he wants to get rid of his symptoms or to obtain the relief that will allow his return to work or to other desired activities. From the doctor who performs the experiment, the patient requests the drugs, operations, communication, and compassion that will achieve these ends. In that achievement, the diagnostic names that a doctor employs and the doctor's concepts of etiology and pathogenesis are interesting, impressive, and useful. But the nomenclature and mechanistic explanations of disease are of secondary importance to a sick person; they are the means to his primary goal, which is treatment.

Because the experimental "material" of treatment is a patient, and because the patient has a definite purpose in soliciting the experiment, every aspect of the design and evaluation of therapeutic activities must be pursued with methods distinctively different from the procedures applied in laboratory experiments. Both types of experiment, at bedside and in laboratory, are rationally planned with exactly the same three-part intellectual sequence: preparation of material, execution of maneuver, and appraisal of response. But a sick person, unlike a laboratory object, chooses the investigator, comes biologically prepared for the experiment, circumscribes its maneuvers, and determines its goals.

The scientific effects of these distinctions in the first aspect of experimental design—preparation of material—have just been discussed in the preceding chapters. The laboratory investigator can manipulate and alter healthy animals or pristine inanimate substances into a selected arrangement before the experiment begins, but a clinician does not decree the state of disease that he treats. He receives a patient whose ailment has already been arranged by the course of nature. Before beginning the experiment of treatment, a clinician must "prepare" his material by classification, not manipulation. Unable to employ the many physical and chemical tactics generally applied to transform laboratory objects into the material of an impending experiment, the clinician, instead, organizes his scientific "preparations" by using the purely intellectual techniques of taxonomic identification.

This difference in laboratory and clinical material has two other important consequences in the design of experiments: repetition and variation. A laboratory investigator can easily repeat his experiments by getting the same material and re-manipulating its preparation. He also can easily alter his basic arrangement in various ways to test the experimental maneuver in a range of different situations. A clinician can neither repeat nor vary his individual preparation. To repeat a major therapeutic experiment, the clinician cannot reproduce the same patient but must find another, similar to the first. To test a therapeutic agent in a varied range of conditions in a specific disease, a clinician cannot readily change individual patents beforehand. Instead, he must collect a populaton of sick people, whose diverse illnesses will constitute the various subgroups that form the clinical spectrum of that disease.

Clinical taxonomy is necessary in the procedures of classification that "prepare" sick people for these experiments, and is particularly important for planning the treatment of individual patients. In selecting treatment for a new patient, the clinician must first evaluate the different results obtained in similar situations of the past. Unless the clinician can effectively classify old and new patients, he cannot identify a *similar situation*. The "design" of the new therapeutic experiment will be inaccurate and unreproducible.

In the second aspect of experimental construction—execution of maneuver—the use of sick people as the "material" imposes many clinical restrictions not present in laboratory work. The laboratory investigator can choose a maneuver without considering the possible adverse effects the maneuver itself may have on the experimental material. Within the boundaries of humane care for animals, a laboratory investigator need not fear that his material will be inconvenienced, damaged, or even destroyed by the experimental procedure. He can use any of the extensive means of maneuver that are available, and can carry an individual maneuver to antipodal extremes for eliciting a wide range of reaction.

In clinical therapy, however, an alive human "material" distinctly limits the choice of available procedures. A therapeutic maneuver that seems indicated by abstract scientific analysis may have to be modified or countermanded by many human events that need not receive paramount consideration in laboratory research. Among such events are pain, vocational incapacitation, scholastic requirements, familial problems, psychic reactions, financial burdens, geographic locations, and many other features of the panorama of human life. These clinical and other personal considerations of sick people necessitate an additional aspect of clinical judgment—the environmental decisions described in Chapter 1. The decisions made during the subsequent "environmental" reasoning may often alter the conclusions reached during the original deliberations that selected an otherwise desirable mode of treatment. Although such distinctively human features of the experimental material may greatly affect the planning of clinical therapy, this type of judgment requires little or no attention in the methodology of the laboratory.

Perhaps the greatest scientific difference between clinical and laboratory experiments, however, occurs in the third aspect of the rational experimental sequence—appraisal of response. The goals of laboratory work are selected arbitrarily by the investigator; the goals of clinical treatment are determined by the patient. In planning therapy, the clinician wants to repeat or surpass a successful result of the past, but the definition of "success" depends largely on what the patient wants done and on what happens to him. A clinician cannot properly estimate a *successful result* without including the effects of treatment on the stimuli that made the patient seek medical assistance, and without noting the patient's general state after treatment. To appraise only what treatment does to "disease" is not enough either for science or for clinical care; the patient must be considered as well as the "disease". Consequently, the *subjective* complaints and responses of sick people are critical scientific variables unique to clinical methodology. Such data are present only in the experiments of human therapy and need not be analyzed in laboratory work.

These clinical attributes are admixed with many other aspects of disease and host in the total response to treatment. To evaluate the accomplishments of treatment, this mixture of disease, host, and illness must be intellectually separated into its constituents, and each constituent must be appraised appropriately. The rest of this chapter is devoted to a citation of the role of these different constituents in the varied goals of treatment, and to a discussion of some defects in the way these goals are evaluated in contemporary therapeutic investigations and reports. The goals can be expressed as targets to be influenced by treatment, and as purposeful actions to be affected on the targets.

THE TARGETS OF TREATMENT

After a particular disease or disorder has been diagnosed, the clinician has three possible targets for treatment:

1) The anatomic lesion, chemical dysfunction, or other basic abnormality of the disease itself.

2) Associated derangements manifested as abnormalities in the concomitant para-clinical tests.

3) Clinical symptoms and signs, attributable either to that disease or to co-existing disorders.

For example, in coronary artery disease, the first type of target would include the narrowed or occluded coronary lumen; the second type would include hypercholesterolemia; the third type of target might be chest pain or anxiety. In carcinoma of the lung, the first type of target is the carcinomatous tissue; the second type would include such entities as hypercalcemia or roentgenographic evidence of hypertrophic periostitis; the third type would include chest pain, clubbing of the fingers, or vocational incapacitation.

THE ACTIONS OF TREATMENT

Treatment can be planned to prevent or to alter any or all of these targets. In prevention, the purpose is to avoid the occurrence of a condition that does not yet exist, or to keep one already present from becoming worse. In alteration, the purpose of therapy is to remove or to modify an existing condition. The methods of appraising how well therapy accomplishes each of these purposes will depend upon the purpose and upon the target.

Since the derangements that occur in laboratory data are not assessed by clinical methods, and since these derangements do not always have direct clinical counterparts, the evaluation of the laboratory targets of therapy will not be further considered here. The discussion will be confined to methods of appraising treatment used for preventing or altering either a disease itself or clinical manifestations.

PREVENTION

In Healthy People

A disease (or pathologic lesion) can be prevented by changing the environmental circumstances conducive to its development; by treating, removing, or otherwise affecting the objects that transmit it; or by increasing the resistance of the potential human host. These effects are accomplished by such maneuvers as sanitation, isolation, nutrition, and vaccination, and sometimes by appropriate pharmaceutical or surgical therapy.

The evaluation of procedures used to prevent a person from getting sick is often much more difficult than the evaluation of those intended to alter a disease that is already established. For the ordinary treatment of an established disease, the pre-therapeutic condition of the sick patient can readily be compared with that of other previous patients similarly affected. In the prevention of disease, however, no pathologic state is immediately available for comparison; the investigation is devoted to essentially healthy people, not sick patients. Thus, in prevention of disease, the statistical appraisals must deal with the problems of defining probabilities and hazards for an event that has not yet occurred, and for hosts of uncertain and varying susceptibilities.

Just as the site of experimental performance for treatment that alters disease is the bedside or clinician's office, the site of such performance for treatment that prevents disease is the healthy community. Only from work in community situations beyond the test tubes, cages, and beds of the medical center can clinicians obtain evidence for adequate studies of disease prevention. These studies require large amounts of data for statistical analysis, and methodologic procedures that can 1) obtain human populations of satisfactory size and content, 2) assess the hosts by appropriate investigative tests, and 3) maintain the population for a follow-up period long enough to ascertain that the disease has, in fact, been prevented.

The methodology required to assess the prevention of disease is therefore a staggering epidemiologic problem. A major part of the problem—adequate personnel for assembling and maintaining the population under investigation—is seldom present to the same degree in other forms of research. To manage material contained in a test tube or cage, the laboratory investigator needs few assistants. To manage patients kept in a hospital bed or recurrently appearing at a clinic, the therapeutic investigator needs nurses and the ancillary personnel of medical settings. To manage a population dispersed in a community, the epidemiologist must have all the personnel just cited, as well as many other collaborators with different skills and talents. The investigative team that attempts to execute the massive, complex human logistics of a satisfactory epidemiologic project not only must include physicians, nurses, social workers, and various non-medical scientific personnel, but also may need receptionists, messengers, chauffeurs, babysitters, clergymen, lawyers, and other functionaries not vital for the research of laboratory or clinic.

The difficulties of recruiting and supporting such epidemiologic teams are probably a major reason why most research physicians in medicine avoid the problems, and prefer laboratories or clinical settings, instead of communities, for their investigative activities. This preference in sites of research helps perpetuate the current absence of scientifically conclusive studies of prevention (as well as of etiology) for almost all human diseases except those transmitted by infectious agents. The chronic degenerative and neoplastic diseases that are prime targets of contemporary research have been carefully studied mainly in the laboratory and at the bedside, but not in the community, which has remained relatively unused as a site of clinical investigation. Consequently, the preventive measures often proposed for such disorders as coronary artery disease, pulmonary emphysema, various cancers, hypertension, and obesity are seldom supported by direct evidence that can withstand critical scientific scrutiny.

In choosing treatment to prevent such diseases, clinicians must currently rely on epidemiologic data of distressingly poor quality, and must draw uncertain conclusions from ambiguous or unsatisfactory evidence, because nothing else is available. Until clinicians improve this situation by devising and executing appropriate epidemiologic techniques to investigate these problems, the therapeutic approaches used for prevention of many common contemporary diseases will remain medical topics distinguished by a plethora of well-publicized theories and a paucity of well-established facts.

In Sick People

A separate issue in methodology is the evaluation of treatment intended to prevent the adverse clinical progression of a disease that is already established. The adverse progression may include such events as acute recrudescence, chronic deterioration, superimposition of new diseases or complications, and the ultimate adversity: death. The therapeutic efforts to prevent these events are prophylactic, rather than remedial, in that treatment is being given not to get rid of something, but to keep something from happening. Such therapeutic maneuvers are illustrated by the use of anti-microbials to prevent recurrences of rheumatic fever, antacids and special diets to prevent recrudescences of peptic ulcer, insulin and special diets to prevent vascular deterioration in diabetes mellitus, anticoagulants to prevent embolic propagation in thrombophlebitis, and antibiotics to prevent a variety of complications in certain patients with stroke or chronic lung disease, and in other patients about to receive dental or surgical operations. In all of these therapeutic situations, the clinician is practicing preventive medicine rather than the traditional remedial form of treatment.

The statistical techniques of classification developed for conventional "preventive" medicine are inadequate for these prophylactic therapeutic situations. In the conventional statistics of "preventive" medicine, the object that receives the treatment (such as vaccination) is a healthy host. Thus, the statistician need make no provision for identifying clinical or para-clinical data of the host, since the host has neither illness nor disease. The classification of the "material" in such preventive experiments can be based exclusively on demographic data. When preventive treatment is given to a diseased host, however, the clinical and para-clinical data must be appropriately classified.

Moreover, in conventional preventive medicine, the target of treatment is easily cited and assessed: the healthy host either does or does not get the disease. When preventive treatment is given to a diseased host, however, both the citation of targets and the assessment of successful prophylaxis become much more complex. In the prophylactic therapeutic experiments that are designed to keep a sick patient from getting worse, the natural course of the disease is a critical feature of the investigation. Unless clinicians can estimate the future course of each instance of the disease, they cannot determine what they are trying to prevent, and how vigorous to make the efforts at prevention. In contemplating natural history as a guide to prognosis, however, clinicans are impeded by the complex clinical spectrum of each disease. The patterns of appearance and of evolution vary so greatly in different hosts with the same pathologic state that no *single* course of natural history can typify the expectations in all the individual patients.

The scientist's usual search for a unifying rule that completely explains and predicts phenomena of nature is generally defeated by the clinical complexity of a human disease. The behavior of the diverse patterns of clinical illness in a single disease can no more be identified accurately by a single rule than can the different species of a single phylum in nature. The taxonomic rule that defines the phylum describes common morphologic properties of all the constituent species, but does not distinguish the different species from one another. Similarly, the diagnosis that defines common morphologic or other pathologic properties in a disease does not distinguish the different sick people who are affected.

As already noted earlier, satisfactory knowledge is not now available either to identify distinctive prognostic subgroups in the clinical spectrum of most major human diseases, or to indicate the subsequent course of the disease in subgroups treated with different modes of therapy. The existing information, although often abundant and quantitative, is usually too non-specific in regard to the critical clinical details. In the absence of this knowledge of diverse "natural histories" for different subgroups of patients with the same "disease", many trials of prophylactic therapy are inevitably designed badly, producing results of dubious validity and uncertain significance.

Proper design of a clinical trial of prophylactic therapy calls first for division of the diseased population into subgroups that have the same prognostic risks; then, the therapeutic agents are allocated randomly within each subgroup. If the agents are merely allocated randomly to the population as a whole, without previous subdivision (or "stratification") according to prognostic distinctions, the subsequent results may be dangerously misleading. Unless prognostic comparability is deliberately established in the groups assigned to different therapeutic agents, the source of diverse therapeutic results is obscure. Many results may be attributed erroneously to the therapy when they actually arise from unrecognized differences in the composition of the original populations.

Suppose, for example, that certain clinical features of diabetic children can be used to divide the population prognostically into two groups, *A* and *B*, whose ultimate natural course shows the development of degenerative vascular disease in 30% of patients in group *A*, and 70% of patients in group *B*. Now suppose that two equally ineffective modes of treatment, *X* and *Y*, are being tested to prevent degenerative vascular complications in two populations of patients, each containing 100 diabetic children, who were selected utterly at random without regard to the prognostic properties that distinguish groups *A* and *B*. Suppose further that the 100 children assigned to treatment *X* happen by chance to comprise 20 patients from group *A* and 80 patients from group *B*, while the population assigned to treatment *Y* contains 80 children from *A* and 20 from *B*. The investigators, of course, will be unaware of these differences in the composition of the two "cohort" populations, because the properties that characterize *A* and *B* were not identified or classified in the allocation of patients. Since treatments *X* and *Y* are equally ineffective, they will not alter the occurrence of degenerative vascular disease, which will appear in 62%* of the patients assigned to *X* and in 38%* of those assigned to *Y*. This difference in outcome of the two treatments is highly significant statistically ($\chi^2 = 10.6$; $P = 0.001$). Unaware that the two base populations were not comparable, and impressed by the statistical difference, the investigators may conclude erroneously that treatment *Y* is much better than *X* for preventing diabetic vascular complications.

The example just presented was deliberately contrived to illustrate the types of error that can arise, and remain unrecognized, because of inadequate classification of the populations used in trials of therapy. The magnitude of the error chosen for illustration may be unusual —but the deficiencies producing such errors are common, and the errors are ubiquitous.

They can occur whenever the clinician or statistician has allocated therapy without appropriate *clinical* classification of the treated population. If the number of patients is large enough, and if principles of "random allocation" are strictly maintained, the problem may be

---

* $62 = (20 \times 0.30) + (80 \times 0.70)$; $38 = (80 \times 0.30) + (20 \times 0.70)$.

avoidable. But clinical samples are seldom large enough for "random-ness" to overcome errors in comparison. Moreover, statisticians are now trying deliberately to *reduce* the size of clinical "samples" by using techniques of "sequential analysis" [139] that bring a therapeutic trial to an end as soon as a "statistically significant" difference is ob-served between the compared groups. If this new statistical technique is used without appropriate pre-therapeutic "stratification" of the compared groups, clinical studies containing the types of error illus-trated in the contrived example will become even more abundant than they are now. The smaller the sample, the greater is the necessity for clinical prognostic comparability in the treated groups.

The problems arising from such errors have impeded the evalua-tion of many therapeutic maneuvers intended to *prevent* the progres-sion of chronic, degenerative, or neoplastic diseases: rigorous glucose regulation in diabetes mellitus, anticoagulants in myocardial in-farction, portacaval shunts in hepatic cirrhosis, steroids in rheumatic fever, corrective surgery in patients with congenital or rheumatic heart disease, radical surgery or irradiation for neoplasms, and many other *prophylactic* treatments of disease. The patient populations in most of the reported investigations of these prophylactic therapeutic agents were classified mainly according to laboratory and personal data, but not according to significant clinical distinctions.

In diabetes mellitus, for example, the risks of future vascular com-plication may be quite different in a patient who came to the doctor because of polydipsia than in one whose disease was asymptomatic and discovered incidentally during a routine urinalysis, or in one whose carbohydrate derangement was not suspected until he entered the hospital semicomatose in acidosis. These differences in the clini-cal mode of discovery of the disease may have prognostic implications more important than variations in the patients' age, serum lipid level, or glucose tolerance curve. Yet these clinical distinctions are seldom noted or used explicitly in analysis of the patients exposed to treat-ment. If the patients of therapeutic investigations are identified only according to demographic and para-clinical data, with no specification of clinical features, the results have dubious scientific value. Neither the investigator, nor the clinician who reads the reported results, could determine how various modes of treatment might affect each of the three different clinical types of diabetic patients just described.

Similar problems exist in evaluating the effects of treatment in neoplasia. What are the *quantitative* differences in prognosis of gastric cancer, for example, between a patient whose lesion was discovered while he was asymptomatic and one who was detected because he had symptoms; between a patient with hematemesis as his only symptom and one with hematemesis and abdominal pain or weight loss; between a patient with hematemesis of 9 days' duration and one with hematemesis for 9 months? Such distinctions may be crucial in determining whether an adverse future course of the disease is best prevented by partial gastrectomy, by total gastrectomy, by radiotherapy, or by combinations of these and other modes of treatment. Yet the existing data on post-therapeutic survival in stomach cancer pay almost no attention to the use of such clinical categories in classifying patients. The clinical data are often cited, but only for their role in diagnosis, not in prognosis. The prognostic results are usually correlated with the morphologic data of structure—cell type, size and location of tumor, lymph node involvement, regional invasion, and distant anatomic dissemination—but not with the symptomatic patterns that represent clinical function.

Without clinically detailed studies of natural and post-therapeutic course of a disease, the results of its prophylactic therapy cannot be effectively evaluated. In cancer, for example, the goal is often to prevent metastasis or to prevent death. (The latter goal is indicated by the frequent use of "survival rates" as an index of therapeutic accomplishment.) Yet the likelihood of metastasis or of death in cancer is known for patients classified only according to the morphologic features of contemporary anatomic "staging". Although each morphologic stage can contain diverse clinical groups with different prognoses, the outcome of these *clinical stages* has been studied only infrequently.[25] Examples of the diverse outcomes for different clinical groups with the same morphologic stage of lung cancer or of rectal cancer were presented earlier in Chapter 11 (pages 194–198).

In cancers and in most of the other principal diseases of contemporary medicine, clinicians have almost no scientifically discriminating evidence to indicate how often or how soon secondary features (or complications) will develop in patients found with primary features only. In patients whose disease is initially detected with *no* clinical features, it is currently impossible to make accurate statistical estimations of the likelihood, or of the time, that any clinical features will develop if the patient is left untreated.

How has such a state of affairs arisen? After receiving a heritage of centuries of observation on the course and treatment of disease, how can contemporary clinicians be so uninformed? Are clinicians naive or stupid to know so little about human illness during an epoch of proliferating scientific precision that has clarified so many other aspects of nature? The answers to these questions are contained in two features of the evolution of science in clinical medicine:

1) At no previous time in medical history was it possible to obtain the diagnostic precision now available from endoscopy, biopsy, roentgenography, and other modern para-clinical tests. Although many prognostic studies of individual portions of the spectrums of disease were performed years ago, the results are generally ineffective or useless by contemporary standards. The definitions and identifications of "disease" have changed, and the past diagnoses were frequently inaccurate, uncertain, or erroneous. Consequently, the populations observed in many past reports of natural history in disease contain so many diagnostic "impurities" that the total data and prognostic correlations cannot be used reliably today.

2) Conversely, the availability of accurate diagnostic tests in contemporary research has led to such emphasis on pathologic and laboratory data that modern studies of natural history have not correlated prognosis with the initial *clinical* manifestations of the patients. Most of the populations studied in recent surveys are thus diagnostically pure, but the clinical diversity of the constituents is inadequately identified.

In making therapeutic judgments about preventing the adverse progress of many diseases, clinicians are thus confronted with a dilemma of data: the older studies were clinically exact, but diagnostically imprecise; the more modern studies have been diagnostically exact, but clinically imprecise. Neither the old nor the more recent data provide clinicians with adequate evidence for sound scientific judgment. The acquisition of such evidence requires new studies of natural (and post-therapeutic) history of the treated diseases, performed with the diagnostic precision that already exists, augmented by precise clinical distinctions of the types just discussed.

ALTERATION

Of Diseases

The pathologic lesion of an anatomic "disease" can often be altered by removal or by modification. Such alterations have become common events only during the last half century. Although surgeons have traditionally used amputation to extirpate disease of limbs, appendages, or skin, the many other types of major alterations performed in modern surgery have become possible only in the past few decades. Total removal can now be accomplished for lesions in such locations as breast, intestine, brain, lung, and heart. Lesions can be directly modified by such procedures as transplantation of tissues, installation of osseous or vascular prostheses, "palliative" excision of parts of neoplasms, and the reparative maneuvers of cardiac surgery. In other circumstances, surgeons leave the basic lesion of a disease intact, but attempt to modify its effects, either by rearranging or by removing apparently normal structures. Examples of such rearrangements are the various "short-circuiting" operations performed for hydrocephalus and for gastrointestinal disease; examples of such removals are splenectomy for spherocytosis and thrombocytopenia, castration for carcinomas of the breast or prostate, and hypophysectomy for diabetic retinopathy.

Compared with the drama of these surgical procedures, the direct medical conquests of structural abnormalities have been less spectacular, being limited to the therapeutic triumphs that physicians produce with antibiotics and radioactivity. Hormones, blood transfusions, electrolytes, fluids, iron, vitamins, and dietary regulation can improve the *manifestations* of a disease, but do not usually affect the pathologic lesion that produced the manifestations. For the many chronic and degenerative diseases whose basic pathologic lesions are not currently amenable to removal or to direct modification by surgery, the target of medical or pharmaceutical treatment is usually to keep the lesion from getting worse, or to prevent or alter the laboratory and clinical manifestations.

The assessment of morphologic change in a pathologic structure usually involves the same anatomic procedures used for the initial diagnostic identification, and these methods of morphologic assessment are beyond the scope of this discussion. The distinctions between pathologic lesions and other targets of treatment, however, are crucial to the methods used for appraisal of therapeutic results. Many studies are often planned and reported in equivocal, ambiguous, or erroneous terms because the appraisal does not adequately distinguish changes in the pathologic lesion itself from changes in the concomitant laboratory and clinical manifestations. For example, clinicians cannot usually determine what medical treatment in living patients has done to the structure of the actual pathologic lesion of such diseases as myocardial infarction, rheumatic carditis, cerebral arteriosclerosis, multiple sclerosis, and pulmonary emphysema. The objects appraised in the treatment of these and many other diseases are *not* the pathologic lesions that give the diseases their names, but the laboratory and clinical manifestations that indicate what the diseases do to the patient.

Of Clinical Manifestations

In saying that a patient is "better" or "worse", "holding his own" or "going downhill", clinicians use the evidence of symptoms and signs more than any other variables in human disease. The evidence includes such items as the expression of a face, the sweat on a brow, the coherence of a statement and the vigor of a gesture, as well as such specific clinical features as pain, fever, swelling, shortness of breath, hiccups, coughing, numbness, palpable enlargement of an organ, and noises in the chest. All of these, and many other clinical and personal phenomena, are critical parts of the data observed, assessed, and analyzed in the appraisal of therapeutic response. These are the features clinicians have in mind when they use the word *sick*.

These human reactions are unique attributes of the material reacting to therapeutic experiment, and must be properly evaluated if the experimental response is to be accurately identified and predictably reproduced. Nevertheless, a therapeutic report that fulfils these clinical requirements is the exception, rather than the rule, in medical literature today. In many reports of therapeutic alterations, contemporary clinicians do not differentiate the laboratory data that indicate a physiologic, microbiologic, pharmacologic, or biochemical effect in a disease, from the clinical data that indicate what happened to the sick patient.

One of the main reasons for the absence of such differentiations in data has been the general belief that a clinical finding can always be correlated with some function expressible in the form of laboratory data. This belief is as fallacious as the concept that every pathologic abnormality produces a specific, constant set of clinical manifestations. Each laboratory abnormality, like each pathologic lesion, is associated with a diverse spectrum, not a single group, of different clinical manifestations in different patients. Consequently, the clinical and laboratory abnormalities in a particular patient will not always be exact counterparts of one another.

For an accurate total identification of human responses to therapy, therefore, the clinical and the laboratory evidence must be assessed separately. The arterial oxygen concentration may rise in cardio-pulmonary disease while cyanosis persists. The sedimentation rate may fall in rheumatic fever, while new murmurs develop. The blood bicarbonate and glucose may reach normal values in diabetic acidosis while gangrene increases in an extremity. A lowered white blood count in chronic leukemia, or a raised hematocrit in renal failure, may not affect fatigue or incapacitation. The roentgenographic crater of a peptic ulcer may grow larger, but the symptoms may disappear. Rheumatoid arthritis may continue to cripple a patient whose serum protein patterns have become normal. The portal vein pressure may drop after vascular operations in cirrhosis, but esophageal varices may continue to bleed. The urine may become sterile in cystitis, while dysuria grows worse.

The neglect of adequate clinical data in the appraisal of responses to treatment is particularly evident in some of the macabre therapeutic triumphs of modern medicine. Successful surgical operations, ingenious restorations in electrolyte balance, or impressive normaliza-tions in blood glucose, cholesterol, or urea nitrogen are often excit-ing improvements marred only by the patient's death soon there-after. Congestive heart failure and renal or hepatic decompensation are often regarded as successfully treated if a patient has a natriuresis even though he may remain dyspneic, edematous, ascitic, or incapaci-tated. A mitral valve deformity is sometimes considered alleviated if the post-operative pressures are reduced in certain cardiac chambers, even though the patient remains fatigued or bed-ridden. Degenerative disorders of the lungs may seem improved when the numbers change in laboratory tests of vital capacity, even though breathlessness still keeps the patient from working or walking.

*   *   *

Although a clinician can be both a healer and a scientist, he cannot be an effective therapist if he merely joins these two roles in tandem by oscillating between them, adding laboratory science to bedside art. A clinician's objective in therapy is not just a conjunction, but a true synthesis, of art and science, fusing the parts into a whole that unifies his work and makes his two roles one: a scientific healer. A clinician is always a healer; the healing function is basic to his care of sick people. The *scientific* performance of that function, however, is what distinguishes a well-trained medical or surgical clinician from other healers whose aid and comfort is given without the rational support of valid evidence, logical analysis, and demonstrable proofs.

No clinician can function as an effective scientist in modern medicine without an adequate knowledge of physiology, microbiology, pharmacology, and biochemistry, and of the data that express these functions in health and in disease. Yet a clinican cannot employ clinical treatment merely as a physiologist, microbiologist, pharmacologist, or biochemist. As a healer, the clinician's purpose is to treat the sick person, not merely the manifestations of disease found in laboratory data. To fulfill this purpose scientifically, the clinician must formally assess the clinical variables of the bedside, as well as the results obtained in the laboratory. The clinical variables are indexes of the effects that occur as responses to therapy; changes in the index variables are ingredients of the criteria by which the effects are evaluated. Clinicians who fail to make adequate use of clinical data for these purposes impede not only the humanistic heritage of medicine, but also the scientific performance of treatment.

14. Indexes and Criteria of Therapeutic Response

Ever since the nosologic concept of "disease" was converted from clinical manifestations into anatomic, chemical, and other pathologic entities, clinicians have searched the clinical evidence of the bedside for clues to the diagnosis of disease. A clinical finding that could be used as a specific indication of diagnosis was given the name pathognomonic, a combination of the Greek words πάθος, *disease,* and γνώμων, *index.*

In diagnostic reasoning, clinicians have now collected a great many pathognomonic clinical findings that are indexes of disease. The symptom of angina pectoris, for example, is usually pathognomonic of coronary artery disease; a post-prandial epigastric distress that subsides with ingestion of alkali usually indicates peptic ulceration. A tophus in a joint or cartilage is a sign pathognomonic of gout; xanthomatous deposits in a tendon indicate hyperlipemia; Koplik's spots denote measles.

In the clinician's eagerness to find pathognomonic clues to diagnosis, many clinical and laboratory indexes have sometimes been erroneously over-emphasized. The ocular sign of lid-lag, for example, although once regarded as pathognomonic of hyperthyroidism, is now recognized as non-specific—an "index" that can be found in other diseases and sometimes in normal people. The cutaneous sign of spider angioma is no longer regarded as a specific indicator of hepatic cirrhosis, since this skin change often occurs during normal pregnancy, and is sometimes found in normal non-pregnant people. Laboratory tests regarded as specific indexes of disease have led to numerous incorrect diagnoses of gout in patients with hyperuricemia, prostatic cancer in patients with an elevated acid phosphatase, liver disease in patients with abnormal serum cephalin flocculation, and—the classic "false positive" diagnostic error—syphilis in patients with positive Wassermann, Venereal Disease Research Laboratory (VDRL), or other serologic tests.

The frequency of diagnostic error caused by falsely positive indexes has led clinicians to re-appraise the criteria for interpreting these "pathognomonic" findings and to recognize that many indexes are often clues to abnormality, but not necessarily characteristic of specific diseases. Thus, the cutaneous spider angioma is now attributed to an endocrine imbalance that may occur occasionally in normal people, and commonly in pregnancy and in cirrhosis. An abnormal cephalin flocculation test may denote deranged protein metabolism in many disorders other than liver disease. Even angina pectoris can, in rare instances, arise when a patient's exertion increases the pressure in a hypertensive pulmonary artery instead of increasing the metabolic demands of a hypoxemic myocardium. What is important about many clinical and laboratory indexes today is not their pathognomonic specificity, but their use as stigmata of abnormality. Every thoughtful clinician has established a series of indexes and criteria that he uses for different diagnoses. Each diagnosis has its own clues, its own indexes, and its own criteria. The concept of the "index" is thus well established in diagnostic reasoning.

The concept of indexes also exists in prognostic reasoning, although generally given much less attention in clinical discussions than the specification of diagnostic clues. The Hippocratic facies, for example, is *prognostognomonic* of impending death; palpable distant lymph node metastases indicate a poor prognosis in a patient with cancer; in acute myocardial infarction, a patient who clinically has either shock or pulmonary edema will generally fare worse than one who has neither, and survival is highly unlikely if the patient has both. One of the main purposes of the clinical taxonomy described in Chapters 8 through 12 is to specify and quantify the prognostic indexes that every clinician uses as part of clinical judgment.

Although clinicians have many indexes with which to diagnose and to prognosticate, no established concept of clinical indexes exists in the reasoning used for evaluating therapeutic accomplishment. By what standard, specific, *clinical* indexes, for example, do we appraise the reactions of patients in such post-therapeutic states as digitalis toxicity, antibiotic sensitivity, insulin shock, or low-salt syndromes? What are the clinical indexes for evaluating the effects of sedatives, tranquilizers, anorexic agents, cathartics, carminatives, anti-spasmodics, oxygen inhalation, positive pressure breathing, diuretics, and anti-coagulants? If indexes exist, do they deal only with morphologic and laboratory changes, or do they make specific provision for clinical effects? Are the clinical effects used in the indexes appropriate and reproducibly defined?

Unfortunately, the contemporary answers to these therapeutic questions give little scientific satisfaction. The clinical indexes, in most instances, are either non-existent, inappropriate, inconsistent, or poorly delineated. Just as the clinical reasoning that designs an act of therapy has frequently lacked an organized formal structure, the reasoning that appraises the results is often the product of amorphous, nondescript judgment, in which clinicians diversely assemble conscious and unconscious background elements, without a uniform or consistent arrangement.

The absence of such indexes—of a *therapognomonic* classification for clinical and laboratory data—often makes the results or reports of treatment impossible to evaluate. In digitalis toxicity, for example, there is clearly a marked difference among such reactions as nausea, syncopal episodes due to an arrhythmia, and asymptomatic electro-cardiographic changes in T waves. Yet "digitalis toxicity" is often assessed and reported with none of these specific distinctions. A shift in cardiac decompensation from pulmonary congestion to peripheral edema may make a patient feel and function much better, but his state may be noted as "unimproved" because no overt diuresis has occurred. Certain diuretic agents may be more effective in pulmonary congestion, whereas others may act best in peripheral edema, but the differences (if they exist) cannot be detected because usually the only indexes assessed are body weight, urine volume, and sodium excretion. The results of treatment for cancer are usually presented as "survival rates", with no indication of whether the treatment relieved or aggravated the patient's clinical state, and with no indication of the treatment's cost to the patient in discomfort, displacement, or despair.

The many available analgesics used in arthropathies may have different effects on small joints than on large, and on peripheral than on vertebral joints, but these distinctions (if present) cannot be recognized because the specific joints are seldom cited among the indexes of response. Many clinicians have shifted their therapeutic tactics from use of sedatives to use of tranquilizers, and from stimulants to "psychic energizers", without having developed any reproducible clinical techniques for effective evaluation of insomnia, tension, anxiety, agitation, lethargy, or depression. Even in such traditional, routine clinical problems as nausea or constipation, there are no satisfactory standard clinical indexes for assessing the effects of therapy, and for ascertaining that the new "physiologic" actions of modern drugs produce clinical effects more desirable than those of the older remedies.

The list of examples is endless. Any clinician can establish his own collection by randomly selecting a few of today's medical journals, reading the reports of "therapeutic" studies, and noting the infrequency and imprecision with which *clinical* features are identified and assessed on either side of the correlations performed in therapeutic appraisal. Most of the studies presented in the literature of contemporary therapeutics and clinical pharmacology contain many superficial virtues available in modern science: treated groups and "controls", "double-blind" procedures, careful assessments of the laboratory data that indicate pharmacologic action, elaborate statistical analyses, and even processing of data by computers. Yet the crux of the investigation often remains unreproducibly documented: the exact clinical state of the patient before and after treatment.

A more pernicious, appalling, and widespread custom is the reporting of therapeutic accomplishment by means of judgmental or interpretive terms for which no criteria are given. Because this custom is so prevalent, and is permitted to continue by so many editors, vast numbers of therapeutic reports have made no distinctions between evidence and inference, between index and interpretation, and between criterion and conclusion. The "methods" sections of publications dealing with therapy are frequently devoid not only of indexes, but also of criteria, for the major clinical variables assessed and correlated in the "results". Seldom do the reports contain statements of the specific elements that entered the judgmental interpretations made in such stock phrases as *mild, moderate, severe, bad, good, fair, excellent, better, worse, downhill, relentless, impending, incipient, progressive, improving, toxic, remission, activation, inoperable, unresectable, indicated, contra-indicated,* and *hopeless.* All of the many statistical and computational techniques used for allocation of patients and for processing data are often wasted because of the simultaneous failure to identify the specific clinical evidence used in appraisal of therapeutic response.

Why have clinicians failed to develop specific clinical indexes and criteria for assessing the accomplishments of therapy? One reason has been the general lack of scientific attention to basic problems in treatment, as contrasted to basic problems in diagnosis, etiology, and pathogenesis of disease. For example, during the 12 years from 1953 to 1964—a period of unprecedented proliferation of new drugs and new surgical procedures—there was a *decline* from 8% to 2% in the percentage of strictly therapeutic projects among the research abstracts reported at the annual Atlantic City meetings of clinical investigators.[36] Although the total number of research abstracts submitted to the American Federation for Clinical Research and to the American Society for Clinical Investigation rose from 359 in 1953 to 729 in 1964, and although the projects included many accounts of new drugs and new operations, the main descriptions in the accounts dealt with physiologic, pharmacologic, biochemical, or other non-clinical effects of the procedures. The *clinical* responses to treatment were noted in only 31 of the 1953 papers, and in 15 of those reported in 1964. Thus, the academic clinical skills that might be used to investigate basic intellectual problems in contemporary therapy have been diverted to other topics in "basic science".

Another reason for the absence of scientific clinical guidelines in treatment has been the fallacious belief (discussed earlier in Chapter 4, pages 66–70) that laboratory or morphologic data can always be used to characterize the details of clinical phenomena. Because our current descriptions of structure do not always correlate with the observed function of the structure, and because different types of function are often dissociated, the diversities of clinical and para-clinical evidence cannot be substituted for each other and must be assessed separately.

There are two other reasons, however, both of them equally fundamental doctrines and equally false. The first doctrine has also been cited earlier (pages 61–64), and is the belief that scientific precision comes only from dimensional measurement, not from verbal description. The second doctrine, a corollary of the first, is the belief that criteria of change cannot be established unless the change is expressed in numerical form. The rest of this chapter is devoted to further discussion of the fallacy of these two doctrines, and to suggestions for filling the scientifically destructive chasm that they produce in clinical therapy.

VERBAL AND DIMENSIONAL PRECISION IN SCIENTIFIC DATA

A statistical analysis depends on numbers but not on dimensional measurement. The numbers used in the analysis are just as numerical if they are obtained by counting, rather than by measuring. Before the entities are counted, they must of course be identified in some way—but the identifications can be verbal descriptions, not dimensional measurements. These scientific distinctions of statistical analysis were described earlier (pages 64–65), together with the comments that precision in science depends not on measurement, but on delineated observation. Precision can come from observations made by oral, visual, tactile, auditory, chemical, mechanical, or electronic procedures, and can be expressed in the form of adjectives, adverbs, nouns, verbs, and numbers. If the precise observation is expressed directly as a number, it can be coded immediately for statistical appraisal. If the observation is expressed in verbal language, its "translation" to statistical form is effected either by assigning an arbitrary code number to the observation (such as "1" for present, and "0" for absent), or by counting and recording the number of such observations made among a population of patients.

Of the clinical variables observed in therapy, some are noted by dimensional measurement and are expressed as numbers; others require verbal description and are expressed as adjectives, adverbs, or nouns. Among the variables expressed in numbers are such direct measurements as age, height, weight, body temperature, length of an extremity, circumference of a limb or surface, depth of a laceration, size of an aperture or of a visible lesion, angulation of a joint, or volume of a fluid. Other variables expressed in numbers come from indirect measurement (for routine blood pressure, intra-ocular tension, or size of a palpable mass), from visual approximation (for angulation of a nail bed), and from counting (for pulse or respiratory rate).

Many other major clinical variables, however, cannot be easily expressed in numerical form, and are reported by verbal descriptions. Among the many physical signs generally expressed by descriptive words, rather than by number, are color, shape, tenderness, texture, moisture, noise, pulsation, movement, and local temperature, as well as such general features of patients as alertness, co-operation, orientation, co-ordination, or distress. All of these verbal descriptions can be numerically coded, of course, when necessary for data processing. For example, a simple numerical code for color can be obtained by assigning the values of *1, 2,* and *4* respectively to the "primary" colors of red, yellow, and blue. Intermediate colors that are combinations of the primary hues could be expressed as sums; thus, orange would be *3,* purple *5,* and green *6.* White could be *0,* gray *7,* and black *8.* As another example, assuming that appropriate criteria were established for the gradations, "non-tender" could be cited as *0,* "slightly tender" as *1,* "moderately tender" as *2,* "very tender" as *3,* and "exquisitely tender" as *4.*

Such numerical scales of clinical coding have long been applied for gradings—usually expressed in scales of 0 to 4+ or some other upper number—of the magnitude of such entities as peripheral edema, palpable arterial pulsations, briskness of reflexes, loudness of murmurs, or size of tonsils. Such numerical codings have even been applied for laboratory data. Many clinicians still prefer to think of urine albumin and urine sugar in terms of 0 to 4+, rather than in the milligram dimensions possible with contemporary tests. The dimensional precision often given to measuring albumin and sugar in *casually* collected urine specimens illustrates the contorted emphasis and spurious quantification possible with modern technology.

The subjective symptoms of patients are major clinical variables that are almost all expressed as non-dimensional descriptions, although numerical dimensions can sometimes be given for such features of symptoms as duration, frequency of recurrence, and rate of increasing or decreasing severity. The severity of a symptom is noted not from just its own description, but from an account of the symptom's concomitant effect on total function of the patient.

Among the other features of symptomatology that require verbal description rather than measurement are the response of each symptom to such maneuvers as respiration, coughing, food intake, defecation, changes in posture of the body, and alterations in exterior climate and temperature. Finally, many important clinical phenomena that are non-dimensional appear as functional clusters, rather than as individual symptoms or signs. Such clusters are manifested in a patient's ability to walk, feed himself, maintain excretory continence, engage in sexual intercourse, work at his usual or some other occupation, participate in athletics, conduct conversation, make intellectual decisions, or perform many other acts of daily living.

These clinical manifestations and functions are specific, distinct, independent evidence of the total state of a patient. The appearance or disappearance of a symptom, a change in duration of a recurrent symptom, a significant alteration in a sign, the loss or return of ability to perform an important function of daily life, or a difference in the frequency of a repetitive clinical event—all these phenomena describe changes in human illness with as much scientific pertinence as alterations in the dimensional measurements of an enzyme, a blood count, a roentgenographic shadow, a flow rate, an antibody titer, or an electrographic wave.

ESTABLISHMENT OF INDEXES AND CRITERIA

Anyone who has ever written a progress note in a medical record has used non-dimensional criteria for expressing change. Such phrases as *patient looks better today,* or *slept well last night,* and such evaluations as *chest pain is increased, respiration is more comfortable, mental status is less obtunded,* all represent judgmental decisions in which numbers had little or no role. In all these decisions, clinicians regularly use clinical data as index variables, and regularly use criteria for evaluating a change in the index. The scientific problem is not that verbal data are impossible to evaluate; they are constantly evaluated in clinical medicine. The problem is that every clinician may use different data as his indexes, and different criteria for deciding about changes in each index.

A therapognomonic taxonomy—a specific, standardized collection of indexes and criteria for assessing clinical changes during the progress of an illness—is the post-therapeutic counterpart of the taxonomy needed to classify the pre-therapeutic clinical behavior of a disease. With both types of taxonomy absent, under-developed, or under-utilized in contemporary medicine, the frequently chaotic results of modern therapy are inevitable. Controversies, conflicts, dissensions, ignorance, and self-deception in evaluating treatment can flourish among clinicians because so many therapeutic results are reported unreproducibly, with the sources of disagreement impossible to discern from the lack of details in the recorded data.

The widespread absence of standardized concepts for evaluating treatment has resulted in the recent formation, by special committees or by individual investigators, of *ad hoc* therapognomonic criteria in several major disorders. For example, specific clinical indexes and criteria have been reported during the past few years for therapy of asthma,[140] cerebrovascular accidents,[141] congestive heart failure,[142] coronary artery disease,[143, 144] hay fever,[145] leukemia,[146, 147] lung disease,[148] multiple myeloma,[149] psychiatric disease,[150] rheumatic fever,[7] rheumatoid arthritis,[151, 152] and thyrotoxicosis.[153] Committees of the American Medical Association have proposed a series of ratings to be used as "guides to the evaluation of permanent impairment" of the extremities and back,[154] visual system,[155] cardiovascular system,[156] ear-nose-throat,[157] central nervous system,[158] digestive system,[159a] and endocrine system.[159b] Many of these "ratings" could probably be adapted for use in evaluating *change* in "impairment", rather than permanence alone.

Although these modern attempts at orderly therapeutic evaluation are encouraging and representative of methodologic progress, the progress is long overdue and small. The methods proposed as the consensus of a committee are essentially standardized, but must be tested by general dissemination and uniform use before they can be accepted as reliable and effective. The methods proposed by individual investigators must be appraised by other workers, in committees or in actual usage, before the new techniques can even be regarded as standardized. And for numerous published reports and ongoing projects in many other major diseases, there still remains the problem that appropriate therapeutic indexes and criteria, if existing, are not used, and, if absent, are not contemplated and developed.

Like the construction of Venn diagrams, the preparation of clinical indexes and criteria of therapeutic response is better demonstrated than discussed. Nevertheless, certain general principles can be noted.

CITATION OF OBJECTIVES

The first step, of course, is to cite the objectives of each therapeutic situation. Before any indexes of therapy can be contemplated, the targets of treatment must be specified, together with the anticipated prophylactic or remedial action on each target. After the targets and goals are cited, the clinician can select the index variables by noting the particular clinical or other features that suitably describe the objectives. At the conclusion of treatment, the changes in the index variables are compared with the initial objectives for each target, and the total effects are then evaluated.

TYPES OF CRITERIA

These evaluations may require the establishment and use of four different types of criteria:

Existence Criteria

For citing whether a particular manifestation (or target) is present or absent. For example, *orthopnea* and *angina pectoris* are manifestations whose existence must be designated by specific criteria that differentiate them from other types of respiratory distress or chest pain. (Such criteria are discussed further in Chapter 19.)

Gradation Criteria

For citing the quantity, severity, or degree of a manifestation. For example, *dyspnea* can be graded as mild, moderate, or severe; *angina pectoris* can be graded in classes of ascending severity from 1 to 4, or higher; the briskness of *neurologic reflexes* can be graded as 0 to 4+; the loudness of *cardiac murmurs,* in a scale of 0 to 6. Each of these gradations will then require criteria for its classification. Thus, for the sake of arbitrary example, dyspnea might be graded as *severe* if the patient is unable to walk on flat ground more than a few yards; as *moderate,* if the patient can walk on level ground, but is unable to climb one flight of stairs; and as *mild,* if the patient can climb one flight of stairs but not two. (These criteria would need sub-criteria to define the rate of walking and the size and steepness of a "flight" of stairs.) Criteria for grading the severity of angina pectoris have been listed by Proudfit, Shirey, and Sones,[112] and criteria for neurologic reflexes are stated in many textbooks of neurology.

Transition Criteria

For citing significant change (or lack of change) in a manifestation. These criteria will indicate the appearance or disappearance of a manifestation cited only by existence, and distinctions such as "better" or "worse", or "larger" or "smaller", for a manifestation cited according to gradation. For many manifestations, a change will be indicated by a transition from one category of gradation to the next. For other manifestations, however, a change in two categories of gradation, rather than one, may be demanded for the increment to be regarded as significant. Thus, in one recent study[12] in which cardiac enlargement had been graded on a scale of 0 to 4+, "incremental cardiomegaly" was defined as a 2+ change from one cardiac size to another. In some circumstances, the decision that a particular manifestation has "appeared" or "disappeared" may depend on transition criteria. For example, the occurrence of a streptococcal infection has been defined as a rise of two tube dilutions in titer of an appropriate antibody, as measured in sequential specimens of sera tested simultaneously with the same reagent system.[2]

Aggregate Criteria

For combining a series of individual changes into a cluster designation that represents a total effect. Words such as *improved, deteriorated,* or *excellent* represent such a cluster designation. For example, the targets of remedial treatment in a particular patient with congestive heart failure may be dyspnea, râles, hepatomegaly, anorexia, peripheral edema, and tachycardia. Each of these indexes may change individually in response to treatment. The total post-therapeutic response of the congestive failure might be called *excellent* if all these manifestations disappeared, *good* if both of the symptoms but not all the signs disappeared, *fair* if only one symptom disappeared, *poor* if none of the symptoms disappeared, and *very poor* if no changes of any type were affected. In prophylactic treatment, *success* or *failure* will depend on the continuing absence or the *de novo* appearance of the target that was to be prevented.

SELECTION OF APPROPRIATE TARGETS
AND INDEXES

The selection of targets to act as indexes of remedial therapy will require perceptive clinical knowledge. In any particular therapeutic situation, the selector must know the appropriate targets, the effects to be expected from the agents of treatment, and the methods to be used for appraising the effects. For example, the array of clinical findings in a patient with acute myocardial infarction may include severe substernal chest pain, a history of post-prandial epigastric distress, supraventricular tachycardia with a rate of 160, and diminished vibratory sense in both legs. In treating the patient with morphine, digitalis, and anticoagulants, the clinician must know that morphine is expected to affect only the chest pain, and digitalis only the ventricular rate, while anticoagulants, being prophylactic rather than remedial in this situation, would affect none of these targets. The clinician must also know that the chest pain can be assessed only as a subjective symptom and that the cardiac rate can be assessed as a physical or electrocardiographic sign, but that subtle changes in the rhythm of the heart would require electrocardiographic observation. If antacids are given for the post-prandial epigastric distress, the clinician must evaluate their results separately, not as part of the therapy for "myocardial infarction", but must also recognize that the distress might have been due to vascular rather than peptic problems. Finally, since the diminished peripheral vibratory sense is not important in this clinical situation and is not affected by the proposed drugs, the neurologic finding would not be a suitable index of therapy here.

DESCRIPTION OF INDEX VARIABLES

After selection of the targets to be remedied, the index variables must be described in terms of observed evidence, not rational inference. As will be discussed later (Chapter 18), many concepts and terms used in "clinical" description today are not the evidence of observation, but the conclusions of physiologic interpretations, pathologic deductions, or clinical gestalts. A clinician for example, often talks about the disappearance of *pulmonary edema,* but he does not observe the disappearance of pulmonary edema; he observes the presence or absence of râles and of respiratory distress. A clinician does not observe the subsidence of *biliary colic;* he hears the patient say that certain discomforts have disappeared and the clinician finds, on examining the patient, that certain physical signs have been altered.

Unless the observations are reported in terms of evidence, the clinician will later have difficulty establishing satisfactory criteria of progress. Is *pulmonary edema* better if râles disappear but respiratory distress persists? Is *biliary colic* improved if fever persists while pain disappears, or vice versa? How much is the biliary illness improved if pain and fever subside but jaundice remains? For establishment of criteria that are adequately detailed and reproducibly applied, every unit of information used as a clinical description must be dissected into its basic constituents, and the criteria must make provision for each constituent. Every inferential clinical judgment must be broken into its observational ingredients, which are then reconstructed as components of the criteria. To establish such clinical criteria in a scientific manner, clinicians must apply at the bedside the celebrated dictum promulgated in the physiology laboratories of the late A. J. Carlson: "What is the evidence?".

PROBLEMS IN CHOICE OF CLINICAL AND LABORATORY CRITERIA

Because the verbal index variables are classified in discrete gradations (e.g., present or absent; none, mild, moderate, or severe; better, unchanged, or worse; 0, 1+, 2+, 3+, or 4+), criteria of change are often easier to establish for verbally described data than for dimensional measurements. In contrast to the specific categories of the verbal variables, the numerical range of dimensional data must be demarcated and interpreted before decisions can be made that a significant alteration has occurred. For example, is a 15-point decrease in the Westergren sedimentation rate significant if the original value was 160 mm. per hour? If not significant, does the decrement become significant if the original value was 30 mm. per hour? How much variation in the decremental index shall be allowed for technologic discrepancies? To illustrate the distinctions in evaluating change in verbal and dimensional data, consider the example of a patient with pain in the ankle and a Westergren sedimentation rate of 110 mm. per hour. After treatment, the ankle pain disappears and the sedimentation rate falls to 102 mm. per hour. The loss of the pain is clearly an improvement, but is an 8-point drop in sedimentation rate an important change?

When clinical phenomena are described by their basic ingredients, the presence or absence of one or more of the ingredients becomes a specific, discrete index easily used in the establishment of criteria. On the other hand, the problems of appraising technologic discrepancies, ranges of variability, and incremental differences in the measurements of laboratory data are often so difficult that dimensional units can frequently cause major inconsistencies when their alteration must be assessed by specific standards. In forming criteria for assessing *change* in verbally described clinical variables, a thoughtful clinician will therefore often have an easier task than his laboratory colleagues have with dimensional numbers.

PATHOGNOMONIC VERSUS THERAPOGNOMONIC INDEXES

Many important therapognomonic data, obtained by either clinical or laboratory observation, are now under-rated, disregarded, or dismissed as important index variables in clinical medicine because they have little or no pathognomonic value. For example, a clinician does not get much *diagnostic* help from the physical finding of inspiratory basilar crepitations in the lungs. To make an anatomic diagnostic decision about the state of the pulmonary parenchyma, a modern clinician will give much more attention to roentgenographic findings than to crepitations. Yet the crepitations, although perhaps unimportant diagnostically, may be a valuable index of therapeutic accomplishment. A significant change in the crepitations, their total disappearance, or their later re-appearance may indicate a therapeutic effect that cannot be discerned via X-ray. Similarly, the symptom of dyspnea is often of paramount importance as a therapeutic index, although its diagnostic specificity is limited.

The laboratory test of erythrocyte sedimentation rate is often disdained by many young clinicians today because it is abnormal in so many diverse circumstances that it is diagnostically non-specific. Yet the sedimentation rate is often an excellent index of therapeutic progress in the treatment of rheumatic fever, rheumatoid arthritis, and many other acute inflammatory conditions, in which the change from a high sedimentation rate to a low one is a valuable guide to the state of systemic inflammation.

In some instances, the sedimentation rate may be the best or the only therapeutic index at the clinician's disposal. For example, antibiotic treatment for suspected subacute bacterial endocarditis is sometimes given to patients without a positive blood culture. In this circumstance, the available clinical indexes of progress—fever and heart murmurs—may not be striking enough or changed enough to be useful guides to therapy. The clinician, without a positive blood culture as a laboratory index, may be uncertain about when to stop treatment or whether treatment accomplished anything. If the sedimentation rate was initially high, however, and then gradually declined to normal values during the antibiotic therapy, the clinician can use the test both to indicate accomplishment and to suggest a time of cessation for the treatment.

STATISTICAL COLLABORATION

In the choices of indexes of therapeutic response, non-clinical statisticians have sometimes given clinicians misleading advice. An ordinary statistician, whose primary skill is in analyzing numbers rather than clinical descriptions, generally prefers to work with basic data that come in the form of numbers. Some statisticians, moreover, are unfamiliar with the ways in which modern mathematical techniques— such as Boolean algebra—can be used for a precise, quantified organization of descriptive verbal data. Consequently, the statisticians who help clinicians design clinical studies often concentrate on the use of conventional numerical variables and of conventional mathematics.

Limited by the boundaries of his own familiarity and professional comfort, a statistician may therefore urge that the chief variables of assessment and correlation be such personal properties as age, race, and sex, and the dimensional values of laboratory data, which can be structured by conventional mathematical equations. Awed by his own ignorance of statistical methods, and impressed by the proposed statistical formulations, the clinician often denigrates his own basic knowledge and judgment, assumes that the clinical variables he uses in his reasoning have no scientific value, and accedes to a plan of therapeutic appraisal that may be statistically elegant, but clinically useless. To solve this problem, clinicians and statisticians need more familiarity with one another's domain, and, when collaborating, must always recall that their purpose is medical meaning rather than mere statistical significance.

*   *   *

In the inanimate laboratory technology of natural science, the basic procedures are isolation of the entity and calibration of the scale. In the human mental technology of clinical science, the basic procedures are observation of attributes and establishment of criteria for classification. The clinician who seeks precise scientific measurement at the bedside can find the necessary apparatus inside his own mind. With delineated observation, consistent criteria, and careful enumeration, he can fulfill every demand of the "scientific method".

He may need help, however, from several external sources in formulating and communicating his improved scientific activities. The establishment of satisfactory criteria for judging clinical variables may require investigative clinicians to hold special meetings and conferences, sometimes of international scope. Such sessions have often been held in the past by anatomists, biochemists, physicists, and other scientific workers attempting to standardize nomenclature and criteria. The procedure is equally applicable and necessary in therapeutic science.

Moreover, the communication of new criteria—whether prepared by individual investigators or by committees—may require a change in the attitude of many editors of medical journals. In a report of research done with established laboratory techniques, the "methods" section of the manuscript will often contain brief citations of existing references, since no new techniques are described. Even if a new laboratory method is reported, its description can still be relatively short. Accustomed to giving only small amounts of space to the methodologic aspects of laboratory research, editors of medical journals may insist that descriptions of new clinical methods receive an equally small spatial allotment. Unfortunately, however, a careful account of reproducible clinical methods requires considerable space to describe the "painstaking, and sometimes very dull, attention to every detail" that Hill[160] has called "the essence of a successful clinical trial". Many existing clinical methods, as already noted, are too defective for scientific use. In new studies that improve the old clinical methods, the authors cannot cite the main techniques by reference to published literature, and will therefore require much more space than the amounts traditionally allotted in medical journals for "clinical material and methods".

Must all these improvements come from editors, committees, international conferences, and massive clinical trials? Is there something an individual investigator can do without a large congregation of human and technologic assistance? Can a single clinician make significant contributions to modern clinical science without assembling hordes of grants, equipment, personnel, and populations of new patients? He can. He has only to look in the right place and to use suitable methods.

There exists today, in every doctor's office and particularly in every hospital, a mine of data whose gold awaits removal. Work in the mine has been deliberately rejected or thoughtlessly avoided, and the ore, inadequately or improperly extracted, has not been recognized as a source of gold. Instead, scientific clinicians in modern research have worked in other mines—the hospital laboratories—whose ore is shinier, more easily refined, and seemingly more golden. After hard labors in these mines and frequent discouragements when the "gold" turned out to be pyrite, many clinicians have mistakenly concluded that they were poor miners, instead of recognizing that they were in the wrong mine.

The individual clinician in contemporary medical research still has an exciting opportunity to use his skills and talents for significant scientific investigation. He can learn the answers to many old questions in clinical taxonomy, in establishment of clinical indexes and criteria, and in evaluation of treatment. He can acquire the background information essential for a valid scientific approach to many new questions in therapy. He is the only scientist who has the training to do this work, and he can do it without traveling vast distances, purchasing elaborate devices, or learning complex new methodologies. With the intellectual equipment already at his disposal, a clinician can extract the scientific gold to be found in the untapped lodes of the mine of patients' medical records.

15. Retrospection, Experience, and Medical Records

Like the results of laboratory experiments, the data of clinical therapy are inscribed in a notebook. The notebook is called the patient's medical record, and it contains an account of the design, maneuver and responses observed in the individual therapeutic experiments performed in that patient's clinical care. From studying a collection of such notebooks, an investigator should be able to discern the patterns of diverse patients who constitute the spectrum of a disease, and to assemble the results of the varied therapeutic experiments to which the patients were subjected. The investigator can then evaluate the success or failure of individual experiments, and can decide how to improve future performances.

The data of these accounts of clinical investigation fill huge volumes of paper and space in the medical record rooms of every hospital. The collected records at a large medical center for a single year contain descriptions of more experiences in disease than a single clinician may observe in a lifetime. Within the abundant reports of these manifold therapeutic experiences are the answers to many perplexing questions in contemporary prognosis and treatment. Yet the answers are not usually sought from analysis of medical records, which often remain disregarded or spurned as sources of data in clinical science.

Medical records are used frequently for many other purposes. The records are recalled and reviewed as memoranda of the past when an individual patient returns to the hospital, or when information must be extracted for financial, legal, insurance, and other administrative purposes. Collections of records are often surveyed for isolated research projects and for studies of administrative or of individual medical phenomena. Nevertheless, no consistent, systematic techniques have been established for dealing with medical records as scientific documents that can be directly, constructively, and constantly assessed to provide prognostic and therapeutic knowledge about human illness.

The reasons for the neglect are conceptual and pragmatic. Conceptually, many clinicians believe that prognosis and therapy cannot be studied advantageously from medical records because the research is retrospective. Pragmatically, the belief is that the data contained in the records are too diverse, unstandardized, or inadequate for scientific quality. These two beliefs about research with medical records—that the work is made scientifically useless both by retrospection and by poor quality of data—are almost universally accepted. Nevertheless, as indicated in the comments that follow, neither belief need be correct.

THE PROBLEMS OF RETROSPECTION

The words *retrospective* and *prospective* are often used in statistical epidemiologic research to refer to two completely different phenomena: pursuit of a population and collection of data.

In the populational sense, the main feature of "spective" is the temporal direction in which the investigator pursues the *index* (or initial) population. In a prospective study, he follows the population forward from its "index" state to see what happens in its future course. In a retrospective study, he follows the population backward to see what had happened before it reached its "index" state. For example, suppose our index population is a group of patients with cancer of the lung. If we study each patient's subsequent clinical course after diagnosis, and analyze the effects of various forms of treatment, we perform a *prospective* study. If we ask each patient about his previous smoking history, and try to decide whether his past consumption of tobacco caused his cancer of the lung, we perform a *retrospective* study. Thus, the state of the index population is correlated in a retrospective study with a former state, and, in a prospective study, with a subsequent state.

In the data sense, the main feature of "spective" is the time at which the investigator begins to collect the research data. In a prospective study, the investigator has planned, in advance, to use the population's data for research; the information is therefore collected from each person with specific, planned techniques to ensure that all details are adequately described. In a retrospective study, the people have already been examined, and their data have already been recorded in diverse ways before the investigator begins to retrieve the data for research analysis; the investigator gets the information from the medical records and various other sources in which the data were initially transcribed. For example, in our index population of patients with lung cancer, we collect the research data retrospectively if we use the patients' routine medical records to find out about their smoking histories. If we talk to the patients directly, asking a series of questions planned specifically for our research, we collect the data prospectively.

It is possible, therefore, for an investigation to be retrospective in population but prospective in data, prospective in population but retrospective in data, prospective in both aspects, or retrospective in both aspects. For example, if we assembled a population of lung cancer patients tomorrow, and if we obtained their smoking histories with carefully designed research questionnaires, the study would be retrospective in population but prospective in data. We would be retrospecting to something that occurred in the population before the patients reached the index state at which we begin to look at them, although we use special research techniques for getting their data prospectively. Conversely, if we assembled a population of patients who all had lung cancer in 1930, and if we studied their medical records to find out what later happened to them after treatment, the study would be prospective in population but retrospective in data. We would be prospecting to something that occurred in the population after the patients reached the index state at which we begin to look at them, but we would get the data retrospectively, from information recorded before we started our investigation.

These retrospective-prospective distinctions in the temporal pursuit of a population and in the time of data collection are critical features of science in clinical statistics. Of the two features, the pursuit of the population is scientifically much more important, since the logical validity of the investigation depends on the direction in which the population was followed.

This issue of logical validity is particularly important in studying *etiology* of disease, where the issue becomes a matter of deciding *cause* and *effect*. Such decisions constantly occur in human reasoning, and an understanding of the logic of these decisions is prerequisite to any investigation of etiology of disease.

The general issue of how to prove "cause" is neither clinical nor statistical, and neither "retrospective" nor "prospective". It is a matter of logic, and of what constitutes a valid form of proof in deductive reasoning with statistics. If we want to conclude that event *A* is likely to cause event *B*, we must observe a series of the *A* events, see how many times they are followed by *B*s, and compare this frequency rate with the number of times that *B* occurs *without* being preceded by *A*. The proposed temporal sequence for these occurrences is (event *A*) → (event *B*), and (not event *A*) → (event *B*).

The pertinent reasoning may be demonstrated by the Venn diagram in Figure 35. We have a universe that comprises the set of all occurrences of event *A*, and its complement set, the occurrences of *not A*. Event *B* may then occur as a subset of *A* or as a subset of *not A*. Our object is to count the number of members in each of the four sets, $A, \overline{A}, B \cap A$, and $B \cap \overline{A}$. We then compare the ratios

$$\frac{\text{No. of } (B \cap A)}{\text{No. of } A} \quad \text{and} \quad \frac{\text{No. of } (B \cap \overline{A})}{\text{No. of } \overline{A}}$$

If the first of these ratios is significantly greater than the second, we have demonstrated that *B* occurs more frequently after *A* than in the absence of *A*. This calculation does not *prove* that *A* causes *B*. No

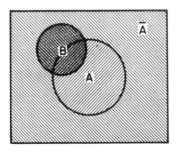

FIGURE 35
The occurrence of event *B* in an enumerated universe of events *A* and $\overline{A}$.

statistical calculations are ever a *proof* of cause. All they can do is give logical support to our suspicions of a cause. If the statistics contradict our hypothesis, we can usually conclude that it was incorrect and that our "suspect" is innocent. If the statistics support the hypothesis, they still do not prove guilt.* This type of reasoning—in which a hypothesis is either excluded or supported, without necessarily being confirmed—often occurs during ordinary diagnostic "work-ups" that do not employ statistics. For example, we may suspect a sick patient of having untreated pernicious anemia. If the hematocrit value is found to be normal, we can usually rule out pernicious anemia as the diagnosis. If the hematocrit value is abnormally low, we have confirmed that the patient is *anemic*, but we still have not proved that the anemia is *pernicious*.

The concept of sequence is a critical feature in the statistical reasoning about cause—the idea that B follows A, or that B arises as a subset of A. Because of that sequence, the members of the A and $\overline{A}$ sets were put into the denominators of the ratios, while the members of the B sets went into the numerators. This is the distinction that is "prospective" for a study of "cause": the "exposed" and "non-exposed" groups are placed in the denominators of the compared ratios.

Suppose, for example, that we want to test the hypothesis that a medical parentage may "cause" the desire to enter medicine. For this test, we would need to find the following data: the number of doctors' children; the number of doctors' children who have entered medical school; the number of children of non-doctors; and the number of non-doctors' children who have entered medical school.

We would then calculate two percentages:

$$\frac{\text{No. of doctors' children in medical school}}{\text{No. of doctors' children}} \times 100$$

and

$$\frac{\text{No. of non-doctors' children in medical school}}{\text{No. of non-doctors' children}} \times 100$$

* Throughout history, doctors have gotten into profound intellectual trouble in dealing with "cause" of disease, and I want to avoid any prolonged discussion of the issue here. The main reason for bringing it up is to exonerate medical records for careful retrospective investigation of prognosis and treatment while demonstrating their insurmountable defects for retrospective studies of etiology. More intensive analyses of the logic of "cause" are provided by Pearson[161] and by Popper.[162]

Note the construction of those percentages in this logical, "prospective" form of comparison. The "effect"—going to medical school—was separated into two appropriate parts and placed in the numerators. The tested "cause" and its absence—being or not being a doctor's child—were in the denominators. In this comparison of percentages, if the first is significantly greater than the second, we would not, of course, *prove* that doctors "cause" their children to go to medical school. Doctors' children might be no more stimulated to go to medical school than the children of anyone else, but the ratio might be higher because admission committees of the medical schools might exert a preferential bias in favor of candidates with medical ancestry. Nevertheless, although our study cannot prove "cause", we at least conducted its calculations in a logical manner.

Such a study, however, might be difficult to do. The registrars of medical schools could easily provide the data for our numerators— how many medical students are children of doctors or of non-doctors —but we might have great difficulty in determining our denominators —the total number of children of doctors and of non-doctors. We might be able to get such information from the national census bureau, but let us assume for the moment that the census data are not available.

Lacking such data, we might use a different approach to the investigation. We might select a "sample" of doctors and non-doctors in the community, interview them, find out how many children they have, and how many of those children have gone to medical school. We might have some problems with both the "sample" and the data: whether the "sample" is representative, how under-age children should be counted, and so on—but at least our fundamental logic would still be correct. In this epidemiologic approach, we would still put the right type of people into the numerators and denominators.

To do such an epidemiologic survey, however, would also be difficult. We would have to leave our office, and start asking questions in the outside community. Besides, with such an approach for getting "new" data, we would not use existing information readily available to us in the office of the medical school registrars. So we look for a simpler way.

We find a "control" group. The law schools and their registrars' records are also readily available, so we decide to use the law students as a "control" group. Thus, we determine the number of students in medical schools and in law schools, and their parentage.

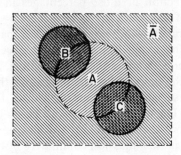

FIGURE 36

The occurrence of event A in an enumerated universe of events B and C. (In sets encompassed by *solid lines*, the number of members has been counted. In sets with *dashed outlines*, the number of members is unknown.)

The composition of our new "universe" in this study is shown in Figure 36, where A is the set of doctors' children; $\overline{A}$, the set of non-doctors' children; B, the set of medical students; and C, the set of law students. What we have counted in this study is a collection of numbers entirely different from what we looked at before. In this new "universe", we have counted the members of sets B, C, $A \cap B$, and $A \cap C$. Since we have not determined the real magnitude of A and $\overline{A}$ in this "universe", their uncounted sections are outlined with dashed lines.

We now might calculate the following percentages:

$$\frac{\text{No. of doctors' children in medical school}}{\text{No. of medical students}} \times 100$$

and

$$\frac{\text{No. of doctors' children in law school}}{\text{No. of law students}} \times 100$$

Because these data have taken us into a line of reasoning quite different from the one we used before, however, we do not know what to make of the two percentages. They can tell us only that medical schools are more or less likely than law schools to contain the children of doctors. We have not determined what we wanted to know: the number of children of doctors (set A) and its complement (set $\overline{A}$). The magnitude of these two fundamental sets was not assessed in the "universe" that we actually counted.

Consequently, the calculations cannot answer our original question. Even if more medical students than law students are doctors' children, we would have learned nothing about the likelihood of medical school attendance by the children of doctors and non-doctors. The "exposed" and "non-exposed" groups that we wanted to assess have disappeared from the calculation. Moreover, the "cause" has entered the numerators, and the "effect" has entered one of the denominators.

This type of comparison of an affected group and a "control" group is often called a *retrospective study of etiology*, but the reasoning is neither "retrospective" nor "prospective". It is simply illogical. We got into this error because we wanted to find an easy way out of an epidemiologic problem. Instead of getting new data in a population that might be difficult to study, we chose to compare substitute populations that were easily studied, readily available—and wrong.

Such illogical comparisons have been frequently performed by statisticians and clinicians in *retrospective* attempts to demonstrate causes of disease. For example, suppose we suspected that drinking coffee causes cancer of the stomach. For logical prospective validity, we would have to compare the prevalence of gastric cancer in populations of people who do or do not drink coffee. With such data, we could put the putative "cause" and its absence in the denominators of our compared percentages. To get such data, however, we would have to leave the hospital and determine the number of coffee drinkers and non-coffee drinkers in the community.

Instead, we prefer to work within the confines of the hospital. We select some sort of a "control" group—perhaps patients with infectious hepatitis. We then find out how many coffee drinkers there were among the patients with gastric cancer, and also among the patients with hepatitis. If the percentage of coffee drinkers is significantly higher in the gastric cancer group than in the hepatitis "controls", we might conclude that coffee drinking may cause cancer of the stomach.

This departure from logic is traditional among doctors studying etiology, and has occurred in every era of recorded history in medicine. The main difference between the inappropriate etiologic speculations of the past and those of the present is that the contemporary errors are accompanied by "statistics". A "retrospective" study of people who already have a disease is always a first step, of course, whenever we begin to suspect that a particular agent is causing that disease. If we do not find frequent enough evidence of that agent among the diseased people, a "prospective" study will be a waste of time. All that the "retrospection" can do, however, is to give us some ideas of what might be the cause. Once our ideas are aroused enough to make us look for statistics, we can even attempt a "retrospective control" comparison, just as a preliminary check. But we can go no further with retrospection. All we can do is get ideas. These ideas are neither logical nor valid suspicions until they have been tested in a population studied "prospectively".

No matter when or how the data are collected, a retrospective study of *etiology* for a disease cannot be logically valid because the investigator is pursuing the wrong population. The study is inherently flawed by his inability to know the "exposed" and "non-exposed" populations from which his "diseased" population has emerged.

There is no problem in logic, however, when an investigator studies prognosis and therapy, rather than etiology, of a disease. Such a study is prospective, because he follows the patients forward in time, and they appear in the denominators of any percentages that he later calculates. The main problem in "validity" is to be sure that he has followed all the patients long enough. For example, he should not report "10-year survival rates" unless all members of the initial population have had the opportunity to survive 10 years.

In such a prospective populational study (often called a "cohort" study), the data may be collected prospectively from the patients directly, or retrospectively from medical records. The "retrospective" data may have many flaws, as a result of imprecision of information in the medical records, but the logical design of such a study is still valid. A retrospective populational study of *etiology* is not logically designed.

Thus, in retrospecting a population for a new study of etiology, the investigator may get good data, but he studies the wrong people. In retrospecting medical records for a new study of prognosis and treatment, the investigator studies the right population, but may get bad data. These distinctions in populational observation and data collection are further illustrated in Figure 37.

During the past few decades, clinicians and statisticians concerned with *etiology* of disease have performed many investigations that

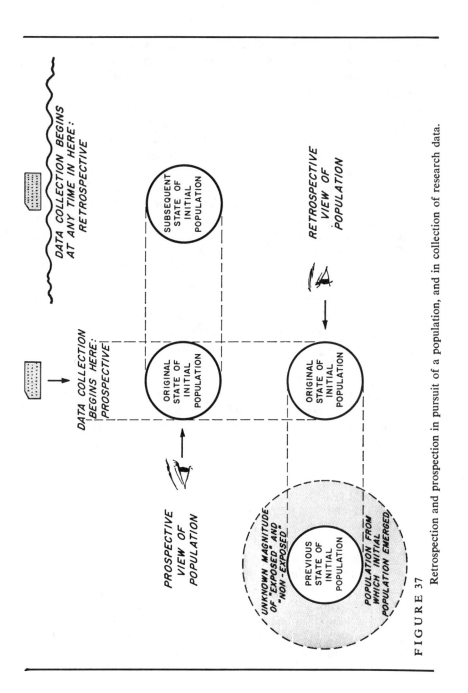

FIGURE 37   Retrospection and prospection in pursuit of a population, and in collection of research data.

were populationally retrospective. When the research was subsequently condemned for its improper logical design, the condemnation was somehow extended to include investigations in which the data are collected retrospectively. The contemporary clamor against any type of "retrospection" often comes loudest from the same etiologically oriented investigators whose defective populational research gave the word *retrospective* its current "evil" connotation.

Frightened by the statistical clamor, unfamiliar with the logical distinctions of the two different types of "retrospection", and unaware of the populational features that make "retrospection" faulty for studies of etiology but valid for studies of prognosis, clinicians have become reluctant to analyze their own clinical experience. Although a study of prognosis and treatment derived from medical records can deal prospectively with the correct population, clinicians fear that the investigations cannot be valid because the data are collected retrospectively. As a consequence of this investigative neglect of medical records, contemporary clinicians lack good information about the natural course of illness, and are often unable to design effective experimental trials of new therapeutic agents.

The merits of a well-designed, well-executed, doubly-prospective therapeutic study (i.e., prospective in both populational pursuit and data collection) are beyond any scientific dispute, and such studies are clearly the ideal way to investigate prognosis and treatment. Unfortunately, however, such studies are seldom possible. When well designed, the studies are rarely well executed, and when well executed, they are rarely well designed. The reasons for this dilemma are discussed in the section that follows.

PROBLEMS IN EXECUTION AND DESIGN OF DOUBLY-PROSPECTIVE THERAPEUTIC STUDIES

The effective execution of a doubly-prospective study of therapy depends on the investigator's opportunity to assemble a population of patients large enough for statistical analysis, and to maintain the patients long enough for observation of their full post-therapeutic course. Assembly of a large number of patients is difficult if the disease is uncommon; long-term maintenance of the population is difficult if the disease is chronic. Uncommon diseases may occur so infrequently that no single investigator or medical center can obtain adequate numbers of patients for study. Chronic diseases present the arduous problem of continuing to observe a large out-patient population for a long period of time. Because the ultimate outcome of therapy cannot be determined for many years, a study of a chronic disease often must go on for so long that the project begins to suffer an attrition of patients or of investigators, who may abandon their participation either because of disinterest, or because of geographic changes. The loss of information or of investigative incentive in these circumstances produces unsatisfactory results, incomplete in numbers or in time. Such problems in population maintenance are particularly common in the prospective investigation of natural history and therapy for diabetes mellitus, cerebral arteriosclerosis, hypertension, renal disease, coronary disease, and many neurologic and neoplastic disorders. Few of these diseases can be studied adequately with wholly prospective observations because the initial population cannot be maintained long enough or intact enough in a single research project for the investigators to procure all the necessary data by direct first-hand observation. Many prospective studies, therefore, currently cannot be well executed, even when well designed.

Good design of a doubly-prospective study depends on the investigator's knowledge of the different clinical distinctions to be used for dividing the population into subgroups with comparable prognoses. This type of prognostic stratification is imperative (as described earlier on pages 238–239) for a satisfactory allocation of different therapeutic regimens. If the research is to be well designed, these prognostic distinctions must be known *before the investigation begins.* The distinctions are currently not known, however, for most of the common, complex diseases that are often studied in contemporary therapeutic trials. In most of these diseases, as discussed earlier (pages 239–241), satisfactory information does not exist about the clinical identification of the populations exposed to therapy. In many cancers, for example, and in diabetes mellitus, coronary artery disease, and other long-term illnesses, the existing data are inadequate for reproducible, effective division of the patients into clinical subgroups with comparable prognoses. In the absence of such data, many investigations now being planned or executed cannot be designed well enough to solve the therapeutic problems for which they are intended. The research, at best, will yield only vague clarification of the clinical prognostic features that should have been known and included beforehand. Consequently, many prospective studies, even when well executed, cannot be well designed.

Because of these two simultaneous problems in design and in execution, contemporary doubly-prospective therapeutic studies in many major diseases can seldom be satisfactory. Defective clinical specifications impede good design; troublesome long-term logistics impede effective execution. To solve these problems, clinicians can improve the *execution* of future research by enlarging the numbers, scope, and capacities of personnel who work in epidemiologic teams. The *design* of future research can be improved from what might be learned during appropriate retrospective surveys, planned not for direct comparison of therapeutic agents, but for appraising clinical experience to recognize the critical clinical variables of prognosis and treatment. With appropriate techniques, such surveys—retrospective in data but prospective in population—can identify the clinical categorizations necessary for effective design of future studies that are wholly prospective. By ignoring what can be learned from data examined retrospectively, a clinician studying prognosis and treatment of human illness incurs a visual impairment that is partly self-imposed. The nature of disease and of people makes it difficult for him to see well when he looks forward, but he closes his own eyes when he fails to look back.

THE USE OF MEDICAL RECORDS IN THERAPEUTIC RESEARCH

For the type of retrospective therapeutic survey that has just been described, medical records are the best, the inevitable, and the only starting point. The records are the only way of obtaining numbers of patients large enough to discern clinical patterns and to perform statistical analyses, and the only way of regularly being able to "follow" each patient long enough to discern the ultimate outcome. Although not appropriate for many types of clinical research, medical records are well suited for studies of prognosis and therapy, since these are the events for which the records are planned, kept, and preserved. A patient's medical record is not necessarily designed as a notebook of general investigations in etiology, pathogenesis, or diagnosis of disease, but *is* always intended as an account of the experiments performed in prognosis and therapy.

Retrospective analysis of the data in medical records can often be dismissed as scientifically valueless not because such research is inherently unscientific, but because so many investigations have been done in an unscientific manner. With removal of some of the existing defects, cited in the list that follows, analyses of medical records can yield important, crucial contributions to clinical knowledge.

ATTEMPTS TO COMPARE DIFFERENT THERAPEUTIC AGENTS

Comparisons of different therapeutic agents are not wholly satisfactory unless performed in a completely prospective study. The retrospective investigation of data in medical records cannot suffice for such comparisons, but can, as already noted, provide significant clinical information for identifying the natural and post-therapeutic history of illness, and for organizing the classification techniques to be used in future prospective research. If the retrospective survey is well planned, if the patients are appropriately stratified according to clinical severity and other categories of comparable prognostic "risks", and if the data are sufficiently reliable, however, the therapeutic conclusions may be so correct, or so striking, that a wholly prospective future study may be unnecessary. Nevertheless, the *prospective* collection of data is critical for settling any doubts or ambiguities that may remain after the retrospective analysis is completed.

CHOICE OF A "ZERO TIME"

An important chronologic feature of retrospective surveys is the choice of a common reference date, or "zero time", for each patient. The date is the point in time at which each patient's "index" state is to be identified, and from which the duration of associated and subsequent events can be measured. The problems of choosing this reference date and of cataloging its co-existent data are responsible for many of the defects that have given retrospective surveys so unsavory a reputation.

In many studies of treatment, the selection of a reference time for the population has been governed more by features of the hospital than by features of the patients. The population under investigation has frequently consisted of all patients admitted to a hospital during a particular interval of time (such as a 3-year period), and the common reference point chosen for each patient has been his date of admission to, or discharge from, the hospital. This chronologic approach is unsatisfactory because it produces a factitious comparison of diverse phases of the disease. Many patients who may already have received diagnosis and one or more courses of treatment for the disease before this admission to the hospital are thereby given the same reference date as other patients who are in their first admission or in their first course of treatment.

A better choice of a reference date for getting a mutually comparable phase of illness in all patients is to classify each patient according to his state when the disease was first diagnosed. This chronologic classification, although oriented to the patient rather than to the hospital, still has many defects. Among the defects, particularly in surveys concerned with treatment, are the problems of deciding which piece of evidence, or which act of reasoning, should be considered definitive enough to be used for the date of diagnosis. Another set of hazards, when the reference date is that of diagnosis, arises in trying to account for delays in treatment, and for clinical and other changes in the patient during the interval between diagnosis and treatment.

Another possible choice of "zero time" for the disease in each patient is the date at which symptoms began. Such a chronologic choice creates three main difficulties: some patients are asymptomatic; some patients cannot give a precise date for onset of symptoms; and in other patients, the clinician may have difficulty deciding which symptoms to attribute to that particular disease.

The best "zero time" for many surveys of treatment is the date of the first main therapeutic procedure directed at the disease. The date of first treatment is easily determined, is readily documented in medical records, and is a common, mutual property of all patients with the disease (except for untreated patients, in whom an appropriate alternate time can be chosen—such as the date of decision against treatment). This choice of a reference date is particularly useful for studies intended to appraise natural history of disease and the evidence used in therapeutic judgment. The date of first treatment represents a comparable "zero time" for all patients, since it is the point at which the natural evolution of the disease is first affected by therapeutic intervention. The clinical conditions that exist in diverse patients at this "zero time" have not been altered by treatment, and can be temporally compared regardless of the reasons for delay in diagnosis or in treatment. With this "zero time" established, appropriate durations can then be calculated for the events that preceded and those that followed the treatment.

CLASSIFICATION AT "ZERO TIME"

The choice of a reference date is important not only for the chronologic aspects just noted, but also for the temporal boundary it places on the permissible information that can be used in each patient's classification at that "zero time". The medical record, investigatively reviewed months or years afterward, will contain an account of the patient's complete subsequent clinical course, and may thus include reports of many events that occurred *after* the initial reference date. The investigator exposed to additional information accrued after "zero time" must not allow it to influence his selection and interpretation of the recorded evidence available *on or before* the reference date. Otherwise, the true state of the patient at "zero time" will be classified improperly, and the retrospection will produce a false account of what was known at that time. For example, in an elderly patient who has a carcinoma of the lung and who later has a stroke, the clinical evidence during life may not have been adequate to denote whether or not the cerebral lesion was a metastasis. The therapeutic decisions in this situation may have been made while the clinicians were uncertain about the true pathologic condition. When the medical record is subsequently reviewed for classifying this patient's state during life, the investigator may know the results later provided by necropsy, and may be tempted to use the results in classifying the patient's pre-mortem state. For accurate classification, however, the necropsy data should not be permitted to influence the notation that diagnosis was uncertain at the time of treatment.

CLASSIFICATION OF THE SEVERITY OF ILLNESS

The severity of a patient's clinical state is usually determined not from morphologic or laboratory data, but from the associated clinical manifestations and co-morbidity. Because symptoms, signs, general clinical condition, and associated diseases have been omitted from most previous retrospective surveys of data in therapy, the subsequent comparison of patients often has not been valid. Two patients with a marked difference in severity of illness might have been associated in an improper comparison because they had similar features of "disease".

This problem makes many investigators reluctant to do retrospective surveys of the therapeutic information in medical records. The investigator may fear that the necessary data to denote "severity" are either absent or unreliable. Moreover, even when satisfactory information seems available, the investigator may be uncertain about how to use it.

In approaching this problem, the investigator should recall that one of the main purposes of analyzing medical records retrospectively is to determine (as noted in Chapters 11 and 14) how to classify the severity of illness. As long as clinicians are uncertain about decisions of "severity", we cannot properly design any prospective studies, either to compare groups of patients or to select pairs of individual patients for comparison in trials conducted by "sequential analysis".[139] A knowledge of severity of illness is prerequisite to a well-designed prospective study and can be obtained only from the "retrospective" type of examination proposed here. Without such previous "retrospection", a prospective study may be based on comparisons less valid and more capricious than those derived from medical records.

Aware of the importance of clinical manifestations and co-morbidity, an investigator can usually find the appropriate information cited in the records, or can acquire the information, when necessary, from other sources. When medical records have been used in the past to note severity of illness, the main difficulty has not been the absence of suitable data, but the absence of the investigator's attention to the suitable data. Investigators who considered only the demographic data of hosts and the para-clinical data of "disease" while ignoring the clinical data of illness were unable to classify severity effectively—but then often concluded that the defect was in the data of the medical records rather than in the investigator's concept of what data to analyze.

ACQUISITION OF COMPLETE DATA

Since "zero time" may occur at a hospital different from the one at which a survey is performed, and since pre-therapeutic and post-therapeutic events may also occur in many different medical localities, the clinicians who use medical records for surveys of disease will often have to obtain information from many sources outside their own medical center. The acquisition of enough evidence for a complete clinical chronology of each patient's illness is often neglected in many surveys, either because the data are not solicited from the external sources or because the requests are not answered. The transmission of such pre- and post-therapeutic information from one medical center to another, and from practitioner to research worker, is a necessary aspect of scientific investigation. Knowing that research workers may later ask him for information about his patients, a clinical practitioner has more incentive for keeping careful medical records than he does when the work of "clinical investigators" seldom impinges on his own daily practice. By maintaining circumspect medical records, and by sending requested information to investigators studying prognosis and treatment, practitioners who now feel alienated from the research activities of laboratory medicine can actively contribute to progress in clinical science.

MANAGEMENT OF UNCERTAIN DATA

Although most people expect life to contain many gray areas in addition to its blacks and whites, the investigators of medical records often become frustrated by information that is uncertain, ambiguous, contradictory, or absent. In many such instances, the defect lies with the investigator, not with the records. As described in the next section, he may have planned an inappropriate study, and may be making unwarranted demands on the recorded data. In many other instances, however, the recorded data are indeed unsatisfactory, lacking precision, verification, and many other attributes of science. Nevertheless, the inadequacies are neither insurmountable nor unmanageable. By communication with sources external to the immediate medical record (e.g., patients, families, doctors, other hospitals), the investigator can often obtain missing information or can clarify points that are doubtful. By thoughtful analysis of sources within the record, the investigator can often easily decide which data to accept and which to reject. For example, of the various notes contained in the medical records, a medical student's report is not likely to be the best account of the patient's physical findings. Nevertheless, the student's note is often the most reliable presentation of the history, because the student has not yet learned to condense, interpret, or distort what the patient tells him. Conversely, the resident house officer or attending physician is most likely to record a reliable physical examination but may shorten or omit many important details of history.

Finally, when these external and internal procedures fail to solve problems in the medical record, the investigator can still manage to categorize the dubious data by using designations such as "uncertain" or "unknown". If the investigator's coding system contains shades of gray, as well as black and white, he can readily classify any of the data he encounters in medical records.

CHOICE OF APPROPRIATE TOPICS FOR INVESTIGATION

Another important source of the current low esteem for medical records as research data has been the disillusionment of investigators who found the records unsatisfactory in studies for which the records were actually not a proper choice of research material. Medical records are inherently unsuitable for many types of investigation in which they have been used; when they were "failures" in such projects, the records were often unjustly blamed for faults that were actually attributable to the investigator who planned his research inappropriately.

Ordinary medical records are an excellent choice of research material, as described earlier, for investigations of natural history, prognosis, and overt aspects of therapy. For certain other types of research, however, routine medical records are not well qualified, and may be quite improper, as the "material" of the investigation. The records of hospitalized patients are usually unsuitable for studies of etiology of disease, for reasons already cited. Moreover, when some new factor becomes suspected as a causal agent in a disease, we cannot reasonably expect to find the factor always described as present or absent in the patients whose routine medical record data were compiled long before the factor was suspected as having any clinical importance. For example, if we really had the idea that coffee drinking may cause stomach cancer, we would get no *pro* or *con* evidence from ordinary medical records. Information about coffee drinking is not recorded in most patients' records.

Ordinary medical records are also often unsuitable for certain studies in which specific clinical events are to be directly correlated with biochemical, immunologic, pharmacologic, and other phenomena expressed in laboratory data. In many instances, neither the clinical nor the laboratory data have been cited in the routine medical record with the detailed precision necessary for satisfactory correlations. The absence of such details is often not surprising, however, and its condemnation is not always justified, since the clinicians executing and recording the procedures of *ordinary therapy* could not be expected to know in advance about all the data that might be selected for intensive analysis months or even years later. For example, an investigator who uses medical records to correlate degree of exophthalmos with the uptake of radioactive iodine in hyperthyroidism may be chagrined to find that the data are not available in the records of many of the patients in his survey. The attending clinicians, able to establish diagnosis and give treatment effectively in many situations without a precise measurement of exophthalmos and without knowing the radio-iodine data, may have had no incentive to obtain or record the information.

No scientific investigator reviews the notes of one of his laboratory experiments and expects to find detailed answers to questions of other experiments that he did not ask or consider in the original investigation. Yet many investigators approach the data of medical records with just this type of unwarranted demand. When the data in the records are then found inadequate, the investigator seldom considers the propriety of his demand or of his own "design" for research. He concludes erroneously that the defects of medical records are so insurmountable that no significant research, including his own inappropriate study, can be done in this medium.

RESEARCH METHODS AND PERSONNEL

The procedures used for analytic surveys of the massive, intricate data contained in medical records offer fundamental research challenges in contemporary clinical methodology. The techniques, and the appropriate technicians, are almost wholly non-existent. Although excellent statistical and computational devices exist for processing the data, these devices contribute little to solving the basic problems of assessing the records, and extracting and organizing the data to be processed. The laboratory data and certain demographic data of medical records are relatively easy to manage; the data of clinical manifestations—which are often the crucial features of prognostic and therapeutic surveys—are much more complicated and difficult. The surveys must therefore be performed or directed by clinicians aware of the complexity of clinical data, and able to exercise subtle clinical judgments in sifting evidence and labeling it as definite, probable, uncertain, or unknown.

Such surveys offer clinicians an excellent opportunity to use their clinical talents in modern research. A clinician is the only investigator who has the necessary background to direct this type of investigation. He is the only scientist whose previous training prepares him to study the experiences recorded by other clinicians; to perceive the nuances of clinical situations; to comprehend esoteric aspects of handwriting, vocabulary, strategy, and tactics; to recognize qualitative differences in sources of the recorded notes; to develop methods for extracting, verifying, completing, and classifying the necessary information; and to maintain a broad view of the total means and ends of the survey.

Moreover, the analysis of medical records is a form of research that can be done in the clinician's office or at home—at a desk, or in an armchair. And it is a form of research whose methodology makes optimal use of what the clinician already knows, instead of forcing him to learn the operation of complex new technical equipment. Medical records contain notes of the vast experience that clinicians have had with human illness, and clinicians are the investigators who can convert this recorded experience into the orderly knowledge of science.

This type of contemplative, circumspect, taxonomic investigation can be just as intellectually dynamic and exciting as experiments in the laboratory. A few of the methodologic techniques have already been described here; most of the general procedures, and those individualized for specific surveys, will need development as part of future research. With such surveys of medical records, clinicians can perform the tabulations and clinical correlations necessary for constructing pre-therapeutic taxonomic classifications, and for identifying appropriate index variables in the appraisal of post-therapeutic response. In getting "technicians" to help in this type of investigation, clinicians may need to call upon medical record librarians, nurses, statisticians, people with training in public health, and other personnel whose previous background is quite different from that of the conventional "technician" who assists in laboratory research.

Although the data and methods will be complex, as befits the intricacy of human disease, the performance of such research surveys is imperative. They are the only way in which clinicians can conveniently and quickly clarify many current obscurities in the natural behavior, prognosis, and therapy of human illness. To clinicians who want to apply clinical rather than laboratory talents in basic problems of medical research today, such activities offer a valuable outlet for investigative energy, and a creative intellectual challenge of major magnitude.

THE QUALITY OF DATA IN MEDICAL RECORDS

Even when investigative clinicians recognize the importance, necessity, techniques, and proper design for retrospective surveys of the clinical data in medical records, a major deterrent to the surveys is the quality of the data encountered. Almost anyone who has performed such a survey has been dismayed by the diversity of the recorded clinical data and by the frequency with which crucial information is omitted or inadequate. To seekers of precision, objectivity, and standardization, the clinical data of medical records often appear to be a huge scientific wasteland.

The data are indeed diverse, their organization is often chaotic, the information is seldom objective, and the necessary details of precision and thoroughness are often omitted. Nevertheless, the quality of the data can easily be improved, and even in their existing state, clinical data are often no less reliable, and are frequently better, than much of the non-clinical information used for other types of investigative analyses.

A peculiar corollary of the contemporary scientific skepticism of symptoms and signs described by clinicians is the ready acceptance of other types of data—usually numerical—obtained by nurses, laboratory technicians, secretaries, and other non-medical personnel with much less scientific background and training than the scorned clinicians. Despite the well-known discrepancies that may exist in performance of the same test by different laboratories, or by different technicians in the same laboratory, a numerical laboratory result frequently receives almost instantaneous acceptance as scientific evidence. Often without knowledge of the accuracy and care of the technician who did the test, and sometimes without awareness of the reliability of the test itself, many clinicians may nevertheless put unswerving faith in the validity of laboratory data, while remaining scientifically incredulous about the qualitative or semi-quantitative data of clinical observation.

As trained, experienced observers of human illness, clinicians record the symptomatic and physical evidence of disease that often cannot be discerned from laboratory tests or perceived by any apparatus other than a human observer. A careful clinical description of symptoms and signs may frequently have more meaning and precision than many of the variables recorded as laboratory data. Moreover, a clinician's descriptive contributions to the data of medical records are sometimes more consistent and better organized than the observations of his colleagues in radiology and pathology.

The clinician is no less competent or wise an observer of *his* data than his laboratory or other colleagues are of theirs—and, like his colleagues, he is often deluded into errors of omission or commission in his observations and in his reasoning. The basic reliability of his primary clinical observations and of his recorded notes can be markedly improved by techniques discussed in the next part of this book. To apply those techniques, however, clinicians must first recognize the importance and scientific value of the reasoning they do with their observations of symptoms, signs, and people.

The diminished attention to clinical observation that characterizes contemporary "science" in clinical therapy has been the product not of a dehumanized disregard by doctors for patients, but of the false assumption that scientific reasoning in the performance of therapy was best done by replacing clinical observations with other types of data. In assessing the condition of sick people, laboratory data are supplements, not replacements, of clinical data. Clinical data provide unique and basic evidence, unobtainable from the laboratory, that must be used for scientific identification of the human beings and human reactions seen in clinical therapy. As long as clinicians continue to treat people, the information learned from direct observation of the people will yield integral data that cannot be superseded as elements of therapeutic science.

*   *   *

With perception of these distinctions, and with recognition of the *scientific* necessity for humanism and for clinical skills in the treatment of human illness, clinicians can once again give major attention to making the observations that are theirs alone to make, and to recording the results. The clinician can organize, classify, process, and analyze his data with exactly the same intellectual, statistical, and computational procedures available in every other branch of science. For these procedures to yield valuable scientific results, however, the clinician must also improve the scientific validity of the primary clinical data.

PART IV

Acquisition of Clinical Data

Chapter 16. Art, Science, and Clinical Observation

Chapter 17. Art in Clinical Examination

History-Taking
Physical Examination
   Concern for the Patient
   Focus and Emphasis in Teaching

Chapter 18. Science in Clinical Examination: Objectivity and Precision

Objectivity
   History-Taking
   Physical Examination
Precision
   Communication
      History-Taking
      Physical Examination
   Specification
      History-Taking
         Iatrotropic Stimulus
         Characterization of Symptomatic Sensations
         Sequence of Clinical Manifestations
         Timing of Manifestations
      Physical Examination
         Use of Additional Equipment
         Separation of Description, Designation, and Diagnosis

Chapter 19. Science in Clinical Examination: Standardization

Consistency
Uniformity
   History-Taking
   Physical Examination
Reliability
   History-Taking
      Direct Supervision of Students
      Direct Review of History by Attending Physician
      Review of History with Other Sources
      Review of History at Re-admission to Hospital
      Standardization in Research Studies
   Physical Examination
      At Teaching Rounds
      Self-Standardization
      Standardization of Multiple Observers in Research Studies

16. Art, Science, and Clinical Observation

So many expostulations, revelations, and platitudes have been written during the traditional art-science debate of clinical medicine that the subject may need burial rather than revival. The old dispute is renewed here, however, because it recently seems to have been settled. The settlement, as in many other disputes, is a partition. The partition, which ends the argument about whether clinical medicine is art or science, separates medicine into two parts: one, called *art,* is a specifically clinical portion done at the bedside; the other, called *science,* is done in the laboratory.

The terms of this settlement have been comfortably accepted by leaders in medical education, research, and practice. Their acceptance of the partition has led to the current fashion of making the words *research* and *science* synonymous with laboratory activity, while the words *healing* and *art* are reserved for bedside care.

As a consequence of this partition, clinicians have come to believe that clinical science consists of correlating or applying, in the care of sick people, the knowledge gained from "basic scientific research" in the laboratory, and that clinical art is the knowledge gained empirically from practical experience at the bedside. This bedside experience is seldom considered to be a scholarly activity with distinctive scientific principles of thought and action. Instead, clinicians regard their own clinical observation and reasoning as a form of artistry—an exercise in human concern and intelligence that is motivated by vocational necessity, tradition, humanism, or sentiment, but not by science. The

291

implication is that when a clinician observes and reasons with the data of the bedside, his work is mere artistic healing; when he observes and reasons with the data of the laboratory, his work is scientific research.

There are many other implications also. The partition suggests that scientific discipline is needed to manipulate laboratory objects with microtomes, centrifuges, and electrical currents, but that only artistic intuition is needed to manipulate clinical objects (i.e., patients) with diets, drugs, and surgical operations. The effects of the partition extend through every aspect of written and oral communication in clinical medicine today. Medical journals and conferences are divided into "clinical" sections and "scientific" sections, as though the contents of the two sections were mutually exclusive. A published account of events in the course of nature is given different names according to the object whose course is described. The account of the ailment of a single sick person is called a *case report;* of the metabolic enzymes of the cheek pouch of a hamster, *investigative medicine;* of the ailments of many sick persons, a *clinical series;* of the metabolic enzymes of the cheek pouches of many hamsters, *basic science.*

The schism is reflected in national meetings of the clinical research societies that so profoundly influence the content of medical activities. The leaders of these investigative groups make public addresses urging the members not to abandon their interest in sick people; the addresses are then followed by a program of research presentations that often have nothing to do with people or sickness.[36] The leaders of these societies tell us, with their hearts, that we must remain attentive to our patients, but the leaders then act, with their minds, to select a program of "clinical research" in which patients were not regarded as satisfactory sources of scientific data. The clinician is urged to listen closely to what a patient says, but only because the words are a legacy of human artistry; they have no real meaning in science. The clinician is urged to perform a thorough physical examination, but only to fulfill the old tradition of intimacy in the laying-on of hands; the physical findings can be disregarded as reliable scientific information. This partition of clinical medicine thus tells the clinician, as an act of art, to examine the patient carefully, and, as an act of science, to ignore what is learned during the examination.

Is this the kind of settlement clinicians want to live with? When we do our work at the bed that gives us our name, are we really so mentally weak, and if so, is it fair to da Vinci, Rembrandt, Mozart, and Shakespeare to call us "artists"? Do we want our clinical reasoning to oscillate schizophrenically between the "two cultures" of art and science, respected by neither? Must the clinician himself be partitioned into healer *and* scientist; can he not be a whole person who is a scientific healer or a healing scientist? Is it fair to our patients—the *raison d'être* of our work—for clinical care to be only a mystic act of intuitional judgment, imposed upon a background barrage of scientific laboratory data? Must the clinician, seeking science, always look exclusively to the laboratory; is there only art in his own work at the bedside?

In the first place, of course, there is nothing *scientifically* shameful in the label of *art*. Although mathematics is often called "queen of the sciences", most good mathematicians regard themselves as artists. They ask no questions of nature and seek no challenges in nature; mathematics works with its own imagery. The mathematician sets up rules for a game that may have nothing to do with reality; he insists only that the basic rules be internally consistent, and that the game be played thereafter with cohesive logic. The "pure" mathematician may work in such unnatural realms as Banach space and algebraic topology; he is concerned not with nature, not with observation, and certainly not with experiment. He thinks of himself as an artist, and may sometimes lament that his work is "soiled by practical application" [163] in science.

If mathematicians are proud to be artists, clinicians should surely not feel degraded by the name. No, the objection to the label of *art* for clinical work is not because of any pejorative scientific connotation, but because the label is inaccurate. Nothing done with nature can be all *art* or all *science*. Everything that man conceives and produces with the entities of nature is inevitably, simultaneously a mixture of art and science. There is "science" in art, and "art" in science.

In the realm of art, "science" is used when a painter combines selected colors to make a specific shade or plans the angles of spatial perspective; when a composer of music apportions the timing of each measure or chooses notes to fit the range of his selected instruments; and when a writer obeys established rules of grammar or applies acknowledged principles of style. In the realm of science, "art" is used as the skill that handles delicate living tissues, as the intuition that converts serendipity into insight, as the imagination that senses excitement in the midst of drab routine, and as the esthetic taste that brings elegance to the conception, execution, evaluation, and communication of experiments.

In getting, organizing, and expressing the observations of biologic science, clinicians and laboratory workers constantly make use of art. In getting data, a clinician uses a skillful art for examining a patient, just as a laboratory worker uses an analogous art for calming a rabbit, injecting the tail vein of a rat, suspending the bladder of a toad, or cutting the sections to be photographed through an electron microscope. In organizing data, the clinician needs artistic taste to design an important therapeutic experiment, just as a laboratory worker's artistic flair will determine whether his idea is brilliant or pedestrian, and his experiment an elucidation of nature or a compendium of trivia. In expressing data, both the clinician and the laboratory worker need artistry with words to create an exciting literature of communicated science, rather than an excreted litany of compiled statistics.

If "art" and "science" differ, the difference is *not* in such human attributes as perception, wisdom, imagination, and discipline. The difference is in the materials and methods. "Art" and "science" have overt disparities in 1) the type of raw material, 2) the way the raw material is verified, 3) the arrangement of the material, 4) the way in which the arrangement is preserved, and 5) the reproducibility of both the material and the arrangement.

1) In the arts, the raw material consists of such entities as colored pigments, musical sounds, and words. In the sciences, the raw material consists of observations made upon substances or phenomena.

2) The artist either receives his material already verified, by manufacturers of colored pigments or musical equipment, or he can easily verify it from color charts, tuning devices, or dictionaries. The scientist must develop his own special methods and equipment for verifying the primary observations.

3) In the arts, the arrangement of raw material creates a painting, symphony, or poem. In the sciences, the arrangement creates the design and interpretation of an experiment.

4) In the arts, the finished arrangement is preserved as a canvas, musical score, or manuscript; the artist "preserves" as he creates, and the raw material, which can usually be recognized in the final product or duplicated whenever necessary, need seldom be saved. In the sciences, the finished arrangement is preserved as measurements, symbols, tabulations, graphs, or other analyses and syntheses in which the original observations are often no longer maintained. Since the observed entity may not be easy to duplicate, and may not be recognizable after the observations are arranged, the scientist must attempt

to preserve it, either by keeping all or part of what was observed, or by saving descriptions of what could not be kept.

5) A creative artist seldom wants an exact reproduction of his initial arrangement of raw material, but he can easily achieve it, if he wishes, by copying the existing arrangement. For a scientist, the ability to reproduce the arrangement is obligatory, and requires careful attention to the manner in which the work is conceived, conducted, and reported.

These features of verification, preservation, and reproducibility provide the confirmation which, although relatively unimportant in the arts, is a *sine qua non* of science. Without significant problems in confirmability, the artist is free to concentrate his major creative efforts on designing the arrangement of his raw material. The scientist's creative efforts, however, must include not only design of arrangements, but also the establishment of techniques for verifying, preserving, and reproducing both the raw material and the arrangements.

Despite these fundamental distinctions in confirmability of raw material and arrangement, the arrangement itself—the design—is often regarded as the main difference between the arts and the sciences. Compared with the precision and reasoning of scientific procedures, the creative design of work in the arts is usually more intuitive than rational, more imaginative than disciplined, and more a product of esthetics than of logic. Yet this division of cognitive processes is never absolute, since all works of art must contain elements of "science", and all works of science, elements of "art". Each activity contains different proportions of these elements, but always has mixtures of both types. Moreover, a painter, composer, or writer does not become an *artist,* nor does a physicist, biochemist, or clinician become a *scientist,* merely because of the medium in which he works. A productively creative act of *art* or *science* must be conceived, designed, and executed with the intuition and rationality, the imagination and discipline, the esthetics and logic that are both "art" and "science". Without intuition, imagination, or esthetics, the "scientist" is a dullard. Without rationality, discipline, or logic, the "artist" is a dawdler.

Clinical medicine, therefore, like most other human activities, is an indivisible mixture of both art and science. In clinical medicine, the raw material consists of observations made upon sick people; the arrangement of the observations creates experiments in the identification and management of human ailments; the arrangement and the observations are preserved as data entered in clinicians' memories, medical records, clinical publications, libraries, and other storehouses of information; the arrangement is reproduced when the stored information is applied in the care of a new patient.

These aspects of material and method pose major difficulties in the confirmability of clinical work. The observations the clinician makes at the bedside are seldom verified, and the actual entities he observes—the symptoms, signs, and personal attributes of sick people —cannot be preserved. The clinician's arrangement of the material— the rational human judgment with which he interprets the observations—is seldom organized in a way that is specific, precise, preservable, and reproducible.

These impediments, which are inherent in the use of human beings as both the observers and the observed, often make clinical medicine seem to be neither an art nor a science, but a mystique. In the ability to reproduce its rational arrangements, clinical medicine seems inferior to most sciences; in the ability to preserve and verify its raw material, clinical medicine (along with many sciences) is inferior to the arts.

During the past few decades, many traditional deficiencies in the arrangement of clinical experiments have been improved by advances in modern technology. The availability of roentgenography, endoscopy, biopsy, and laboratory tests has made pathologic diagnosis more accurate than ever before, and mechanisms of disease better understood. The refinements of modern pharmacology and surgery have provided both specificity and potency for the maneuvers used in treatment. Although these powerful new modes of therapy are still applied with persistent doubts, dissensions, and conflicts about when and how to use them, these intellectual defects can be helped by the rational techniques of judgmental analysis suggested earlier in this book.

No matter what rational and other improvements are given to the *arrangement* of data, however, there still remains the fundamental problem of the data—the basic clinical observations of the bedside. Modern technology has also helped many of these observations, making them verifiable and permanent. In the direct examination of patients, clinicians have been assisted and sometimes supplanted by inanimate devices that have no subjective variability and that produce their evidence as permanent documents. An electrocardiogram, for example, indicates cardiac arrhythmias better than a clinician's palpation of pulse, and leaves a formal tracing for the record. The sugary sweetness of urine, once assessed only by the taste buds of the clinician's tongue, can now be measured simply and chemically by dropping a tablet or dipping a stick into the urine. Many other bedside observations, however, have not yet been removed from the clinician's domain, and still others cannot be removed. The more distinctly human the phenomenon, the more necessary is a human observer to discern the phenomenon adequately. Whatever can be distinguished only by human speech, sight, smell, touch, hearing, taste, movement, and cerebration cannot be discerned by inanimate devices, which lack the perception of human sensory organs and the ingenuity of a human brain.

As long as clinicians continue to treat sick people, many entities unique to people will continue to require observation and assessment by clinicians. Yet, surrounded by a world of scientific standardization and precision, the clinician continues to get his primary data—the basic observations of the bedside—by the same unstandardized, imprecise methods he has always used. The modern clinician may have become even worse than his ancestors in his bedside observational techniques, because his attention is so often diverted to data observed in the laboratory.

If the irreplaceable clinical material of the bedside is a sick person, then the irreplaceable equipment for observing a sick person is a clinician. Many contemporary functions of this human observational equipment are antiquated, defective, and performed with built-in sources of error. The contemporary clinician needs a complete reappraisal of the techniques with which he exercises the skill that distinguishes him from all other artists, biologists, and scientific scholars: the ability to examine a sick person and to reason with the information thereby obtained.

The next few chapters of this book are devoted to the problems of making, verifying, and preserving the primary observations of clinical examination—to the art and science with which clinicians acquire the fundamental data of clinical medicine. As an observer of human beings and human reactions, the clinician can benefit from any inanimate device that improves his sensory acuity. But he must first recognize that he is a talented, effective, and unique apparatus for perceiving the attributes that distinguish people from each other, from animals, and from all other objects of investigation. To advance art and science in clinical examination, the equipment a clinician most needs to improve is himself.

17. Art in Clinical Examination

The art of clinical examination comes from attitudes and qualities that are neither obtained nor easily detected by scientific procedures: the clinician's awareness of people and of human needs; his ability to temper the rational aspects of his work with a tolerant acceptance of the irrationalities of mankind; his perception of faith, hope, charity, love, and other elements of human spirit and human emotion. These properties of care and of compassion, although sometimes dismissed as *merely* "bedside manner", are the fundamental and most important tools of any clinician. With them, he can often give healing or comfort where science fails or does not exist. Without them, his science is unsatisfactory, no matter how excellent.

The *what* of clinical science is provided by the clinician's observations and subsequent reasoning. The *how* of clinical art depends on the human intelligence and concern with which those scientific activities are performed. One of the main purposes of improving science in clinical examination, and of transmitting the improved science in clinical training, is to separate the false art from the true. The clinician who becomes adept at scientific clinical examination and reasoning may no longer need to preserve irrational barricades of the intellect to defend his old "art" against apparent assaults from the new "science". As he begins to improve the way he works scientifically, he can also improve the highest human aspects of his work: the artistry with which it is done.

Although the art of clinical examination cannot be demonstrated or evaluated by ordinary logical analyses, certain aspects of the artistry can be improved by increased attention to the way they are taught and performed in contemporary medicine.

HISTORY-TAKING

History-taking, the most clinically sophisticated procedure of medicine, is an extraordinary investigative technique: in few other forms of scientific research does the observed object talk. The acquisition of data by this verbal process is far more complex than by the techniques of physical examination or of laboratory tests, and the function of the history-taking apparatus cannot be learned from didactic lectures or textbooks. The student physician must be able to see and hear the subtle exchange of information in the intricate human relationship between patient and clinician. Yet history-taking is demonstrated to students less often than almost any other technologic aspect of the medical curriculum.

Described briefly in textbooks that concentrate on "physical diagnosis", and taught to medical students at a time when they can least comprehend clinical subtleties, history-taking usually remains untaught and infrequently demonstrated thereafter. The student is often left to learn its structure from a printed outline, its content from his growing knowledge of medicine, and its skillful application from random observation of diverse performances by house officers. At bedside teaching rounds, attending physicians seldom give prominent display to their talents in history-taking lest too much time be taken from scientific contemplation of the data. The student is thus often taught what to do with the evidence, but not how to get it.

The art and science of history-taking are symbiotic: the form, content, and skills of the procedure are therefore best shown simultaneously. Yet modern academic physicians often ignore this concurrence, by discussing scientific content without considering the form and skills with which the questions are asked. Many psychiatrists teach the humanistic form and skills of an interview but neglect the scientific features of the content. These two separate approaches tend to fragment the patient into a "soma", attended by one group of doctors, and a "psyche", attended by another. In such approaches, the physician deals with the disease, the psychiatrist deals with the person, and neither deals with the combination of disease and person that constitutes a patient.

The form, content, and skills of history-taking must be demonstrated, explicitly and concomitantly, by clinicians who apply the science while illustrating the art. Only from suitable examples can students learn the integration of art in the scientific human apparatus that acquires the data of a medical history.

PHYSICAL EXAMINATION

CONCERN FOR THE PATIENT

A vanishing aspect of art in physical examination, particularly at modern academic centers, is concern for the patient's welfare or comfort during the procedure.

At the beginning of the individual examination, patients are often not properly introduced to the examiner or told what he proposes to do. Examinations on open wards may be conducted without the closing of curtains at potentially embarrassing times. Painful regions are sometimes manipulated thoughtlessly. Rectal examinations, and otoscopic or other endoscopic procedures, are occasionally performed as though they were attacks on a target instead of gentle entrances into delicate orifices. The pharynx is sometimes inspected with the stick placed posteriorly on the tongue in positions where discomfort or gagging is inevitable. No effort may be made to warm the cold metal of the stethoscope, or the cold hands of the physician, before touching the patient's body. A patient who is asked no questions in the "grand rounds" of a medical center may be asked to travel long distances for the audience merely to have a brief glimpse of him; or, disrobed, he may sit shivering on the unheated "stage" of the amphitheatre.

In addition to the defects in these general procedures of clinical examination and demonstration, several other unfortunate customs have become prevalent in the ordinary bedside teaching rounds that are the mainstay of clinical instruction. The rounds were originally intended to be a walk from one bed to another—a "round"—in which the attending physician reviewed the care being given to each patient on the service. This tradition, which still prevails at many institutions, maintains rounds as a way of checking each patient, and maintains the patient as the focal point of the procedure. At many other institutions today, however, these routine rounds have become a miniature version of "grand rounds": the session is devoted only to two or three patients, selected as "interesting" cases of disease, and most of the discussion takes place, away from the bedside, in a conference room.

The examination of each patient, whenever possible, is a critical aspect of ordinary teaching rounds. To reject certain patients as "uninteresting" implies that rounds are intended to deal with diseases, not people, and with topics that intrigue doctors, not problems that bother patients. The patient with an "uninteresting" disease may be just as ill and distressed, is just as much hospitalized, and, as a sick person, is just as interesting as any other patient. An attending physician who cannot find something interesting in every sick person should re-evaluate the incentives that led him into clinical medicine and clinical teaching. If rounds are confined to patients with the esoteric and often hopelessly tragic diseases that are "interesting" to house officers, the medical students may get a grotesque picture of human ailments. After such distorted medical instruction, the student may emerge a connoisseur of rarities in disease, but ignorant of commonplace problems of sick people.

In recent years, as small conference rooms have become ubiquitously available in teaching hospitals, the discussion of the patient is often conducted away from the bedside. The conference room is excellent for many aspects of clinical instruction: the attending physician can ask questions, make comments, and discuss topics that may be unsuitable for the patient to hear, or that might jeopardize the patient's relationship with the house staff doctor or medical student who is interrogated and criticized during the instruction. The conference room is often used excessively, however, to produce rounds that are either "abstract" or "veterinary".

"Abstract" rounds are totally confined to the conference room. In this situation, which has become particularly prevalent as "scientific" full-time clinical investigators assume increasing responsibility for "bedside" teaching, the attending physician does not see the patient at all. The patient's history and physical findings are reported in the conference room by a student or house officer, and the teaching discussion begins immediately afterward. This abstract type of teaching —bedside rounds *sine* bedside—is detrimental to science as well as to art in clinical medicine. Only a clinician who has no scientific respect for his own observational capacities would rely exclusively on reports from other observers when he can so conveniently examine the patient himself.

In the "veterinary" situation, the patient's clinical account is presented in the conference room; the attending physician, surrounded by the entourage of trainees, then goes to the patient's bed to check the physical findings; the examination is performed in a silence broken only by a few words of direction to the patient; immediately afterward, the entourage departs, in an aura of sagacity, and returns to the conference room for the discussion. The patient is left behind, flustered and often frightened by the lack of any truly human communication. He has, like a caged animal, been removed from the cage, examined, and put back, completely according to the whims and convenience of the animal keeper. The patient has been used as a disease for instruction, and has been observed without being considered.

This dehumanized approach to ordinary teaching rounds is often excused by the belief that any discussion conducted in front of the patient may be harmful to him. The clinician who does not hesitate to use drugs and surgery that may produce many adverse complications is reluctant to use words because he fears their toxic effect. To treat the patient as a veterinary object is a confession of clinical and pedagogic failure: the clinician confesses that he does not know how to talk to people without disturbing them, and that he does not know how to regulate the contents of the discussion he leads. An attending physician who conducts such veterinary rounds does a disservice to students, medicine, and himself, as well as to patients. For students, he suggests the humanistically contemptuous attitude that patients have no intelligence beyond the animal. For the general public, he permits an increase of the belief, now unfortunately too well disseminated, that doctors are interested in only disease, not sick people. For himself, he allows his own clinical ability to remain undeveloped or to wither.

A patient usually regards the attending physician as a consultant; the patient expects and deserves some comment beyond a brief examination and an abrupt departure. A few pertinent remarks should always be made to the patient at the end of the examination, and—with appropriate safeguards—a small part or all of the teaching discussion can be conducted at the bedside. The art of bedside teaching rounds is contained not in the particular techniques of pedagogy, but in the management of a discussion that avoids psychic trauma to the patient. To prevent the patient from being disturbed by thoughtless remarks, the attending physician must insist on selective discretion in the topics to be pursued at the bedside; on appropriate circumlocutions for what the patient (or nearby patients) will overhear; on respectful attention to the sensibility of the clinical trainee whose performance may be questioned; and on careful re-assurance to the patient before, during, and after the rounds.

There is no single formula for prescribing either the optimal contents of routine teaching rounds or the proportionate allocation of time at bedside or in conference room. The conference room is desirable for certain discussions "in depth", and sometimes mainly to allow everyone to sit down for a physical rest from the standing and walking. The one element that cannot be omitted from the prescription, however, is concern for the patient. He must be seen during the rounds and he is their main purpose; the educational aspects of the procedure are perverted if the teaching, however excellent, does not deal with the patient or his problems. The patient is neither a disease to be discussed, nor a showcase of pathologic interest, nor a dispassionate bystander. He is a sick person in the alien environment of the hospital, disturbed by his illness and involved in it at least as much as the doctors. He is anxious to know what is happening, entitled to find out, and generally able to make helpful contributions to all aspects of his clinical management. Whether the teaching rounds be conducted mostly at the bedside or in the conference room, the failure to give adequate concern to the patient is detrimental to the art of medical education and of patient care.

Concern for the patient, not only in physical examination and in teaching rounds, but in all aspects of everything done to and with him, has vital scientific importance as well as its traditional obvious humanistic purpose. A patient will talk more freely, and thus provide better data, to a sympathetic clinician. An out-patient in a long-term study is likely to continue his participation and repeated visits to the clinic (or other medical setting) if he believes that the investigators care for *him*, as well as for his data. If he fails to sense human concern, he will often stop coming, and the absence of his data may be scientifically deleterious to the total investigation.

FOCUS AND EMPHASIS IN TEACHING

A separate aspect of art in physical examination is the way the basic elements are taught. Many contemporary courses in "physical diagnosis" emphasize the "diagnosis" rather than the "physical". The young medical student emerges knowing the significance of a diastolic murmur, basilar râles, retinal exudate, a large spleen, or a swollen joint, but often cannot distinguish the specific noises, sights, or tactile sensations that indicate these entities. Although the physiologic explanations and diagnostic implications of physical findings are important background in the instruction, the main purpose of the elementary course is for the student to learn to identify physical signs precisely and reliably. He has several additional years of clinical training for development of his deductive reasoning, and he learns neither evidence nor inference well if his initial instruction is devoted mainly to inference.

In teaching the acquisition of physical evidence, instructors should emphasize signs and procedures that are most important and meaningful in modern medicine. Students are misled and confused by instruction that does not distinguish between critically useful examination procedures and those that are only of traditional or of academic interest. The limited time available for instruction should not be wasted on tracheal tugs, amphoric breathing, and other esoterica of a departed medical era. In the modern atmosphere of diagnostic and scientific precision, the student should learn to be particularly adept and precise in those aspects of physical examination that provide evidence either unobtainable, or superior to that obtainable, by other methods of examination.

Physical observations yield unique types of evidence in appraising functions of the patient as an entire organism and in identification of disorders in skin, eyes, ears, nose, mouth, pharynx, lymph nodes, joints, bones, muscles, genitalia, abdominal and pelvic viscera, peripheral blood vessels, and neurologic system. In the *diagnostic* assessment of pulmonary anatomy, the precision of evidence obtained by physical examination is usually inferior to that of roentgenograms. Nevertheless, the physical data of pulmonary examination are often particularly pertinent and useful for evaluating *treatment.* Changes in râles, wheezes, thoracic dullness, cyanosis, and respiratory distress can all be indexes of therapeutic response not discernible by radiographic or other techniques.

Physical examination is inferior to roentgenograms for observing heart size and to electrocardiograms for cardiac arrhythmias. For these particular assessments, physical findings are of academic interest but do not yield the scientific precision of the other tests that are now almost routine. Many other aspects of cardiac examination, however, receive their only, or their best, appraisals from physical procedures. The palpation of a thrill or of a parasternal heave can often provide evidence of valvular deformity, septal defect, or right ventricular enlargement that cannot be discerned from an electrocardiogram or from a standard posteroanterior roentgenogram. In the appraisal of cardiac murmurs, the clinician's auscultation is the best available simple technique for performing a clinical "biopsy" on valvular and septal defects. The ordinary phonocardiographic equipment in current use (as discussed later) is helpful in the timing of low-pitched noises and in various other properties of sound, but cannot record certain high-pitched noises, distinguish nuances of sonorous quality, or produce standardized microphonic pressure for the critical discernment of thoracic sites of maximal acoustic loudness.

For teaching contemporary physical examination, therefore, the instructors of the neophyte physician should reappraise the techniques, evaluate the purposes of the data, and focus upon those procedures that are most pertinent and useful. Exotic and obsolete techniques, and those yielding evidence better obtained by other means, should be eliminated or relegated to subsequent and specialized training.

*   *   *

All these aspects of clinical and pedagogic artistry can flourish, however, only if there is a reason for them. Just as a laboratory investigator does not bother to learn the artful operation of a mechanical technique that gives him scientifically valueless data, the young or old clinician will give little attention to an examining art perpetuated only by tradition or sentiment. To improve the artistry of clinical examination, clinicians must first recognize that the data have a scientific function and can be given scientific quality. Without this recognition, clinicians will have no real incentive for acquiring the data and no real purpose for improving the methods of acquisition.

The scientific function of clinical data has been demonstrated in the preceding chapters of this book; symptoms and signs are not just clues to pathologic diagnosis, but are crucial evidence for designing, executing, and appraising the experiments of clinical therapy. The scientific quality of the basic data, however, still remains to be considered. No matter how artfully the data are acquired, they cannot fulfill their scientific functions if they are facts, but not truth.

18. Science in Clinical Examination: Objectivity and Precision

Among the many traditional concepts cited earlier as barriers to clinical science, the one that most affects a clinician when he acts as an observer is his frequent inability to use numbers for expressing the observations. In contemporary thought, numbers are generally accorded the magical aura and quantified garb of science, but words are usually regarded as imperfect and nude.

A number, of course, does not arise spontaneously. In order to get a number as the result of a dimensional measurement, an observer must prepare some type of measuring system, use it, and interpret the actual entity he observes. As the end product of these activities, a number will be only as good as the way the observer made the system ready to work, and the way he obtained and presented the result. If these aspects of the measuring system are managed scientifically, the number will be accurate and significant; if not, the number may be worthless, no matter how many digits it contains.

Since the operation of the measuring system, rather than the resulting numerical expression, is the hallmark of scientific assessment, an analysis of these dimensional operations is prerequisite to a clinician's attempt to make science out of words.

We begin our preparation of a dimensional measuring system by trying to make it objective—undistorted by any subjective attributes of its human operation. For example, if a ruler is used to measure the length of a line, we want to be sure that the user will not distort the results by bending the ruler, by placing it improperly, or by misreading the numbers on the scale.

306

Next, we try to make the observations precise, both qualitatively and quantitatively. Qualitative precision depends on a correct identification (or qualification) of the observed entity. Thus, if we want to measure a single line among a group of many lines, we must make sure we have picked out the correct line. Moreover, we must use the correct measuring device; a thermometer and a wrist-watch both have numerical scales, but are clearly not satisfactory for measuring length of a line. Quantitative precision depends on a detailed specification of the selected entity; the more or better the details we can specify, the more quantitatively precise will be the characterization.

In the numerical specifications of a dimension, these quantitative details are called "significant figures". Thus, the number *3* has only one significant figure and is a quantitatively imprecise expression for π, the ratio of the circumference and diameter of a circle. The number *3.14,* with three significant figures, is more precise and is satisfactory for many scientific calculations using π; the number *3.14159* is even more precise. The number of significant figures our ruler can give us depends on the fine detail of its scalar delineations. If the unit interval between lines is a millimeter, the ruler is more quantitatively precise than one in which the unit interval is a centimeter.

We must also decide about how much precision we want, in both the qualitative and quantitative aspects of the assessment. This decision depends upon the purpose of the measurement. For example, Benedict's reagent is qualitatively imprecise for measuring glycosuria, because the chemical reacts with any reducing substance in the urine—certain amino acids, galactose, and many sugars other than glucose. Nevertheless, although glucose is not the only substance identified, the reagent is satisfactory for most routine medical assessments of glycosuria. In quantitative precision, a ruler scaled in units of miles might be excellent for measuring the distance between cities but unsatisfactory for height of people; a ruler scaled in units of millimeters would be too imprecise for measuring the size of a red blood cell, and excessively precise for interurban distances.

For our next step, in interpreting the observations, we want to know about the consistency, uniformity, and reliability of the system. To obtain consistency, we want the system to give the same result each time we use it for the same measurement. Do the lines of our ruler's scale remain unchanged between one measurement and the next? Are lines of the same incremental distinction placed equidistant from each other? When we read the scale, do we assign the same values to increments of equal magnitude, or do we vary our values with each new measurement?

For uniformity, we want the system to be homogeneous in its results. Are all the units in our ruler's scale expressed in terms of length, or are some of them units of weight, temperature, or time? If the units are all expressed in terms of length, are they the same throughout the scale, or are some of the units angstroms, others millimeters, and yet others inches?

Finally, we want the system to be reliable. It may be objective, precise, consistent, and uniform, but is it accurate? Has it given us a correct measurement? Would the measurement we got with this ruler be the same as that obtained with other comparable rulers, or with a specially tested ruler supplied by the Bureau of Standards?

In all these basic procedures of scientific measurement, the number itself was unimportant. The number was the result of the procedures, not the constituent. The scientific constituents of the measurement were objective preparation, delineated precision, and standardized interpretation.

Each of these scientific constituents of measurement is available to a clinician performing the observations of the bedside. He may use words instead of lines for his "scale", and he may express the results as symptoms and signs, rather than numbers, but he can make his verbal "measurements" with the same basic scientific procedures used to obtain numerical dimensions. For objective preparation, the clinician must try to remove his own prejudices and preconceptions before he observes. For delineated precision, he must make maximal use of the unique observational capacities of his sensory organs. For standardized interpretation, he must apply the intelligence of his human brain with logic and order.

Unlike other types of scientific equipment, a clinician is not easily tested, compared, or calibrated in the act of getting clinical evidence. He can markedly improve the scientific quality of his performance, however, if he is willing to recognize the importance of what he does, to acknowledge himself as the apparatus to be improved, and to revise many minor and some major aspects of the way he works.

The rest of this chapter is devoted to methods of improving the objectivity with which a clinician begins the examination, and the precision with which he makes the observations. The problems of standardized interpretation will be discussed in the next chapter.

OBJECTIVITY

HISTORY-TAKING

A major source of error in history-taking is the bias or preconception that a clinician brings to his observations when he expects each instance of a disease to behave in a "typical" way. Since every pathologic entity (or disease) has the complex clinical spectrum discussed earlier, clinicians will frequently encounter patients from diverse portions of this spectrum. When the disease in a particular patient is asymptomatic, atypical, or discovered accidentally, the clinician must beware that his anticipation of the more common "typical" clinical events does not evoke distortion of past or present symptoms to fill in the gaps. Streptococcal infections, for example, can occur without sore throat; hepatitis without jaundice; rheumatic fever without joint pain; peptic ulcer without digestive or abdominal symptoms; myocardial infarction without chest pain; and carcinoma of the lung without hemoptysis. The failure of such patients to describe "typical" symptoms is attributable to the biologic behavior of the disease, and does not necessarily indicate observational ineptness in either patient or clinician. Similarly, symptoms that are nondescript or that develop insidiously are also often due to vagaries of biologic behavior in disease; the *absence* of exact descriptions for the symptoms, or of an exact time of onset, may itself be a specific, precise property of that particular instance of the disease.

Since the main purpose of history-taking is not just a pathologic diagnosis but a distinctive classification of patients, clinicians should not develop intellectual discomfort when a disease is present without "typical" features, without specifically outlined symptoms, or without definite points of timing. These absent or indistinct data may be scientifically *exact* descriptions of the symptomatic events that classify patients whose disease has occurred in the less common portion of its total spectrum. Unless the clinician realizes that such atypical histories can be reliable, and that such apparently imprecise data can be managed scientifically, he may be dissatisfied with anything other than a history that confirms his diagnostic prejudice. He may then badger the patient with inappropriate or leading questions, and may subconsciously manipulate either the patient or the answers to extract a history that is inaccurate, but satisfying because it seems quantified and typical.

PHYSICAL EXAMINATION

Perhaps the most pernicious source of defective science in clinical medicine today is the almost total absence of objectivity in certain examinations performed by specialized consultants. The defect is present in the work of pathologists, radiologists, and electrocardiographers, as well as in examinations done by clinical specialists in such procedures as cardiac auscultation, abdominal palpation, ophthalmoscopy, and endoscopy. Elements of subjectivity are always present in all these examinations because they are done by a human observer, but the "objectivity" of the observer depends on the state of his mind before he begins the examination.

The current custom for consultative examination is traditional, and calls for the referring physician to give the consultant a complete account of the data already assembled, including all the findings and interpretations of other observers. When a patient or substance is to be re-examined, the consultant can look at records that tell him what he or others have previously found and thought. The consultant receives all this information beforehand; then, with his objectivity destroyed by what he has just learned, he performs his examination.

This unscientific sequence of examination has no justification except the inertia of tradition, and, perhaps, some saving of time. In exchange for the time saved, however, clinicians preserve and encourage unwarranted complacency, unverified dogma, and self-perpetuating error. The destruction of a consultant's objectivity is not necessary for a satisfactory examination, and can be prevented by a simple change in the sequence of the examining procedure. The present order is as follows: 1) the consultant is told what region to examine; 2) he is told what other observers, including possibly himself, have previously found there or elsewhere; 3) he examines the region and forms an impression; and 4) he states his conclusion. This sequence can be made objective by altering the order of steps 2 and 3. The new process would be as follows: 1) the consultant is told what region to examine, but not the previous findings; 2) he examines the region and forms a preliminary impression; 3) he receives all the other previous information and may then, if he wishes, re-examine the region or change his preliminary impression; and 4) he states his conclusion.

The consultant's final opinion should always incorporate the total available data, but his first impression as he examines crucial physical findings (or roentgenographic shadows or pathologic tissue) should be formed objectively. To save the time of a detailed search through many unimportant regions, specialist clinicians and necropsy pathologists should be told which sites require particular attention; radiologists, surgical pathologists, and electrocardiographers already have their attention directed to specific regions by the requisitions or material submitted to them. Except for an indication of what to examine, a specialized consultant should avoid learning any other information until he forms his first impression. In many instances, the associated clinical history should also be initially withheld, since it can often create bias as great as a knowledge of previous physical (or other) findings. For example, a consultant auscultator cannot give wholly objective initial appraisal to a systolic murmur of uncertain origin if he knows that the patient has had rheumatic fever or that the heart is enlarged on the roentgenogram; a spleen is often noted as "enlarged" by an observer who has been told the patient has bacterial endocarditis, and as "not palpable" by another examiner deprived of previous clinical information; an objective ophthalmoscopist may consider white spots in the fundus to be "drusen", but might call them "exudate" if first informed that the patient has diabetes mellitus; radiologists and surgical pathologists will sometimes reverse their assessments of the same shadows and tissues, if provided with two different clinical histories beforehand.

A consultant examiner should always receive all additional information before he forms his final opinion—but his first act of looking, listening, or feeling, and his transient interpretation of the initial observations, should be objective. If the consultant is an auscultator, he should first judge the noise as a noise, uninfluenced by the associated symptoms, roentgenographic findings, or opinions of other auscultators. If he is an ophthalmologist asked to examine the retina, he should first look at what is in the retina, not at the requisition or note that tells him the ocular or systemic diagnosis. If he is a roentgenologist, he should first judge the visual entities that he sees in the film or screen; a knowledge of the non-radiologic findings may distort the "insight" with which he looks. If he is a surgical pathologist, he should first judge tissue as tissue, not on the basis of clinical evidence or surgical anatomic descriptions. Having made his first decision objectively, a consultant can then obtain, and, if desirable, apply, all the other ancillary data; he can optionally examine the original entity again and can alter his initial impression; then, he can make the final decision that he submits to his colleagues.

The first complete clinical examination that a patient receives cannot be done "blindly", and needs no immediate changes in its performance. The attainment of objectivity by the subsequent consultant examiners can be achieved so easily, however, that it requires only the intellectual effort. A consultant who says he is not biased by advance information is actually betraying his bias.[164]

PRECISION

Many painstakingly detailed clinical observations are scientifically defective not because they are imprecise, but because they are biased. If the subjective bias of the observer can be removed or minimized, precise clinical observations can often be as exact and accurate as the dimensional data of the laboratory.

The basic elements of clinical observation are the sensations perceived by patient, by clinician, or by both. These elemental sensations are then converted, by subsequent descriptions and interpretations, into the products of clinical examination: the data that are called *symptoms* and *signs*. This observational process of converting bedside sensation into clinical data begins with two descriptive techniques. First, the sensation must be properly noted or qualified, so that subsequent descriptions will focus on the correct sensation. Second, the qualified sensation must be specified with enough descriptive detail to distinguish it from all other types of sensation.

Thus, the clinical counterpart of qualitative precision in measurement is effective *communication* of the sensation; the clinical counterpart of quantitative precision (the "significant figures" of the measurement) is *specification* of detail.

COMMUNICATION

History-Taking

As information given by one human being to another, the sensations recorded as *symptoms* are processed in five ways before emerging as units of scientific data: 1) perception by patient, 2) description by patient to clinician, 3) perception by clinician, 4) interpretation and designation by clinician, and 5) inscription by clinician in medical record. At each step in these procedures, errors of omission or commission can occur inadvertently or deliberately, irregularly or constantly. The clinician's questions may be scientifically designed, but the way he asks them—the attitudes, approaches, and vocabulary he brings to his relationship with the patient—may evoke incomplete, inaccurate, or evasive answers. The questions may be well designed and well asked but the responses may be scientifically useless if they are not true and if the clinician fails to recognize the patient's unreliability. The questions may be good and the responses offered by the patient may be reliable, but the clinician may distort the evidence as he perceives, designates, or records it.

A crucial feature of the oral and written information is the terms used in the exchange. Unless people mean the same thing when they talk to each other, accurate communication is impossible. Yet many clinicians express certain sensations, or accept and record sensations expressed by patients, in symptomatic designations that are "standard" or traditional, but ambiguous and imprecise. Does the symptom of *heartburn,* for example, designate a pressure or a gnawing sensation; is it substernal, precordial, or epigastric? Is *palpitation* a slow pounding, a rapid pounding, a mere awareness of heartbeat, the sensation of a skipped beat, or a fluttery abdominal feeling? Does *fatigue* mean a weakness of muscles, shortness of breath, or the absence of desire for physical activity? Does *diarrhea* refer to loose stools, many stools, or both—and *constipation* to hard stools, few stools, or both? Does *anorexia* signify lack of desire for food, lack of appealing food, or unwillingness to eat lest the intake of food be followed by discomfort? And what does *indigestion* mean? Each of these illustrative terms is a commonly stated symptom; each is frequently used and recorded with no further description; and each can have the different meanings and implications just cited.

The problems of communication are even greater when the symptoms refer to psychic rather than somatic sensations. Such symptomatic designations as *nervous, high-strung, tense, upset, anxious, hostile, agitated,* and *depressed* are constantly used by both patients and clinicians to describe certain sensations. Yet no two people may mean exactly the same thing when they use these words. For example, a patient may dislike the world, his employer, his family, his wife, or the doctor who is examining him, but he may be called *hostile* regardless of the particular object that receives his antipathy and regardless of the possible justification for his feeling. Not a single one of the foregoing psychic terms represents an actual entity that is experienced by a patient or observed by a clinician. Each of these symptomatic designations is either an inference deduced from certain observations, or a label applied to a particular sensation or cluster of sensations. Although no standard criteria exist either for applying the labels or for making the inferences, these symptomatic designations are often used by clinicians as though they were the direct, primary vocabulary of observed evidence. Without precision in the fundamental terms of communication, none of the subsequent interpretations and classifications by psychiatrists can have scientific reliability. Yet a precise use of the vocabulary of human sensations—the words that are the basic elements of any concepts of diagnosis, pathogenesis, and therapy of psychiatric disease—has received almost no attention in the contemporary "basic research" devoted to mental illness.

In all of these somatic and psychic difficulties in precise communication, the problem is that the name of the *symptom* is ambiguous. Each person who uses the name may be designating a different sensation or group of sensations. To avoid ambiguity when a patient uses such terms, clinicians should always ask the patient to describe the particular sensations that are involved. When the terms are used for communication among clinicians, criteria must be established to indicate the sensations designated by each symptomatic label.

A different type of ambiguity arises from certain symptoms whose names clearly denote a particular sensation, but may not indicate what the patient feels, or the location or the circumstances in which the sensation occurs. Such ambiguities are frequent for such symptomatic designations as *chest pain, dyspnea, orthopnea,* and *backache.* Clinicians concentrating on these terms of symptomatic vocabulary may either distort or fail to obtain the patient's true perception of his own sensations. For example, a patient may be marked negative for angina pectoris because he denies having had *chest pain;* when interrogated in different terms, however, he may readily acknowledge that exertion produces a substernal "discomfort" or "funny feeling". A patient may be considered *dyspneic* not because he is truly short of breath, but because pain on inspiration makes him breathe shallowly. Without elevating his upper torso in bed, a patient may be deemed *orthopneic* because he likes to sleep with two pillows under his head. The non-specific designation of *backache* may be given to pain in the scapula, upper thorax, lower thorax, costovertebral area, or lumbosacral region because the clinician has failed to note the exact localization of the symptoms.

These problems can be solved if clinicians insist that the basic elements of medical communication be direct descriptions of sensation, and that the words be understood by each user. A too-hurried interview, a question or an answer phrased in jargon or in ambiguous terms, an assumption that patients have studied medical vocabulary and that clinicians use words uniformly—all impede or prevent the transfer of critical scientific information contained in the presence, absence, or change of important symptoms.

Physical Examination

The main contemporary problem in communicating the data of physical examination is the modern clinician's misdirected preference for the nomenclature of anatomy, pathology, or physiology instead of the vocabulary of clinical observation. Clinicians do not see, feel, or hear many of the things they currently report as physical findings.

A clinician sees pallor, but may say he sees anemia; he sees tears, but may say he sees sorrow or depression; he hears a loud blowing apical systolic murmur that is transmitted to the axilla, but may say he hears mitral regurgitation; he feels a lump, but may say he feels a cancer; he percusses dullness, but may say he percusses a pleural effusion. In many other descriptive examples, clinicians have sacrificed the language and discipline of clinical observation in favor of judgmental interpretations that use the terminology of other domains. Among such examples are the use of "paralyzed", instead of "motionless", to describe a limb; "uremic", instead of "ammoniacal", to describe an odor; "pleuritic", instead of "inspiratory", to describe the timing of a pain; "dehydrated", instead of "dry", to describe skin; "inflamed", instead of "red", "hot", "swollen", or "tender" (or combinations of these), to describe a region; and "atrophic", instead of "small" (or "hypertrophic", instead of "large"), to describe a muscle.

By omitting the exact ingredients of bedside observations, clinicians cannot reproducibly describe what has been observed. Moreover, the inferences that are reported instead of evidence may sometimes be incorrect. Pallor may be due to shock, not anemia; tears may be caused by joy or by some external irritant; the systolic murmur just cited may be physiologic, not pathologic; the lump may be benign; the dullness may be due to many things other than pleural effusion. A patient may keep a limb immobile because of pain, not paralysis; a "uremic" odor may arise from urine in the bedclothes, not urea in the blood; "pleuritic" pain may come from lesions in muscle, rib, or spleen, rather than pleura; a well-hydrated patient may have dry skin; a joint may be swollen from a bursal cyst, not from inflammation; a muscle may be enlarged from inflammation or degeneration, not hypertrophy.

If the data of physical examination are to achieve the quality they must have for prognostic and therapeutic science, the observations must be communicated in terms of evidence, not inference.

SPECIFICATION

Even when qualified enough to describe the correct entity and to be understood by all users, the terms of clinical communication must include enough descriptive detail to specify all the significant properties of the entity under consideration. *Headache* and *abdominal mass,* for example, are clear and unambiguous terms, but they do not adequately delineate the entities they describe. Yet many such imprecise phrases frequently appear, without further modification, as statements of clinical observation. Clinicians who will not tolerate a laboratory report that contains an enumeration of white blood cells without a differential count, or a urinalysis without microscopic inspection of the sediment, will often accept, create, and perpetuate appalling vagueness in the description of clinical features. Some of the most frequently omitted details are listed in the sections that follow.

History-Taking

The role of the history in prognosis and therapy often does not begin until some time after the patient's initial meeting with the doctor. The standard initial history is used mainly to suggest diagnostic impressions and is usually followed by a series of tests that confirm or alter those impressions. At this juncture, with a definite or presumptive diagnosis established, the clinician must make a therapeutic decision. For this decision, a "second" or pre-therapeutic history is often necessary. The "second" history must ascertain or verify details left incomplete or omitted in the first one because the clinician was not initially aware or sure of the diagnosis later established. The additional details are needed for three different purposes: 1) to classify the patient into a clinical subgroup for which prognosis of disease can be estimated and therapy chosen; 2) to determine the symptoms (and signs) that will serve as clinical indexes of response to treatment; and 3) to confirm or expand information (such as social habits or family history) that may have been initially recorded with scant attention, but that may now be particularly germane to the established diagnosis.

Although not deliberately called a *second history,* such post-diagnostic histories are an established feature of modern medicine. A medical record with notes from different consultants will show how each consultant has obtained the additional information, pertinent to his own particular specialty, that may have been unspecified in the standard initial (or diagnostic) history. Many of the details of this information, as discussed in the next few sections, may be unimportant for purposes of pathologic diagnosis, but may be critical features of the clinical data needed for prognosis and therapy.

IATROTROPIC STIMULUS. The *iatrotropic stimulus* is the particular event or series of events that made the patient go to the doctor whose examination led to detection of the disease at its current pre-therapeutic clinical stage. The components and clinical distinctions of iatrotropic stimuli were discussed previously (in Chapters 8 and 9), and were cited for their importance in identifying patients with comparable clinical attributes.

The *exact* reason why a patient chose to seek medical aid at the time he did is important not only for taxonomic purposes of clinical classification, but also for the clinician's therapeutic relationship with the patient. When a clinician decides what to say in explaining diagnosis and care, how to say it, and whom to talk to, he must know just why the patient came to see him. Otherwise, the clinician's discussion may deal with the wrong topic, and he may sometimes talk to the wrong person. For example, to a patient with the chief complaint of headache, the clinician may report that the skull X-ray, neurologic examination, and electroencephalogram are all negative, but the patient may not find the reassurance satisfactory because his iatrotropic stimulus—the recent death of a friend with cerebral metastases—made him want a specific statement that he did not have a brain tumor. If the iatrotropic stimulus in the case just cited was anxiety of the patient's wife, rather than the patient's concern over his headache, the clinician's reassurance of "negative findings" may be inadequate unless communicated specifically to the wife as well as to the patient.

A statement of *chief complaint* is alone unsatisfactory for indicating iatrotropic stimulus, particularly when the patient is asymptomatic, when the symptoms are of long duration, or when the symptoms deal with psychic rather than somatic sensations. When a patient who says he has no significant symptoms suddenly seeks a "routine check-up" that had not been previously scheduled, the clinician must carefully rule out an iatrotropic provocation by important psychologic events or by existing symptoms that are unmentioned because the patient minimizes or fears their implications. When the symptoms are of long duration, the clinician should determine why the patient delayed seeking medical aid sooner or what additional or associated events made the patient finally decide to come in when he did. Such events may be a change in the severity of a symptom, the development of a supervening symptom previously unstated or overlooked by the patient, or a stimulus unrelated to symptoms *per se* (such as a spouse's anxiety or the death of a friend). When a patient with primarily psychic symptoms comes to a physician or psychiatrist, a crucial feature in the patient's management is the discovery of familial, occupational, or other iatrotropic stimuli that may not have been stated.

CHARACTERIZATION OF SYMPTOMATIC SENSATIONS. No clinical training is needed for merely listening to a patient talk about what bothers him. In a wholly non-directive interview, a social worker, clergyman, or newspaper reporter can get information as well as a clinician. The distinctive talent a clinician brings to medical history-taking is his ability to obtain descriptive specifications of the patient's sensations, to elicit important information not volunteered spontaneously, and to ascertain that the features a patient leaves unmentioned are indeed absent. To acquire these details, the clinician should be an active participant, not just a passive recorder, in the exchange of information. He, not the patient, has been trained to know what to look for in the history.

When two different examiners get variations in a history from the same patient, they often assume that the patient is unreliable or perverse. In many instances, however, the fault lies with the examiners, not with the patient. The differences in history may arise from many aspects of the examining procedure. Among the major sources of variability is the specificity with which details of symptoms are noted.

Every symptomatic sensation has its own particular characteristics[165] in such attributes as general description, site of maximal intensity, local region of spread, transmission to distant regions, time of onset, circumstances of onset, rapidity with which maximum severity developed, fluctuations in intensity, frequency of occurrence, and duration of each occurrence. The attributes also include severity—as manifested by the symptom's effects not just locally but on the patient's total function—and the associated features that make the symptom better or worse. Among these features can be weather, temperature, time of day, time of year, general food intake or specific food intake, respiration, movement, position, digestive or excretory functions, medications, and many different acts of the vocational and personal aspects of daily life.

Every time a clinician verbally specifies another one of these attributes, he adds a "significant figure" to the "measurement". Just as each adjacent digit of a number specifies such attributes as tenths, hundredths, and thousandths, the verbal description of a symptom specifies such attributes as location, severity, and responsive variation. These verbal descriptions can even be converted, when desired for coding purposes, into numbers. Each distinctive attribute can be assigned an individual column in a coding form, and a number for 0 to 9 can be entered according to the absence, presence, or some other distinction of that attribute. For a symptom with many different attributes, such numerical coding will produce a conglomerate integer that extends across many adjacent columns—a number with many more "significant figures" than the three traditionally obtained in most dimensional measurements. Each of those "significant figures" would be contributed by another attribute of specification, and the coded number would have the exact counterpart of quantitative precision in a dimensional measurement.

The many different attributes just listed need not be noted for many minor clinical sensations, but all of the attributes, and others not yet cited, may be necessary for a precise distinction and reproducible description of major symptoms. A notation of these many attributes may be particularly important in descriptive specifications of chest pain, headache, abdominal pain, gastrointestinal complaints, respiratory distress, aches in the joints or locomotor system, urinary symptoms, menstrual irregularities, and many other disturbed human sensations commonly encountered in clinical work. Without such specifications, a clinician may not be able to distinguish cardiac disease from lung disease, arthritis from myalgia, peptic ulcer from functional bowel distress, tension headache from migraine, and many other entities in which critical diagnostic evidence comes from symptoms. Even when other para-clinical data produce the necessary diagnostic precision, clinicians still must use symptomatic specifications in order to evaluate prognosis and therapy.

Other types of specificity are needed to document a patient's citation of weight loss, medication, "drug reactions", antecedent illnesses, and previous surgical operations. Many of these findings are often accepted as stated by the patient, and no attempt is made to list the evidence that verifies the statements.

THE SEQUENCE OF CLINICAL MANIFESTATIONS. The exact order of occurrence of symptoms and other clinical events cannot always be established for each patient, but should always be sought, and can often be obtained. In many contemporary histories, however, the sequence of manifestations is frequently unlisted or recorded too vaguely for effective use in classification of the patient's clinical state. The examiner sometimes makes no effort to determine the sequence of events, or even to time their occurrence and duration. In other instances, two events are listed as essentially contemporaneous because they happened at about the same time in the distant past, but their order of precedence is not indicated. A difference of even several days or hours in the sequence of such events as angina pectoris and dyspnea, or hemoptysis and anorexia, might be crucial evidence in classifying patients for estimation of prognosis, respectively, in myocardial infarction or in carcinoma of the lung.

THE TIMING OF MANIFESTATIONS. In an era devoted to "early" diagnosis and treatment, many clinicians often fail to elicit enough information to indicate how "early" a disease is found. The information comes from timing the duration of abnormalities in symptoms, signs, and paraclinical tests. When a symptom has a specific time of onset, its duration is easily measured. The measurement is often neglected, however, when a symptom has an insidious onset, or when the abnormality is a physical sign or a para-clinical test.

The duration of an insidious symptom can be approximated and certain time limits demarcated from determining the most recent date at which the symptom was known to be absent. This date can often be found by reference to national holidays or other public events, or to important personal occurrences (such as birthdays and anniversaries) in the patient's life. The duration of a physical abnormality can be found by consulting other clinicians (or hospitals) with records of previous examinations of the region now noted to be abnormal. For example, signs found unexpectedly by a clinician (such as elevated blood pressure, a cardiac murmur, or a prostatic nodule) or by a patient (such as a lump in the breast or a cutaneous lesion) must be further investigated by comparing results of previous examinations, if any exist, to discover how long the abnormalities have, or could have, been present. The search should go back as far as necessary to determine the nearest date on which the region was examined and found normal, and the first date on which the abnormality was detected.

Similarly, the duration of an unexpected para-clinical abnormality can be approximated from the results found at previous performances of the same test. For example, the discovery of an abnormal roentgenographic chest shadow should be checked by direct comparison with all other previous chest roentgenograms, wherever and whenever taken, to determine the time of the most recent previous film that was negative for that shadow, and the time of the film showing the shadow's earliest onset. Similar procedures should be used to check results of old tests after accidental discovery of such derangements as glycosuria, albuminuria, leukocytosis, and electrocardiographic abnormalities.

The main reason for doing complete physical examinations and para-clinical laboratory tests as a matter of "routine" is to obtain a "baseline", or to discover *unexpected* abnormalities. When negative, the routine results can be used as a reference for timing future positive findings. When positive, the results are incomplete if not timed by comparison with past examinations. The chronometry of abnormal signs and para-clinical tests, as well as the duration of symptoms, is a particularly necessary aspect of classification in comparing patients with such chronic or neoplastic diseases as diabetes mellitus, hypertension, coronary artery disease, and cancers of the lung, breast, colon, and other sites. Without such data, the clinician can never know how "early" or "late" he has found the disease.

Physical Examination

USE OF ADDITIONAL EQUIPMENT. The specificity of physical examination can be helped, when feasible, by such devices as rulers (to supply exact measurements instead of nondescript dimensions like "egg-sized" and "finger-breadths"), by color charts (to ensure that one man's *red* is not another man's *crimson*), by better stethoscopes (to eliminate defects that lie outside the clinician's ears), and by other specialized instruments such as goniometers and ocular tonometers. The rapidity of certain reflex or muscular movements can be measured, on suitable occasions, with electrophysiologic tracings instead of by naked eye. All these technologic advances, however, are peripheral to the more important central problem of how the clinician uses himself, and not just his inanimate aids.

SEPARATION OF DESCRIPTION, DESIGNATION, AND DIAGNOSIS. The main contemporary impediment to detailed specificity in physical examination is the failure of many clinicians to distinguish the three different intellectual disciplines—description, designation, and diagnosis—used for the total procedure. In description, the clinician gives an account of the sensation, substance, or phenomenon that he has actually observed. In designation, he gives a name or classification to the observed entity. In diagnosis, he indicates the anatomic or other abnormality that is responsible for the observed entity.

For example, a clinician uses inspection to describe a blanching red area on the skin, with a non-blanching darker red center; by designation, he calls it a petechia surrounded by erythema; by diagnosis, he attributes it to meningococcemia. By palpation, a clinician describes a hard, fixed, non-tender, non-fluctuant, 8- by 6-cm. lumpy mass in the neck; by designation, he calls it a group of enlarged, matted, non-inflamed lymph nodes; by diagnosis, he attributes it to Hodgkin's disease. By percussion, a clinician describes a thump less resonant than he normally expects in the lower chest; by designation, he calls it basal dullness; by diagnosis (after making other physical observations), he attributes it to a pleural effusion. By auscultation, a clinician describes a noise with various acoustic properties; by designation, he calls it an organic apical systolic murmur; by diagnosis, he attributes it to mitral regurgitation.

Clinicians often fail to distinguish the three separate acts of conceptual reasoning used for these processes, and may inadvertently combine description with designation, or may even fuse all three procedures into a single act. Such fusions obliterate precision in observation and ignore the need for criteria whenever descriptions are converted to designations, and designations to diagnoses. The consequence of the fusions is the development of physical examination by nondescript pattern (or gestalt), rather than by precise observation and specified criteria. Designatory or diagnostic gestalts are used instead of descriptions when the findings of physical examination are reported in such terms as *opening snap of mitral valve, pericardial friction rub, hypertensive retinopathy, choreiform movements, pharyngitis, pulmo-*

nary congestion, bronchospasm, diabetic ulcer, clubbing of fingers, splinter hemorrhages, hyperperistalsis, lymphadenopathy, and many others.

Almost all of these terms are designations or inferences stated mainly in the nomenclature of anatomists, pathologists, and physiologists; the terms are not descriptions of the actual evidence of clinical observers. The terms may be satisfactory for the conclusions made as designation or as diagnosis—but they do not describe what the clinical observer has seen, felt, or heard. Gestalt observations are a major source of error in physical examination and help perpetuate the errors in the clinicians who perform and teach the process. The gestalts have two outstanding scientific defects: 1) they close the observer's mind to the possibility that the described entity may represent something other than the conclusion assumed in the gestalt; 2) they prevent the clinician from recording the evidence that can help him distinguish why he was wrong if his conclusions are later found to be erroneous. If the "basic science" of the laboratory often consists of determining the molecules, atoms, or other elements that compose a biologic substance, the "molecular biology" of the bedside is based on the clinician's dissection of his observational gestalts into their fundamental elements of descriptive evidence.

In other aspects of physical examination, a clinician may avoid gestalt inferences and may report his evidence directly—but may not specify it adequately. For example, the lower margin of palpability is often used to describe enlargement of the liver, but the upper margin of dullness is omitted. A lesion may be reported at "3 o'clock" in the rectal lumen, and no indication given of whether "12 o'clock" is anterior or posterior. Judgmental terms—such as "large", "small", "severe", "soft", and "loud"—are often used without quantification or without criteria.

The replacement of clinicians by inanimate observational devices does not always solve these problems in getting clinical evidence, and may sometimes make things worse. The devices often cannot perceive, or may distort, many of the subtle, distinct characteristics of sights, noises, and tactile sensations that are discernible only by human sensory receptors. An excellent illustration of observational capacities in man versus machine is provided by contemporary problems in teaching and performing cardiac auscultation.

For cardiac auscultation, instead of concentrating on the clinical description of noises as acoustic phenomena, academic clinicians may focus on the physiologic or pathologic significance of the noises, and on apparatus for graphic illustration of the noises. Students learn about the formation of normal noises during valve closure, ventricular filling, turbulent currents, and other events of the cardiac cycle; about the formation of abnormal noises by damaged valves, congenital defects, or other lesions; and about the analysis of the visual portraits given to the noises by phonocardiographic tracings. The student is often not taught, however, to develop and standardize himself as a competent instrument for recognizing, describing, designating, and interpreting the noise as a noise. Consequently, many practicing clinicians, when tested for auscultatory skill,[3] produce mediocre or poor performances with the stethoscope that—probably more than any other single instrument—symbolizes the clinician.

The clinician's attention to cause instead of character of the noise, or to its conversion from auditory to visual entity, is detrimental not only to the auscultatory skill that distinguishes a clinician, but also to the characteristics that distinguish a noise. Like proteins, white cells, and other entities observed in the laboratory, cardiac noises have many different properties. The noises can vary in location; radiation; loudness; pitch; time of onset and of cessation in relation to other noises; duration; thoracic site of maximal loudness; response of loudness and of other properties to procedures that induce changes in heart rate, in blood flow, in pulmonary aeration, and in position of the heart during its own cycle and during excursions of diaphragm or of thoracic wall. Like the phenomena assessed in the laboratory, each of these acoustic properties has its own range of variation, and each property can often vary independently of changes in the others. All the properties must be observed for the noises to be described reproducibly; their range of variation in healthy people must be established to determine physiologic boundaries of normal; and each individual abnormality must be identified in criteria for designating the noise and for diagnosing its pathologic significance. Some of these acoustic properties are distorted or unperceived by existing inanimate devices, and are better assessed by a human ear and mind.

The phenomenon to be evaluated is a noise, not merely a visual image (in phonocardiography), or a magnetic entity (for computer analysis). With each translation of the noise from acoustic to non-acoustic forms, some of the critical properties that distinguish the noise are lost, or altered. The phonocardiograph, for example, is a boon to the timing of noises. A visible graphic tracing is much better than a clinician's ear for indicating a noise's onset, duration, and temporal relation to other cardiac events. Yet, because the writing stylus of ordinary phonocardiographs cannot move quickly enough to inscribe certain high-pitched noises, the graphic tracing may be unable to show soft murmurs of aortic regurgitation or to distinguish between a murmur and a rub. By omitting the high-frequency components of a systolic or diastolic murmur, a graphic tracing may sometimes falsify the actual intensity, duration, and timing of the murmur.

The loss of high frequencies in visual graphic recording can be avoided by inscribing the noise electronically, rather than mechanically, with suitable oscilloscopic devices. But these devices introduce problems of their own. The instrument's increased sensitivity becomes its major disadvantage; oscillations and other variations of the ordinary baseline may be difficult to separate from those of superimposed noises —and, besides, the image is transient. If a permanent record is to be kept of the proceedings, a photograph must be taken of the oscilloscopic tracing. The need for photography then introduces a new set of difficulties. Spectral phonocardiography,[166] like the other techniques, also has its advantages—and disadvantages.

Another problem in the conversion of sound to sight is that the recorded image is a summation of electrical, rather than acoustic, energy. Except when special "spectral" equipment is used to separate contributions of different frequencies, the magnitude of the tracing recorded by the oscillating motion at any moment represents the sum of the amplitudes of all the different frequencies of sound that are present at that moment. Since acoustic events are transmitted as waves that are alternatingly positive and negative, a positive electrical contribution from one frequency may be cancelled by a negative contribution from another. This type of electrical cancellation can cause a "damped beat",[167] in which the graphic record shows zero amplitude, producing the visual illusion that no noise is present although the noise is acoustically evident. Thus, many a clinician who clearly hears only a single heart sound through his stethoscope at a particular moment in the cardiac cycle may begin to doubt his ears, his stethoscope, or his auscultatory skill when the graphic tracing, because of a fallacious "damped beat", shows a sound that looks split.

A further problem in "visual" auscultation has to do with microphonic input, rather than graphic output. This problem arises because the high and low frequencies of noise are attenuated differently in their acoustic transmission upstream or downstream through liquid moving in an enclosed space.[168] Consequently, the same thoracic noise may be sonorously altered in two different ways when transmitted to two distant but diametrically opposite locations. For example, a physiologic pulmonic systolic murmur that is best audible along the left sternal border may be distorted in transmission so that it sounds high-pitched and blowing when heard at the apex, and low-pitched and rumbling when heard at the "aortic" area of auscultation. Perceiving three different noises at three different sites of cardiac auscultation, the unwary observer may conclude that there are three different sources of noise, instead of one.

In the analysis of this acoustic problem, a crucial item of evidence is the place on the chest where the noise is loudest. The site of maximal thoracic loudness is a major point in the clinical decision that two different systolic murmurs heard in the "aortic" and "mitral" areas of auscultation may both come from a physiologic pulmonic murmur and not from aortic stenosis and mitral regurgitation. To discern the site of maximal thoracic loudness, the pressure and position of a chest microphone must be exactly calibrated and standardized. Yet no mechanical technique now in general use for microphone placement satisfies this requirement. The best contemporary servomechanism for integrating receptor pressure with acoustic output is the coordinated ear, mind, and hand of a clinician.

For the sensory perceptions of quality and of certain other critical properties of noises, a clinician is thus often better than inanimate devices. Moreover, he and his stethoscope are always portable, and constantly available. His ability to perceive sensory qualities of noise is apparent in the richness of his vocabulary for describing them; he uses words such as *hums, rasps, squeaks, hisses,* and *coos.* The scientific defect of these observational terms is not their descriptive capacities but the lack of uniformity and standardization in the way the clinician uses them. One observer's *rasp* is often another's *squeak.*

The noises heard during clinical auscultation are often described non-reproducibly, not because of defects in human perceptory apparatus, but because the apparatus is used without adequate care and precision. Clinicians do not generally listen for all the acoustic properties they can distinguish, and do not use sufficient or consistent criteria for designating what they hear. By expanding the detail of their observations, and (as described later) by establishing criteria and "standardizing" themselves, clinicians can reduce their human inconsistencies while preserving their human sensory superiorities. By abandoning their own capacities in favor of inanimate devices, however, clinicians remove the defect of human variability but lose the advantage of human perception. The mechanical instruments may be objective, precise, and standardized—but they can often distinguish neither rasp nor squeak.

*　　　*　　　*

In all the aspects of clinical examination that have just been discussed, the clinician was assembling the basic observational evidence of the bedside. He obtained descriptions of the sensations noted by the patient and by himself. The clinician's next task in the examining procedure is to designate the evidence with the names of symptoms and signs, to record the descriptive evidence and the designations, and to check the reliability of his work. The techniques of scientific standardization available for these interpretive aspects of clinical examination will be discussed in the next chapter.

19. Science in Clinical Examination: Standardization

After performing the examination procedures just described, the clinician has obtained his "raw material": the basic observations of the bedside. He must now convert those observations into *data*.

Not all of the many entities observed during clinical examination are important enough to warrant formal preservation as data, or to receive formal consideration during the subsequent diagnostic and therapeutic reasoning. For example, the clinician may give no further attention to such observed items as cutaneous freckles, or the color of the patient's shoes. From the totality of observed evidence, the clinician therefore chooses a collection of noteworthy entities by making decisions about which ones are abnormal, and which ones are pertinent although normal. These selected entities are then designated with appropriate names, making them the facts (or data) that will be preserved by inscription in the medical record, and that will be used in the subsequent clinical reasoning. Together with these procedures of selection, designation, and preservation, the clinician also engages in acts of verification, to test the reliability of the data.

All of these preliminary interpretations of clinical observation occur before the clinician can begin any of the intellectual "arrangements" of the data in diagnostic and therapeutic reasoning. He must first decide which items of observed evidence to think about; what to call them; how to record them; and how to check them. These are the procedures of interpretive reasoning that convert bedside observations into clinical data.

To improve the standardization of these procedures, the clinician

328

must develop methods for becoming more consistent in designating, more uniform in recording, and more reliable in verifying the symptoms and signs that are the main units of clinical measurement.

CONSISTENCY

During the many interpretations that occur in human reasoning, observations of facts are converted from one state to another: a name is given to an entity or collection of entities; a category label is assigned to a representative sample; and evidence is transformed into inference, or witnessed effect into deduced cause. For example, a certain type of respiratory distress may be named *orthopnea,* categorized as abnormal, and inferred as due to a failing heart, which is deduced as having an atrial septal defect.

Just as the agents of metabolic conversion for chemical substances are called *enzymes,* the agents of rational transformations for human thought are called *criteria.* Criteria are the prerequisites of consistency in any type of intellectual reasoning. The initial evidence may be described objectively and precisely, but it must be converted with specific criteria if the subsequent interpretations are to be consistent. Without criteria, a rational transformation is unstandardized, and may produce many discrepancies and inaccuracies. Without criteria, the clinical conversions of observation to designation, and of designation to diagnosis, cannot be reproducible.

The first main set of criteria needed in bedside work are those used for designating the abnormal (and some normal) entities with the names of symptoms and signs. For example, observing that the liver edge is palpable 10 cm. below the right costal margin, the clinician may designate this sign as *hepatomegaly;* indentation of the skin and subcutaneous tissue after firm palpation of the pre-tibial region may be called the sign of *peripheral edema;* the patient's description of a substernal discomfort that occurs with exertion and subsides with rest may be called the symptom of *angina pectoris;* a twitch of the mouth muscles when the facial nerve is tapped in the parotid area is called *Chvostek's sign.* For these designations, the criteria must provide identification of the entities to be included as contents of the label, and also a statement of the acceptable range of normal variation in symptoms and signs of comparable healthy people. Thus, is the liver hepatomegalic if its edge is palpable at 2 cm. rather than 10 cm.? How much or for how long must the skin be indented to be called edematous? Is the exertional discomfort still angina pectoris if the patient feels it in the jaw rather than substernally? Is Chvostek's sign abnormal?

To establish scientific criteria of normality is one of the most difficult tasks in human biology. The observation or test must be performed in a general human population of satisfactory size and diversity, and the data must be demarcated by a satisfactory boundary of variation. Either the epidemiologic or the statistical principles, or both, have been neglected in the concepts of "normal" used today for many clinical data and for most para-clinical tests.

Statistically, a range of normal is chosen by noting the collection of numbers, contemplating their pattern of distribution, calculating an appropriate mean and standard deviation, and then establishing the boundary zone of normality, which is often two standard deviations on either side of the mean. Epidemiologically, the group of people who comprise the "sample" population must be: demographically diverse enough in such features as age, race, and occupation for ordinary human variability to be present; abundant enough for their differences to be statistically useful and for uncommon variations to be encountered; and representative enough of the "general population" for the results to be applicable to people other than the observed sample.

An epidemiologic sample of ordinary human variation may not be valid if the sample is too small, if it is confined by demographic restrictions to a limited age or occupational group, or if the base population is either self-selected or pre-selected by any procedures related to health or sickness before the investigator chooses his sample. For instance, people who elect to answer a mailed questionnaire, who volunteer for a study of a new diet, or who decide to apply for life insurance are a self-selected population. People who are members of the armed forces, or who are given life insurance, were subjected to significant selection procedures, based on their state of health, before being admitted to the military or insured populations. The best type of epidemiologic sample for human variability in a particular country is the population of a national census; all the people of the country are included, so no distorted sampling selections are made. Since this type of "total sample" is generally unfeasible in contemporary medicine, the next best general epidemiologic sample is an entire community—provided that people in the community are sufficiently representative of the "general population". A community composed mainly of young people, wealthy people, or people of a restricted ethnic group would not be a good choice as a general epidemiologic sample.

These statistical and epidemiologic principles have not been fulfilled in the development of most contemporary concepts of normality in clinical data. For clinical data that are not expressed as numbers, no statistical calculations of means and standard deviations are possible. For clinical data that are numerical, most of the sampled populations have been epidemiologically unsatisfactory: insurance company clients, members of the armed forces, college students, or factory workers. For example, current standards of normal weight are based mainly on data from a base population of people accepted by life insurance companies; current standards of normal blood pressure are based on other populations that lack valid epidemiologic generality. Only recently have results of the clinical range of normality begun to come from appropriate epidemiologic samples of entire communities, but the data are not yet large enough or analyzed in enough detail for the results to be accepted as general standards.

Because of these deficiencies, there now exist almost no satisfactory absolute criteria for designating a clinical manifestation as normal or abnormal. Many relative criteria are used for physical signs—comparing one side or part of the body against another—and many judgmental assessments of absolute normality are constantly made, but the relative criteria and absolute judgments are different for each individual clinician. For example, by what exact criteria do we decide whether ocular lid-lag, splinter hemorrhages in the finger-nails, or a Chvostek's sign are normal or abnormal? What are the criteria for concluding that pains in the region of a joint represent arthritis, arthralgia, or myalgia? What are the specific standards for concluding that lymph nodes are hypertrophied, a pharynx inflamed, a reflex hyperactive, a movement choreic, a liver enlarged, a chest pain anginal, or a type of breathing asthmatic? What specific populational data have been assembled to demonstrate the ranges of normal in these observations, and what are the exact criteria for abnormality in many other interpretations of clinical evidence? The criteria usually exist—but only as individual concepts of individual clinicians, not as universal standards.

Moreover, such criteria as do exist are often inadequate because they fail to provide for all the different attributes of variation in the observed entity. For example, in a child or adolescent, an apical systolic murmur is often called abnormal (or *organic*) if it is loud, high-pitched, blowing, and audible in the axilla. These four attributes (loudness, pitch, quality, and transmission) are the acoustic components generally listed in most statements of criteria for distinguishing the "organicity" of the murmur. Yet the particular distinctions just cited in these attributes can be present in many normal (or physiologic) systolic murmurs that are heard at the cardiac apex of young people.[14, 169, 170] To distinguish an organic from a physiologic apical systolic murmur, the criteria must account not only for the four acoustic properties just cited, but also for the variations in such additional attributes as exact time of onset and cessation in relation to the surrounding heart sounds, thoracic site of maximal loudness, and response of apical loudness to respiratory and positional maneuvers that make the heart vertical.[7, 14, 170]

In the absence of satisfactory standardized criteria, inconsistencies are rampant today in the clinical designation of abnormal symptoms and signs. What is surprising about these inconsistencies, however, is not that they exist, but that they are not worse. Despite many minor variations and some major disagreements, experienced clinicians can generally reach good agreement with themselves or with other clinicians in most of the important designations of clinical evidence. The clinicians have allowed their many examinations of normal regions to serve as an "epidemiologic" background, and have formulated many effective standards of judgment for deciding about the range of normal in non-dimensional clinical observations. With specific attention to the problem, clinicians should easily be able to formulate appropriate criteria for designating most of their non-dimensional observations.

To establish criteria for range of normal in verbally described clinical evidence, clinicians need not rely on purely numerical statistical assessments. In an approach analogous to that described earlier (pages 254–260) for therapeutic indexes and criteria, clinicians can use each of the different attributes of observation as "significant figures" that are either absent or present in degrees of gradation. As a deliberate epidemiologic background, clinicians can select special new populations, and can also incorporate the results obtained during the many routine examinations of healthy patients or of healthy regions in sick patients. With these data at hand, clinicians can then make decisions about criteria for normality and for other clinical designations. For example, by routinely testing all patients for lid-lag and Chvostek's sign, clinicians can quickly discover that these entities occur often enough in healthy people to disqualify the signs from being regarded *per se* as abnormal.

Although the consistency of clinical data is hampered by the absence of designatory criteria, the situation is much worse in regard to many concepts of normal range in laboratory data. Generally aware of the inconsistencies in bedside statements, clinicians are usually skeptical and cautious about the use of clinical data. On the other hand, clinicians often gullibly assume that the numerical specifications of laboratory data are validated for their statements of normal or abnormal results.

Although standardized *clinical* criteria for range of normal are generally non-existent, the standards of *laboratory* criteria are generally spurious. Statistical calculations have been used to get the means, standard deviations, and boundaries of normality in the data of many laboratory procedures, but the data, in most cases, were obtained epidemiologically from a population that consisted of a small group of house officers, technicians, and other personnel of the hospital staff. Although such a population is inadequate in size and in demographic diversity, many important standards of normality in contemporary laboratory tests have been calculated in this unsatisfactory way.

Consequently, when the same laboratory test at two different hospitals is done on the same specimen using the same methods, with the same qualitative and quantitative precision, and yielding the same number, the result may be called *normal* at one hospital and *abnormal* at the other. The epidemiologic deficiencies in range-of-normal criteria for contemporary laboratory tests are responsible for many diagnostic errors, some with tragic sequelae, in modern medicine. Patients have been falsely diagnosed as having infectious hepatitis, coronary artery disease, diabetes mellitus, rheumatic carditis, or prostatic carcinoma because of "abnormalities", respectively, in cephalin flocculation, electrocardiographic T waves, blood sugar, P-R interval, or serum acid phosphatase tests that might have been called "normal" if a better epidemiologic sampling had been used for establishing the basic range of normal.

The "statistical childishness" that Norbert Wiener[35] decried in clinical therapy is often matched by an epidemiologic naïveté in laboratory diagnosis. A new laboratory test is developed; its range of normal is determined in a restricted population of hospital employees; the test is then applied mainly to patients with a particular disease; when found to be frequently abnormal in those patients, the test is then reported as "specific" for that disease. Later on, the test is applied to patients with other diseases, and many "false positive" results are encountered. The test is then reduced in specificity; it becomes regarded not as diagnostic of a particular disease, but as indicative of a distinct abnormality. The test then comes into widespread use for "screening" or other diagnostic purposes. It is now, for the first time, tried out in a wide range of healthy people, some of whom are then found to have unexplained "abnormalities". The unwise clinician accepts the "abnormal" result and regards his patient as having the associated "disease" or other disorder; the wise clinician ignores the result if no other confirmatory evidence exists; the scientific clinician looks into the background of the test, finds that it is epidemiologically unstandardized, and either searches for better data elsewhere or demands a better epidemiologic investigation.

Satisfactory epidemiologic assessment is a critical aspect of any new para-clinical test. The clinician's daily practice brings him in contact with many relatively healthy people from whom he can establish a working range of normal for clinical observations. But new para-clinical tests are usually developed in hospital laboratories where a satisfactory general population is not readily available. In recent years, such new tests as C-reactive protein and serum transaminase measurements were widely disseminated and led to many instances of "iatrogenic" disease, before their epidemiologic (and diagnostic) limitations were recognized. The literature of contemporary genetics contains an increasing threnody of new chromosomal "abnormalities", although the fundamental concepts of morphologic normality in human chromosomes still depend on an inadequately small sampling of healthy people. Amid the many investigations of contemporary "basic research" in clinical science, almost no attention has been given to the basic epidemiologic and statistical deficiencies in the criteria used for designating normality in laboratory data, as well as in clinical symptoms and signs.

The need for standardized criteria is equally great when the designated abnormalities in symptoms, signs, and para-clinical data are converted to diagnoses. The establishment of diagnostic criteria, as discussed earlier (pages 93–102), involves no additional epidemiologic or statistical difficulties. Once the abnormal evidence is designated, all that is necessary is an arbitrary decision about which abnormality or collection of abnormalities will be regarded as diagnostic. The decision is arbitrary, because most "diseases" are defined arbitrarily from evidence observed either by a pathologist, by a clinician, or by both. Although such diagnostic criteria are relatively easy to form, very few standardized formulations have been established. Each doctor uses his own criteria, and different doctors may often reach confusing or contradictory conclusions about the same set of abnormalities.

Much of the perennial confusion about the identification of rheumatic fever, for example, was removed when Jones[65] established arbitrary but specific diagnostic criteria for the disease. That "criteriology" is a young and changing science was demonstrated by a later modification[5] of the criteria, intended to clarify and improve Jones' original standards. The later modification, in turn, has now been noted[17] to have deficiencies that will need subsequent attention, and some of these deficiencies were corrected in a recent "modification" of the "modified" original criteria.[66] In rheumatoid arthritis—after decades of investigation devoted to etiology, pathogenesis, prognosis, and therapy —the population to be studied has finally been explicitly defined by recent establishment of specific clinical diagnostic criteria.[64] Deficiencies have now also been noted[171] in these criteria, and subsequent modifications will be needed.

In the diseases just mentioned, great progress has been made— although belatedly—by the institution of rigorous diagnostic criteria. In many other chronic and degenerative diseases, however, universally accepted and universally used diagnostic clinical criteria still do not exist. Standardized rigorous criteria are absent, as described in Chapter 6, for the clinical diagnosis of myocardial infarction, cerebrovascular thrombosis, pulmonary emphysema, bronchial asthma, pancreatitis, herniated lumbar disc, and many other common disorders. The establishment of the criteria requires only suitable attention and thought by appropriate authorities.

Specific standard criteria are a prerequisite in clinical science not only for distinguishing the normal from the abnormal (in designation), and the source of abnormality (in diagnosis), but also for appraising the significance of clinical changes after therapy. The importance of such post-therapeutic criteria has already been discussed. Unless a clinician uses deliberate overt criteria for all these procedures of rational "metabolism", he may convert objective, precise observations into disorderly, non-reproducible conclusions.

UNIFORMITY

Since symptoms and signs are transient and cannot be directly removed for storage, they become permanent evidence only by the way in which they are "preserved". For a symptom, no preservation is possible. A symptom exists as an element of subjective sensation, and its conversion to scientific data occurs as an act of verbal communication and intellectual designation. Certain signs can be "preserved" by photographs, tape recordings, or contour models, but these methods of preservation are not always convenient, exact, or available. Moreover, they cannot preserve evidence derived from percussion or from nuances of palpation. For symptoms and for most signs, therefore, the permanent evidence is the descriptive data entered in a medical record.

A patient's medical record is thus a unique object of clinical science. In many aspects of laboratory research, the investigator's notebook has a secondary role as evidence. The notebook contains descriptions and assessments of evidence, but the substances that were actually observed can often be saved and stored for subsequent review. In clinical work, the medical record is, for all practical purposes, the only permanent evidence. This feature of medical records gives them an importance greater than that of any other notebook in scientific investigation. Since a patient's record contains the permanent evidence, as well as the assessments of the evidence, the quality and uniformity of the data transcribed in the records form a crucial scientific aspect of clinical medicine.

Yet, like the taking of a history, the maintenance of a patient's clinical record is seldom taught in either graduate or undergraduate medical education. At most medical institutions, the content of the initial (admission) history and physical examination is outlined by established tradition, or by a formal set of instructions—but the people who compile the records are seldom exposed to critical inspection of the way they execute the tradition or the instructions. As for the record of what happens *after* the patient's admission, the content and frequency of clinical "progress notes" appear to be governed almost entirely by the principle of *laissez faire*. There are no standard rules or traditions for what the notes should contain or when they should be written. Many years ago, the "progress notes" of medical records reflected changes in clinical state, but many contemporary notes contain few remarks that indicate clinical skill in the observer. The notes written by modern clinicians and house officers often merely state the results of the laboratory tests, changes in therapeutic agents, or nonspecific general comments, such as "patient looks better today".

This lamentable state can be improved if academic clinical investigators, who usually keep impeccable records in the laboratory, will teach and demand the same quality in the clinical records of the bed-side. A clinician should note and inscribe not only all the pertinent clinical variables and their successive alteration, but also the events and reasoning that led to changes in therapeutic tactics. A competent secretary can record laboratory reports and changes in medication, and call the entries "progress notes". A student nurse or observant relative can state that a patient is better or worse, comfortable or distressed. The clinician's role is to make and record the *specific* clinical observations that serve as evidence of the patient's progress, and as basis for changes in therapeutic strategy.

The problem of uniformity in recording clinical data involves both their acquisition and their transcription.

HISTORY-TAKING

If the patient writes answers to printed questions, the variability of a clinician's interrogation can be eliminated. The written arrangement can allow the patient a free (and hence non-uniform) response to a blank space, or he can select uniform answers from stated multiple choices or from "yes" or "no" alternatives. Many clinicians in office practice now use such forms for the routine initial history, probably as much for the time saved as for scientific standardization.

Although these techniques provide considerable uniformity of data, a printed form (or a computer program) used for the *routine initial* history cannot be adequate for obtaining all the descriptions of "present illness" needed for diagnosis, prognosis, and therapy:

1) The more standard a question and the more rigid the response it permits, the narrower is its scope.

2) A fixed sequence of questions prohibits pursuit of implications and extensions of individual responses.

3) A specific, finite set of written questions can hardly detect nuances or reliability of answers.

To obtain the scope and breadth of a complete initial history that will encompass all possible combinations of circumstance while simul-taneously evaluating emotional state and reliability of patients, a printed form and its questions would need enormous, almost infinite, length. Even if such a form were feasible, the precision and uniformity of data thereby acquired would hardly be worth either the huge amount of extraneous information or the exhaustion of the patient who had to provide it.

What the clinician brings to history-taking, and what any printed form for routine initial history lacks, is the ability to change focus. The clinician can intensify or digress, combine or dissect, choose what to accept and amplify, or what to reject and ignore. As instruments for general history-taking—for sensing quality and content of responses and integrating them with subsequent questions—astute, thoughtful clinicians cannot be surpassed by any inanimate method of interrogation.

Not all clinicians, however, are equally astute and thoughtful. They may occasionally forget, omit, overlook, distort, or fail to record important data. At many medical centers where the clinical records are later used for investigative purposes, the young resident, the younger intern, and the embryonic student-clinicians usually serve as the main sources of the recorded histories. As these observers get more experience, they may increase their skill and reliability, but the amount they write decreases. The medical records then used for scientific appraisals of disease thus have most of their clinical data entered by persons whose capability is least developed. For these reasons, printed forms for the routine initial history would provide a way of ensuring that certain essential data are always obtained and recorded.

No routine standard form can be adequate for establishing *accurate diagnosis* from the initial history. Forms used mainly for diagnosis are too inflexible to offer more than clues; the information obtained will inevitably be too much or too little for diagnostic precision. When diagnosis depends mainly on the history, the clinician usually needs much more detail than any standard initial form can provide. When diagnosis depends on laboratory and other tests, the clinician can often choose those tests after receiving answers to a few brief questions, without recourse to all the data contained in a comprehensive form.

Printed forms can make valuable contributions to medical records, however, for two major scientific purposes beyond diagnosis:

1) In the initial history, the forms can be used to obtain specific information that sometimes is omitted because it may seem unrelated to the present illness. Such information would include accounts of familial disorders, occupational history, previous hospitalizations or diseases, review of apparently uninvolved systems, social status, and drinking and smoking habits. Such data may often be important not for the immediate diagnosis of the patient's current situation, but as critical ancillary evidence when the patient's record is reviewed at a later date for

genetic, environmental, epidemiologic, or other research studies that may not have been contemplated when the initial history was obtained.

2) A second major role for printed forms would come *after* diagnostic tests are completed and a pre-therapeutic focus is established. Here the forms would implement the second history, described earlier, whose contents deal with all the clinical and other data pertinent to classifying the patient about to be treated. Designed specifically for each particular disease or therapeutic situation, such forms could augment the initial history and remind the clinician of the information necessary for proper classification of patients.

To avoid extreme length, the pre-therapeutic forms just described should arrange for "fill-in" replies rather than for choices among fixed answers. Hence, the forms should be completed by the clinician interviewing the patient, rather than by patient alone, since the clinician will bring more uniformity to the process. Such forms, although seemingly impersonal, may sometimes actually increase the amount of communication between clinician and patient. To obtain the information needed for completing the blanks, a clinician may have to spend more time talking with patients than he might have done otherwise.

Such forms, and other rigorous procedures for collecting information, will become increasingly used as more attention is given to storing, processing, and analyzing data with computers and other devices of modern informational technology. The forms must be long enough to get the necessary data, but concise enough for practical use; and detailed enough for significant nuances to be recorded, but not crammed with so many minutiae that the user of the form becomes inattentive. The directions for completing the form must be indicated precisely, but not so meticulously that the user must read great gobs of instructions before each move. To design questionnaires and other informational forms complex enough for the demands of science, yet simple enough for the arts of man, will be a major intellectual challenge in the clinical research of the future.

PHYSICAL EXAMINATION

The use of specific printed forms for recording the evidence of physical examination has advantages and disadvantages analogous to those just noted for forms in history-taking. In the routine initial examination, many normal regions can be conveniently described in relatively brief phrases, and the filling of a detailed form may only add needless length to the clinician's scientific task. After a pre-therapeutic diagnostic focus is established, however, the precise details of pertinent negative (as well as positive) findings in appropriate regions are imperative for proper classification of the patient. The use of forms specifically adapted to each particular pre-therapeutic situation would ensure that all the requisite observations are made and recorded. The techniques of observation, and choice of properties to be observed and inscribed, would be determined by the methods already discussed.

RELIABILITY

The reliability of an examining apparatus is established by checking it repeatedly against itself and against other apparatus than can perform the same examination. In the repeat examinations, of course, the same substance and the same apparatus must be used. This type of standardization is easy and performed routinely for laboratory materials and equipment that do not change from one examination to the next. When the "substance" is a patient, however, and the "examining apparatus" a clinician, neither the "substance" nor the "apparatus" remains the same when an examination is repeated. The patient may be affected by changes in himself, in the disease, or in the examiner. The clinician's recall of his first set of observations will inevitably bias his second.

Since both the patient and the clinician must be checked, the establishment of reliability in clinical examination is a difficult task.

HISTORY-TAKING

In history-taking, a clinician cannot check himself against himself. It is impossible for him to repeat two histories with the *same* patient under identical observational circumstances. To compare results in history-taking, therefore, a clinician would have to check his data with those obtained by others. When different clinicians successively take a history from the same patient, however, the patient may change. If repetitively examined in a short period of time by too many examiners, the patient may become exhausted or unco-operative. If the interval between examinations is too long, the evolving illness may make him gain or lose symptoms, or otherwise change his story. If the successive examiners affect his perception of his own sensations, the patient may report different information from one examination to the next. For example, a skillful second clinical examiner may elicit much more detailed description of certain symptoms by prompting the patient with more specific questions than those asked by the first examiner. After the second history-taking session, the patient may then spontaneously volunteer the extra details when subsequent histories are taken. Consequently, a third examiner, although less adept at history-taking than the first, may be falsely credited with better technique because he fortuitously obtained additional details omitted by the first examiner.

The inherent reliability of a patient is even more difficult to gauge than that of a clinician. A patient can give unreliable information because of defects that are transient or permanent, deliberate or inadvertent, perceptive or expressive, organic or psychic. In the absence of specific tests for determining reliability of a patient's story, the clinician can seek confirmation by consulting other sources (as discussed later) and by testing the internal consistency of the data. These tests consist of assessing 1) the patient's memory and general sensorial state, 2) the patient's possible motivations for deceiving either himself or the clinician, and 3) the logical and clinical coherence between the patient's story and the objective data noted in physical findings and laboratory tests. Clinicians must beware, however, that they do not label a patient as unreliable when the disease appears with atypical or unexpected clinical manifestations (as discussed earlier), or when discrepancies occur in the content of two histories taken with different techniques of history-taking.

The reliability of histories and of history-takers can be considerably improved by a number of procedures that are readily available, but not generally or adequately applied. Among them are the following:

Direct Supervision of Students

As noted earlier, a medical student seldom watches his teachers take a history. His teachers also seldom watch him. They often check that he has acquired salient information; they check his ability to reason with the information; but they almost never check his competence in the act of getting the primary data at the bedside. A few hours of direct supervision and enlightened criticism early in his career as a history-taker could greatly improve a student's subsequent attitudes and abilities as a clinician.

History-taking is also unsupervised even in procedures that assess the competence of clinical specialists. The contemporary tests for certification by specialty boards contain methods for checking surgeons, anesthesiologists, pathologists, and radiologists in their actual performance of the major skills of the specialty, but internists are not observed *while* they take a history. Since verbal data are more important in internal medicine than in any other specialty of organic disease, an internist's ability to communicate with sick people is as basic a tool of his craft as his knowledge of molecular biology. Yet this communicative ability is not tested by the examining boards that certify him as a specialist. (The direct assessment of history-taking was recently attempted during the third part of National Board Examinations of *interns,* but the procedure has now been abandoned.)

These defects of teaching and testing, present in physical examination as well as in history-taking, have many serious consequences that have been discussed here and elsewhere.[172] The situation can be improved easily. It needs only the appropriate attention, time, and effort.

Direct Review of History by Attending Physician

A corollary of the failure to demonstrate and to supervise history-taking is the frequent failure of academic clinicians to verify it. The clinical investigator who checks his laboratory equipment with scientific care and skepticism may be hasty and credulous at bedside teaching rounds. He may often accept brief histories as presented (sometimes without even seeing the patient) and he may fail to confirm the most pertinent points *directly with the patient.* The confirmation, always desirable, is especially necessary for such symptoms as chest pain, dizziness, fatigue, headache, and gastrointestinal distress. In these situations, all other examinations may be negative, and diagnosis may often rest upon history alone. An attending physician's failure to take concise histories at the bedside is detrimental to both art and science in clinical medicine. He leaves the art undemonstrated, and he allows possible inaccuracies to pass unchallenged.

Review of History with Other Sources

In the era of the telephone, clinicians can easily confirm and augment details of a history by communicating with a patient's relatives, friends, previous physicians, or employers, and with medical record librarians or other sources of information. The past details may often correct important errors in data and may sometimes prevent unnecessary diagnostic and therapeutic procedures.

These efforts to authenticate the data of a history are seldom carried out with care or consistency. House officers (and practicing clinicians) may ask a secretarial clerk to ask another clerk to write to a third clerk who then sends a "summary" which, when it arrives in time, often lacks the details that only a specific telephoned request from the physician might have elicited. A patient's relatives or hospital visitors are seldom invited to contribute important information that only they may know. A referring or previous physician—who may not have had time to write a detailed referral note and who may not even know that the patient has been admitted to a hospital—is sometimes dismissed as an *LMD,** and the significant data he might provide are thus ignored. The *LMD,* not consulted because his information is expected to be useless, might keep better records if he knew the "medical center" regarded him as a source not merely of patients, but of data.

Review of History at Re-admission to Hospital

When a patient re-enters the same hospital, the new physicians and students should go over his entire history with him, not merely the "interval" history. The old medical record, which is generally reviewed and summarized to save time, may have been incomplete or inaccurate; a direct survey of the total history may disclose omissions or errors in previous observations.

Standardization in Research Studies

When the innumerable opportunities for error are contemplated, the most remarkable feature of history-taking is not its occasional inaccuracies but the frequency with which it is correct, reliable, and of paramount clinical importance. Every competent clinician recognizes the history as his most valuable tool in the strategy of diagnosis and management, and every clinician has used his clinical experience to standardize his own techniques for verifying the data.

In research studies that depend on symptoms as critical scientific evidence, however, a more formal standardization of clinical history-taking is necessary. For example, in trials of anticoagulant therapy for coronary artery disease, an exact description of chest pain is often crucial not only for entering the patient into the study, but also for classi-

* Local Medical Doctor.

fying him into an appropriate clinical subgroup for therapeutic allocation and assessment. Despite the many investigations already devoted
to anticoagulants, the different clinical examiners have never been
tested for their comparability in obtaining the fundamental symptomatic evidence upon which all the other work depends. Discrepancies
of history-taking in the patients receiving anticoagulants may well be
responsible for many of the currently unidentified populational inconsistencies in the investigations whose unreproducible results have led
to so much confusion and controversy.

Although special forms for history-taking can remove some of the
inconsistencies in such research studies, certain types of symptoms require direct confirmation by a clinician interviewing each patient. For
such situations, different observers in the same study or in different
studies should assemble together, *before the investigation begins,* to
agree on the approaches they will use for history-taking, and to observe one another's performance. Although they cannot attain the type
of standardization possible for physical examination (as described
later), they can at least ensure that their performance of history-taking
has been given this additional element of consistency.

PHYSICAL EXAMINATION

Unlike the evidence of history-taking, the findings of physical examination are objective and usually unchanged by the examination process. To test reliability in physical examination, the methodologic problems therefore deal not only with the standardization of observers, but
also with the assessment of accuracy. (A group of different observers
may be standardized in that each gets the same results, but the results
may be inaccurate.) Problems of accuracy occur in each separate act
of physical examination: description, designation, and diagnosis.

For confirmation of diagnoses, which are usually expressed as conclusions about deranged anatomy, the accuracy of the conclusions is
assessed from direct anatomic evidence obtained by biopsy, surgery, or
necropsy. (Roentgenograms, electrophysiologic tracings, and other laboratory tests are useful adjuncts in morphologic diagnosis but are also
inferential; they are never an *exact* confirmation of pathologic anatomy.) Pathologic confirmation of diagnosis, however, often cannot be
obtained in circumstances where biopsy is unfeasible, surgery unjusti-
fied, and necropsy either impossible or performed too late to be helpful
in the preceding clinical situation. The treatment of patients with path-

ologically unconfirmed diagnoses is the rule, rather than the exception, in ordinary clinical practice. No *exact* proof of diagnosis is available during life for most of man's minor ailments, and for many important chronic and degenerative diseases of heart, lungs, blood vessels, and brain.

Many designations of clinical abnormality are expressed as the names of deranged physiologic functions, and can be confirmed when appropriate techniques are available. For example, electrocardiograms can confirm the designation of an irregular pulse as *atrial fibrillation;* roentgenograms may confirm the designation that abdominal distention and other findings represent *intestinal obstruction.* Many other designations, however, cannot be confirmed by any exact mechanism other than a clinician's reasoning. Among such designations are the decisions that a patient has choreic movements, tension headaches, angina pectoris, intermittent claudication, or congestive heart failure.

The description of the clinical evidence itself can occasionally be confirmed precisely, but the confirmatory mechanism is usually inconvenient or hazardous. For example, cutaneous thermocouples can verify that skin is warm; intra-arterial sphygmomanometry can measure the exact blood pressure. No exact confirmation can be used, however, for such physical evidence as descriptions of texture (firmness or fluctuance), resonance, noise, and tenderness.

Consequently, a clinician generally works with descriptive, designative, and diagnostic data for which absolute accuracy cannot be established. This impediment to science, however, is more apparent than real. Physicists and astronomers often also have this same difficulty, but manage to produce works of science without being able to get an *exact* confirmation of the basic evidence they assess. No one has ever directly seen an atom, an electron, or a meson, and no one has ever, as yet, had a close-up direct view of the moon or stars; nevertheless, the absence of primary confirmation of evidence has not impeded progress in the "exact" physical sciences.

The critical quality of scientific data is not accuracy, but reproducibility. There is no such thing as absolute accuracy, any more than there is an absolute vacuum, an absolute number of chemical elements, an absolute limit to the size of particles into which matter can be finely divided, or absolute truth. The Bureau of Standards establishes an arbitrary concept, called *accuracy*, that enables dimensional measurements to be made reproducibly with different copies of the measuring instrument. Clinicians can establish similar concepts (and similar Bureaus) that will enable clinical assessments to be *reproducible*.

To attain reproducibility, clinicians have many opportunities for improving the reliability of physical examination. Among the opportunities are the following:

At Teaching Rounds

As part of routine bedside instruction to house officers and students, the attending clinician should examine selected areas *before* he is told what has been found there. He often cannot take time for a complete physical survey of the patient, and his examination should be directed to particular regions chosen by the house officers for positive, pertinent negative, or controversial findings. If the attending clinician's observations should disagree with those of the house officers or students, the differences will be desirable, not deplorable. His confirmation increases the validity of the initial observations; his dissensions, and exploration of the reasons for them, will help teach him and his younger colleagues the range of variation and the development of precision in the use of human clinical examination apparatus.

Self-Standardization

A practicing clinician, regardless of specialty, has an excellent and constant opportunity for self-standardization. This process is particularly necessary for consultants whose specialty stresses the examination of a particular region. As long as the clinician has forgotten his previous findings in an individual patient—a situation that often occurs in a busy practice—he can always re-examine certain regions "blindly" and compare his present observations with those he recorded before. Such assessments, possible only if the physical properties have not changed between examinations, can often be applied in the repetitive examination of patients with retinopathy, cardiac murmurs, prostatic enlargement, peripheral vascular lesions, locomotor restrictions, and neurologic abnormalities. The frequency of these opportunities for self-standardization will depend on the state of the patient, the interval between the two examinations, and the circumstances that affect the clinician's memory.

Standardization of Multiple Observers in Research Studies

The type of self-standardization just described can indicate only whether an individual observer is internally consistent. It tells whether he agrees with himself, but not whether he agrees with others. For the external standardization required in scientific research, the different observers who perform physical examination must be tested against each other. For such procedures, the same selected "unknown" patients should be examined for the observers to standardize one another and to arrive at a consensus of technique and criteria. The standardization cannot be achieved merely from written or oral efforts to agree about the components of observation, or about the criteria used for interpretation. The observers must meet in the same place, at the same time, and examine the same patients to be certain that the actual performance, perception, and interpretation of the observations do not occur with subtle, unrecognized discrepancies.

Such discrepancies are responsible for some of the dissensions and contradictory conclusions that currently exist after, and despite, many contemporary investigations of clinical therapy. For example, the prevention and treatment of complications in diabetes mellitus cannot be compared if different observers have not standardized their observation of retinopathy or of peripheral vascular lesions. Anticoagulant and surgical therapy for neurologic disorders cannot be appraised if the neurologists at one institution use observational standards different from those at another. The value of prophylactic vascular shunts in hepatic cirrhosis cannot be determined if esophageal varices are identified non-reproducibly.

Examiners in comparable or "co-operative" studies often believe they have used the same techniques, terms, and criteria for their examinations, but have actually differed in crucial, undetected nuances that create disparate results. Conflicts in conclusions by two sets of investigators are then attributed to differences in therapy or to the unreliability of patients, when the conflicts are actually due to unrecognized inconsistencies in the unstandardized examiners.

In rheumatic fever, for example, a program of repeated examination, by multiple objective observers, of the cardiac noises and shadows of the same patients helped to demonstrate unsuspected observational errors whose sources could then be explored. The explorations enabled the clinicians to recognize the need for observing attributes of the noises and shadows that had previously been unspecified, to eliminate many inconsistencies, to establish reproducible descriptions and precise criteria, and to increase the uniformity and standardization of observational skills.[7] The consequences of these improvements in basic observational science at the bedside were a recognition of major errors in therapeutic appraisals and even in pathogenetic concepts. In therapy, many previous triumphs over "carditis" had been falsely attributed to treatment: the "organic" systolic murmur that "disappeared" had actually been a physiologic systolic murmur made louder while the patient was febrile; and the "cardiac enlargement" that "vanished" actually consisted of erroneously interpreted normal variations in the mobile cardiac silhouette.[14] In pathogenesis, many patients had been falsely believed to have "developed" rheumatic heart disease either insidiously or in recurrences of rheumatic fever, because of errors in the interpretation of auscultation.[173]

Standardization in laboratory science is obtained by sending the specimens to the equipment. In clinical science, the order of movement is reversed. The different clinicians who are the "equipment" must travel—across a continent or hemisphere, if necessary—to the various selected patients at the place where the observers will standardize themselves. The process may seem strange, inconvenient, or expensive— but no more so than the frequent repetition or new inception of large-scale clinical research studies doomed to failure before they begin because the basic procedures of clinical examination are unstandardized and unreproducible.

*   *   *

In his timeless, compassionate prescription for the clinician's work in therapy, Francis Peabody[174] wrote that "the secret of patient care is in caring for the patient." This secret is also the prescription for improving the activities of clinical examination. For the art needed to obtain the data and to preserve the humanistic tradition of clinical medicine, the patient must be examined artfully. For the exacting requirements the data and the therapy must fulfill in modern science, the patient must be examined scientifically.

Clinical medicine is more than just an analysis, dissection, division, or partition of sick people into parts assessed by other domains of investigation, and clinical methods cannot be a mere application of the techniques used in those domains. The clinician deals with a synthesis of human parts into an entire, whole organism having all the additional properties and new variations present in the whole. To observe that whole, the clinician must examine it as its own unit: the patient.

In the observational acquisition of raw data and in the subsequent intellectual arrangements, clinical medicine is neither art nor science.

It is not divided between them nor does it divide them. Its every function contains and unites elements of both. Of all man's activities, clinical medicine is the most scientific art and the most humanistic science. The art and science are intermingled, symbiotic, and inseparable. Without the art, there can be no data for the science. Without the science, there can be no reason for the art.

PART V

Conclusions

352

20. The Human Regulation of Technology

A clinician today often eats a breakfast that was stored in a refrigerator and cooked on an electric stove; he drives his automobile to a multi-storied building, where he takes a self-service elevator to his office; he checks the telephoned reports of results obtained via X-ray, electrocardiograph, or spectrophotometer; he looks at his television set and sees pictures sent instantaneously via artificial satellite from the other side of the earth; he then takes the microphone of his dictation equipment and composes a letter that will be transcribed with the aid of an electric typewriter. In the letter, he deplores the destruction of human values by technology.

Confronted with the problems of technology, people have always reacted incongruously, condemning the abuses of the mechanism whose products they happily use. From the most ancient civilizations to the modern, the recorded attitudes about the ethical consequences of technologic advance indicate that man has been alarmed but assimilating, concerned but consuming. The very media of mass communication made possible by technology—the printed page, the broadcast voice, the transmitted image—have often been employed to denounce its dehumanizing effects.

No era in recorded history and no valuable new technologic device have been spared the problem of acceptance and abuse in man's long struggle to live with the artifacts he creates. The human invention of the spear, so important in hunting animals for food, was followed by its use as a weapon for killing other humans. The discovery of fire, so effective for heat and light, was later applied to torture people or to burn them at the stake. The discovery of radiation, which enables man to see and label what he cannot otherwise recognize, has led to explosives that can maim or murder large human populations.

Nor has any era of man been spared the occupational disruptions of new technology. The invention of the wheel must have put many laborers out of work; illumination from natural gas, and later from electricity, ruined the tallow and candle industry; the automobile abolished the village smithy; the neighborhood corner grocer is fighting a losing battle against the supermarket chain stores.

Whenever introduced, a new technologic advance has been initially rejected and feared: rejected, because of the belief that it could not work as well as existing devices; feared, because of the suspicion that it might. A constant source of wry amusement in any era is to read the deprecations of the initial reception given to technology developed in a previous era. For example, Laënnec's introduction of the stethoscope was not greeted as the universal symbol of the clinician that it has now become. Said the London *Times,* in 1834,

> That it will ever come into general use notwithstanding its value . . . [is] extremely doubtful; because its beneficial application requires much time and gives a good bit of trouble both to the patient and the practitioner; because its hue and character are foreign, and opposed to all our habits and associations. . . . There is something even ludicrous in the picture of a grave physician proudly listening through a long tube applied to the patient's thorax.[175]

Since man may be frightened out of his wits transiently, but does not remain witless permanently, every new device or method that is useful becomes accepted ultimately. Once the new advance has won its battle for acceptance, however, man's real problems then begin. During the acceptance period and afterward, the technologic procedure is inevitably abused. As the procedure becomes disseminated, the device(s) may be copied or constructed incorrectly, or the procedure may be applied in ways that are technologically improper or humanistically destructive.

Consequently, man's main problem with a new and accepted technique is its regulation. He must adapt, control, and govern the new procedures or devices that he has now made part of his environment in nature. The infinite imagination of the human mind will always create new technology; the wonder of a child can constantly invent new devices or new applications for old devices, but only the wisdom of an adult can decide how best to use them. Man's fundamental un-

derstanding of nature—his basic science—is incomplete and imma-
ture until he has regulated his artifacts, mastered his inanimate machinery, and incorporated technology harmoniously into his natural
daily existence.

The characteristic sequence of rejection, acceptance, abuse, regulation, and incorporation of new technology in modern life is particularly well illustrated by what has happened to electricity. The first
observers of electricity were ridiculed, and those who devised a way
to generate it were initially rebuffed. When this new source of power
finally became accepted, many people were electrocuted by open wires
and many homes were destroyed by fires from improperly designed
circuits, before satisfactory wiring insulation and better circuit designs
were developed. Urban man has now regulated electricity so well,
incorporating it into daily acts of living, that we need a massive failure
of a regional power supply to remind us of the extent to which electricity has now become almost a natural part of human existence.
When the power fails, we discover that our regulation is incomplete;
we still need better circuit-breakers or other ways of governing the
flow of current so that enormous rural and urban areas will not suddenly be plunged into suspended animation.

Regulating the abuse of technology is a chronic problem for which
man's solutions always come late. The acceptance lag enables the
abuses to become well established long before man's main efforts are
converted from rejecting the technology to deciding that it should be
regulated. When the technology is finally accepted and its abuses are
noted, the regulations can seldom be completely successful: 1) the
regulations themselves may create new abuses—such as the lawless-
ness that followed prohibition of commercially distilled alcoholic
beverages; 2) the regulations, although seemingly adequate, may omit
a crucial point—as with the regional electrical circuit-breakers; or 3)
the technology may later be applied for nefarious new purposes, not
covered in the initial regulations. For example, after many centuries
of regulation, man had learned to live well with fire and the wheel.
The harmony was broken, however, by the technologic revolution of
the past century, which changed the application of these agents so
that they now require additional control: fire has become a frequent
aerial incendiary weapon against innocent people, and the wheel, via
automobile crashes, has become a frequent source of mutilation and
death.

Although the occupational disruptions of technology are not solved easily or immediately, solutions always become available because the new technology, while obliterating old occupations, inevitably creates new ones. The blacksmith becomes an automotive worker; the candler, an electrician; the whaler makes, sells, or repairs sailboats for the automotive worker and electrician to use during the extra leisure time provided by technology and affluence.

There is almost no evidence to support the contention that technology has reduced man's ethical standards toward his fellow man. Throughout history, people have been exploiting, stabbing, dismembering, burning, or slaughtering other people; technology has changed only the means, not the principle. Nor is there evidence to prove that technology has reduced man's appreciation of nature and of human artifact. Encountering the pristine, the beautiful, or the historic, people have always polluted, pillaged, sacked, or destroyed; technology has changed the means, not the principle. If technology has made man less self-reliant in his contacts with nature (for example, how would the average contemporary urbanite manage the problem of starting a fire in the woods on a damp day?), man has also become able to add his arts and architecture to the beauties of nature.

The current outcry about the evils of technology seems, therefore, to be a repetition of man's constant response to a persistent or recurrent difficulty. The problems of today, however, include three drastic distinctions that have not occurred before at any time in man's long past, and that make contemporary fears more reasonable. We now have much better grounds for fright about modern technology than the old human xenophobia for the different and the new:

1) Man now has the capacity to mutilate the unborn. In the past, the injuries of conventional weapons were always confined to the lifetime of the recipient. A person might be killed, maimed, or economically incapacitated, but his genes were unharmed; he could hope that his children would have a fresh start. In contemporary society, however, generations of children that are yet unborn may be adversely affected if irradiation from atomic weapons alters sperm and ova in the gonads of the survivors, or if biologists cannot suitably control the impending possibilities for molecular modification of human genes.

2) Machines now have the capacity to simulate some of man's ability to think. All the preceding advances in technology have been devices that extended man's sensory and motor capacities—his ability to see, hear, move, and build—but his cerebration was left alone. The

technology of computers has now invaded the realm of thought. The machines can store information more effectively than the memory of man, and can perform calculations and certain analyses more rapidly and more accurately than human minds.

3) Man has begun to spurn or to neglect the regulation of technology. The invention or discovery of new knowledge and technologic procedures in science is often called "basic" research, while the development and regulation is called "applied". In the rapid advances of modern science, many "applied" regulations have a short life. For example, commercial illumination with gas was antiquated when electricity became the main source of power; many modern airports have needed total re-design to deal with the new jet airplanes; existing railroad facilities may need complete revision as new forms of mass ground transportation are developed. The fear of early obsolescence is one belief, therefore, that makes "applied" research unattractive to many good scientists today. Another current belief diverting outstanding scientific minds from regulatory activities is that "basic" research is superior to "applied" research. Because of these two beliefs, contemporary and subsequent new technology may be left unregulated or regulated inadequately, bereft of attention from the best minds man can bring to the challenges.

Although "basic" research deserves abundant support purely on its own merits, the current prejudices about the superiority of "basic" research are relatively new, beginning mainly after the success of physicists in producing an atomic bomb. In a society devoted to practical accomplishment, this achievement showed that "basic" research was important and needed support. The magnitude of contemporary support has now almost compensated "basic" investigators for their many previous years of neglect and deprecation; they are now well recognized and well endowed with funds from federal and other sources. For the past decade in physical and biologic science, "basic" research has been given intellectual and financial encouragement exceeding anything of the past, and often well beyond the support given to concomitant "applied" activities.

This reversal of attitude toward research has not entirely solved the problem of defining what is "basic" or "applied", and has led to many unvalidated decisions about what type of research should be regarded as "science". The definition of "basic" has often depended on the minuteness of the material rather than the magnitude of the problem. Thus, physicists become regarded as more "basic" than chemists, and people who study paramecia are more "basic" than those who study rats. People who study man rather than man's cells, in this definition, can never do "basic" research. "Science" has often been defined by goal rather than by method. As long as the purpose is to understand nature rather than to change it, or to find new devices rather than to regulate existing technology, the activity is regarded as science. Thus, the engineer and the clinician, who remedy and regulate, are excluded from "science" in this definition, no matter how well they design their experiments or do their work.

The fallacy of the intellectual prejudices contained in these definitions is that many "basic" problems in science may be solved during "applied" research, just as "basic" research may bring eventual solution for many "applied" problems. This distinction is well illustrated by considering the fate of commercial illumination with natural gas.

In the days when public streets were lit with gas, "applied" researchers were scientifically investigating such issues as the types of pipe to use for transporting the gas, the optimal mixture of gas and air to reduce the risk of explosions, the construction of the lamp in which the gas was burned, and the optimal position of the lamp for lighting the allocated portion of the street. While all this "applied" work was taking place, a "basic" researcher was developing a means to generate a substance called electricity that would eventually make gas lights obsolete.

The first reaction to this story is to conclude that all the "applied" research was wasted. Nevertheless, if the work was done well, most of it is still important today because it provided solutions for fundamental problems in science. Although we no longer need gas lamps, we still use pipes to transport gas for other purposes, and we still must know how best to design those pipes, regardless of what they lead to. The best method of mixing gas and air is a basic problem in combustion, regardless of how the mixture is used, and the optimal position of a street lamp is a basic problem in illumination, regardless of how the light gets its power. These aspects of transportation, combustion, and illumination are basic scientific problems, and their solutions are important contributions to human knowledge, regardless of whether the solutions were developed during "applied" or "basic" research.

The qualifying aspect of "basic research" is the basic importance of the problem, not the material, incentive, or possible applications of the investigation. What makes it "science" is how well the work is conceived, performed, and analyzed, not the particular technologic methods or devices that are used.

Some of the leading scientists of our time have spoken out against the limited intellectual horizon of many fashions in current "basic research":

Norbert Wiener[176]—

> We need to cultivate fertility of thought as we have cultivated efficiency in administration. We need to find some mechanism by which an invention of interest to the public may effectively be dedicated to the public. . . . To throw the problem of [man's] responsibility on the machine . . . is to cast responsibility to the winds, and to find it coming back seated on the whirlwind.

John R. Platt[177]—

> Measurements and equations are supposed to sharpen thinking, but in my observation, they more often tend to make the thinking non-causal and fuzzy. . . . We become "method-oriented" rather than "problem-oriented."

Leo Szilard[178]—

> If you do stupid experiments and finish one a year, it can take 50 years. . . . But if you stop doing experiments for a little while and *think* . . . , it will only take a few experiments.

Barry Commoner[179]—

> The proper correlation of physics and biology requires that the *integrity of both sciences* be maintained in the collaborative process. . . . We cannot study the property of life without retaining it in our experiments.

René Dubos[180]—

> The time has come to give to the study of the responses that the living organism makes to its total environment the same dignity and support which is being given at present to the science of parts and reactions isolated from the organism. . . . Physicians have the overwhelming advantage that bedside experience gives them an awareness of the fundamental needs and potentialities of the human condition.

> ... Medicine has the opportunity to ... [develop] a science of man
> ... [to] complement the reductionist analysis of structures and mecha-
> nisms.

No matter how we define "basic", "applied", and "science", man's ability to live harmoniously with his own artifacts of nature is surely a fundamental problem in contemporary scientific research. The drastic modern possibilities—mutilation of the unborn, mechanization of thought, and abandonment of attention to regulation—create an imbalance in technologic control that threatens the very foundations of nature and of human existence on earth. Unless man develops better methods for governing his technology, human values may become extinct because man will be extinct. The predicament affects every aspect of human life today, but the rest of this discussion will deal only with certain medical consequences.

With regard to mutilation, clinicians have already become able to deform the unborn or the newly born, even without radiation and molecular genetics. The mutilations have been accomplished by injudicious prescription of such drugs as thalidomide to pregnant women, and by administration of excessive oxygen to premature babies. With regard to the intellectual challenges of computers, clinicians have been reluctant to assume the burden or have been fearful of the consequences. The medical application of computers is now being guided by non-clinical scientists who may understand the machine, but not the problem, and who may produce excellent answers to useless questions. With regard to the regulation of medical technology, many contemporary workers in clinical research believe that the laboratory quest for "basic science" is intellectually superior to the search for solutions to "applied" clinical problems, and that further "basic" advances may eliminate those problems. Clinical investigators have begun to direct their research primarily at causes of disease, mechanisms of disease, new drugs and devices, and the exploration of cellular biology, but have not adequately investigated ways of regulating either the diagnostic or the therapeutic maneuvers now at our disposal.

These fashions in contemporary clinical investigation often produce a hit-and-run type of research. Seeking "basic science", the investigator may devise a new physiologic, biochemical, immunologic, or other laboratory procedure that seems to offer an index of disease, but he may stop at that point, without assembling a satisfactory healthy epidemiologic population or a wide clinical spectrum of patients for determining the test's range of normal values and its most effective usage. The investigator may devise a new drug for treatment of disease, but may confine his research to studies of animals or of short-term metabolic effects in man, avoiding the lengthy clinical trials necessary to decide whether the drug is really beneficial to patients. Instead of studying these "applications", the academic clinician may continue searching for yet newer diagnostic and therapeutic maneuvers, leaving the "applied" investigation to be done at a later date or by a "lesser" scientist. The technology of clinical medicine, thus precociously released from its "basic" sources, becomes augmented as an anarchy of adolescence instead of regulated as an equilibrium of maturity.

We are amused today by the diagnostic uroscopy of the medieval physician. How will the clinician of the future regard our diagnostic failure to regulate the inconsistencies of microscopy, the exorbitance of roentgenograms, and the phantasmagoria of contemporary laboratory tests? We now look with disdain at the "barbarous" blood-letting of the past. How will clinicians of the future regard the radical surgery and radiotherapy with which we have been treating cancers for more than 60 years without truly scientific knowledge of when and whether these treatments have been effective? By applying the advances of technology during the past century, we have saved lives with blood transfusion, but have brought death to mismatched recipients; we have given the blessings of anesthesia to patients undergoing surgery, but we have killed or paralyzed many with untoward reactions to anesthetics; we have prevented the ravages of bacteria by using antibiotics correctly, but we have produced fatal or protracted illness with their abuse; we have made birth easier for the mother, but have injured the child removed untimely from its womb; we have learned to operate successfully upon every part of the human body, but we are not yet sure about when to do so, and in whom. Will clinicians of the future share our infatuation for the technology that makes possible these glories—and these tragedies? Will our clinical successors maintain the scientific urge to "do something" that makes us so often ignore the clinician's sacred law of technologic regulation: *primum non nocere?*

Many of the basic problems requiring diagnostic and therapeutic regulation in modern medical technology have already been cited in previous chapters. The remainder of this chapter is devoted to other aspects of the clinician's co-existence with established technology and with the new computers.

TECHNOLOGY AND CLINICAL SKILLS

Because contemporary clinicians have become pre-occupied with the technology available for pathologic diagnosis, the "science" produced by the technology has often obscured the differences between precise function in a machine and in a human mind.

Many young clinicians have lost (or never acquired) large parts of old clinical skills for interpreting the observations of the bedside. The new clinicians have correctly recognized many situations in which clinical examination need be only brief and incomplete for the appropriate diagnostic tests to be selected. In such situations, the clinical data are not used as precise evidence in the *diagnostic* reasoning, and serve mainly as clues to ordering the appropriate adjunctive tests that provide precise evidence. Extrapolating from these situations, many clinicians have changed their methods of diagnostic reasoning. The reasoning has become not a systematic exercise in deductive logic, but a rapid reflex arc that begins with a few perfunctory observations at the bedside, and ends with a profound list of entries in the nurse's order book. The brief clinical observation of "chest pain", not further specified, often evokes the reflex of a written order for diagnostic tests that may include "ECG, Sputum Pap Smear, Sputum Cultures, 4-Posn. Chest X-ray c̄ Barium, Transaminase, Lactic Dehydrogenase, etc." The brief clinical observation of "palpable liver", also not further specified, may evoke the order-book reflex of "LFTs c̄ BSP, Pro Time, Bleed Time, Clot Time, Serum Electrophoresis, TP c̄ A/G, Liver Scan, Liver Consult for Biopsy, etc."

There is nothing wrong with ordering all these tests—in the situations for which they are appropriate. But the clinician's obsession with diagnostic technology may make him lose the scientific intellectual skills that tell him when the situation is appropriate. After all the tests are ordered, done, and returned with negative results, he may then sometimes discover, by simple muscle testing, that the "chest pain" was in the chest wall, not in the heart or lungs. He may find, by percussing for the upper margin of liver dullness, that the "palpable liver" was proptosed, but not abnormally enlarged.

More significantly, however, after recognizing that technologic evidence is better than clinical evidence for certain pathologic diagnoses, the clinician may begin to think that clinical data have no importance at all. Having begun to abandon his skill in clinical examination because he often did not need that skill for pathologic diagnosis, he may no longer have the skill available, or he may no longer recognize its pertinence, when he needs it for diagnoses that cannot be made technologically, and for his reasoning in the crucial design and appraisal of therapeutic experiments.

The clinician may begin to think that *angina pectoris* is not a symptom, but a sign or a disease discerned from certain electrocardiographic maneuvers. He may become unable to explain, to himself or to patients, many clinical manifestations that do not correlate with morbid anatomy. Frustrated by his inability to find histopathologic explanations for such clinical manifestations as *anxiety* or the *functional bowel distress syndrome,* he may vent his frustration on the patient, who now becomes not a sick person asking for help, but an annoying "crock" who refuses to show a positive result in the technologic tests. A patient complaining of "low back strain" may be put through the expensive, uncomfortable gamut of a complex technologic "work-up", including perhaps even the hazards of a myelogram, before the clinician emerges with the impressive scientific diagnosis of "low back strain; no organic disease". By performing elaborate technologic "work-ups" for minor problems or functional disorders, clinicians often achieve a precise pathologic diagnosis of the "non-disease" that Meador[181] has so incisively described.

Furthermore, after these excursions in technologic diagnosis, the clinician may plan and administer treatment not as a scientific healer, but as a bedside technician. The problem is illustrated by the self-adulation of an intern who believes he has given a patient superb *care,* because he (the intern) stayed up all night treating the patient's diabetic acidosis, ordering all the appropriate blood tests, calculating the quantities of adequate fluids, checking the urine sugars and acetones, getting hourly electrocardiographic tracings while worrying about cellular shifts of potassium, giving the periodic insulin injections, and achieving, by morning, the scientific success of normoglycemia. And all the while, the patient has lain there terrified by an anxiety that has not been assuaged, and parched by an aching dry tongue that has received "nothing by mouth"—not even a few ice chips—in the intern's passion for ascertaining each atom of intake.

The abandonment of treating a patient in favor of treating a pathologic diagnosis is even reflected in the way physicians talk about their cases of disease. A *case* refers to an instance of disease. A patient may represent a case, or an instance, of *myocardial infarction,* but in contemporary clinical vocabulary, the patient has often become the disease. The resident physician may say, "Last night we admitted two myocardial infarctions, a bleeding ulcer, and a viral pneumonia."

The problems of technologic prowess *versus* scientific skill affect the work of surgeons as well as physicians. The physician, because of technology, is often no longer as adept as he used to be in the skills of purely clinical diagnosis. The surgeon, because of technology, no longer has some of his old skills in the operating room. Aided by contemporary anesthesia, heart-lung machines, cardiac pacemakers, blood transfusion, and antibiotics, the surgeon need no longer be as prompt or as proficient as he used to be in handling, cutting, and sewing tissue. If he is excessively rough, he can excise the damage or substitute a graft or perhaps a prosthesis; if he is excessively slow, he can rely on the anesthesiologist to keep the patient asleep, if necessary, for days; if he causes too much loss of blood, he can get replacements from the blood bank; and if the wounds get infected, he can treat them with antibiotics.

Intent upon learning how to do the complex operative maneuvers of modern surgery, the surgical resident begins to study the maneuvers rather than the patients, and begins to lose the insightful knowledge of the natural course of illness that was always the key to good surgical judgment. Moreover, the surgeon, like the internist, has also begun to use a nomenclature of technology for labeling patients. The internist may technologically designate his patients as diseases, and send a *duodenal ulcer* to the surgeon, but the surgeon may call *his* patients by the names of therapeutic maneuvers. The surgical resident may report, for example, that his ward now contains "two gastrectomies, a herniorrhaphy, and a double-barreled colostomy."

With the modern technology of pathologic diagnosis and of therapeutic maneuvers, clinicians can now replace a destroyed mitral valve with a prosthesis; eradicate staphylococcal endocarditis by specifically selected antibiotics; successfully manage Rh blood disparities, in mother and newborn infant, by use of immunologic procedures and blood transfusions; and restore useful function in limbs that had been severed or devastatingly fractured. No patient whose life has been saved or redeemed by these and other procedures of scientific technology would want to trade any of their benefits for all the "bedside manner" of the therapeutically ineffectual clinical practice of the past.

There is no need, however, to exclude human concern and compassion from treatment merely because clinicians have become such excellent technologists. Science and care are completely compatible: the clinician loses no scientific stature by giving a patient the ice chips of care while administering agents for the diabetic acidosis; by reassuring the patient while treating him; by studying the full course of the patient's illness and not just the isolated tableau of disease seen in the hospital; and by thinking of the patient as a person, rather than a disease or a therapeutic maneuver.

The concept of care that makes a clinician lose scientific stature today is not his attention to the patient, but the current belief that this clinical concern is only or merely an act of humane tradition and sentiment. Without appropriate classification of the clinical and personal attributes of sick people, the experiments of therapy cannot be identified reproducibly or assessed effectively. It is precisely because modern clinicians have given inadequate attention to observing and evaluating the *patient* that contemporary clinical therapy has become so scientifically defective—an accepted, but unregulated, technology.

THE USE OF COMPUTERS IN CLINICAL ACTIVITIES

Computers have been proposed for so many different medical purposes that clinicians may have begun to regard the machine as a beast with multiple heads and multiple extremities, all going in diverse directions. A computer is merely a device. To talk about "computers in medicine" is no more specific or enlightening than to talk about "devices in medicine". Just as there are different technologic devices for different functions, there are different types of computer facilities for different purposes, or different sets of instructions (or *programs*) for the functions of a single computer. If clinicians are to regulate the use of these devices in clinical medicine, the first step is to recognize what a computer can do, and what it can't.

At its "input", the computer is attached to sensory organs of observation: an "eye" that can perceive nuances of light and darkness, or variations in magnetic and electrical impulses. At its "output", the computer is attached to kinetic extremities: an "arm" that can effect movements or print numerical and alphabetical characters. These sensory and locomotor appendages will be chosen according to what the device is made to do, and their variations are responsible for the diversity of literature today about "computers in medicine".

The key to understanding computers is not an awareness of these corporeal appurtenances, but a recognition of what goes on inside the computer's "brain". Unlike the many inanimate beasts of burden used in modern technology, a computer is a beast of intellect. It cannot produce new forms of movement, like an automobile, an elevator, or an airplane. It cannot produce new materials or transform tangible substances, like the equipment used in a steel mill, an oil refinery, or a chemistry laboratory. It cannot generate new types of observation and data, like an X-ray, an electrocardiograph, an electrophoresis apparatus, a chemical test, or a person. It is simply a "brain", and nothing else. It must be attached to these observational and locomotive appendages in order to work, and the quality of its work will depend entirely on the quality of input and output in the appendages, and on the quality of the commands it receives.

And it is not a very good "brain", either; it can only do three things. It can co-ordinate the action of the appendages; it can transform the information it receives; and it can store the information in such "memory banks" as punched cards, punched tapes, and magnetized tapes. *Moreover, man must compose the program that tells the computer exactly how to do each of these things.*

After getting its instructions, however, the computer's "brain" can do these three things faster and more accurately than the brain of man. It can accomplish details of mechanical co-ordination with much more precision than a person; for example, a thermostat is essentially a type of computer that can co-ordinate the temperature of a room and the output of a furnace more efficiently than can be done with purely human efforts. A computer can accomplish transformations of data with a rapidity and reliability that are impossible in human intellectual function; for example, a computer in several minutes can make calculations that would require months of human labor and that would contain many inevitable human errors if done by man. A computer, in its "files" when at rest and in its "core" when active, can store or recall the specific details of hordes of information far beyond the capacity of any human memory; for example, computer tapes can preserve each detail of the demographic, clinical, para-clinical, therapeutic, and other data of every patient's complete course in every disease known to man.

In all these features of inanimate co-ordination, calculation, and mnemonics, the computer is completely dependent on man for its program of instruction, but is greatly superior to man in performance. It is a magnificent addition to human technology. Just as man prefers to ride long distances rather than walk, and to use mechanical adjuncts for feats of strength, he will want to use intellectual aids that can free his mind of the need for supervising certain co-ordinations of machinery, for performing the drudgery of massive calculations, and for trying to remember a cerebrally overwhelming amount of detail.

Like the technologic beasts of burden that serve man by doing what he physically cannot do alone, this beast of intellect can excel man in the low-level rational functions that it executes in response to man's instructions. But the computer's "brain" has no aptitude for any high-level functions of a human intellect. A computer cannot recognize new or unfamiliar patterns; it cannot make conceptual abstractions that lead to categorical generalizations; and it cannot make any decisions of judgment, excellence, or other human values. A computer can be instructed to do all these things, but when it does, it always works with the human recognitions, concepts, and judgments that it has been commanded to use.

In pattern recognition, for example, a digital computer ordinarily "reads" its information from alphabetical and numerical characters previously punched, by man, onto a card or tape. Unless the characters are presented in this punched form, the computer cannot recognize them. Certain new computers may be fitted with a sensory appendage that enables them to read a printed or drawn character directly, without previous human transformation, but the ability to recognize variations in a pattern is extremely limited. A child who once has learned to read can thereafter easily recognize the letter *A* when it varies in height or other aspects of its visual pattern. A computer, however, must be programmed to recognize each of the possible patterns separately. Thus, after learning to identify the letter *A* when it appears as an A, the computer would still be unable to recognize it as an A or **A** or as an A, $\mathfrak{A}$, $\mathbb{A}$, *a*, a, *a*, or **a**.

In conceptual abstraction, a computer may distinguish, from appropriate data in cases of cancer of the lung, that prognosis is poor for patients with such entities as a paralyzed vocal cord, dysphagia, or the superior vena cava syndrome, but the computer could not make the categorical generalization—unless given both concept and word by man—that these three entities all arise from metastatic lesions in the mediastinum.

In judgmental decisions, a computer can be instructed to determine statistical significance, to play chess, to conduct an interview with a patient, to make decisions about diagnosis and therapy, or to teach a student—but in all these activities, the computer will merely reflect the criteria, judgments, and values of the man or men who wrote its program. The computer will do these things well or badly, according to whether the assigned statistical test was proper; whether the programmer was a good chess player who knew how to prepare a formulated strategy for anticipating all possible moves; whether the interview program and the computer's appendages were able to attract the patient to initiate and continue a "conversation" with a machine; whether the programmed data and logic for diagnosis and therapy were prepared with clinical wisdom; and whether the teaching information was arranged by a mind that knew how to organize knowledge for pedagogic instruction. Even when the computer is "taught" to "learn" on its own—by analyzing its errors—the method of analysis and learning will be a product of the human intellect that prepared the instructions.

In all these acts, the computer is totally the servant of man. It is obedient, reliable, completely subordinate, and abjectly dependent. It needs only explicit commands, given in a language that it is equipped to understand. But clinicians fear the "beast". And for the wrong reasons.

A clinician fears that he may be replaced by the machine. There is surely nothing in clinical skill that a computer can replace with its capacities for mechanical co-ordination, data processing, and mnemonic storage. The thermostat co-ordinates heat but has not replaced the furnace; an abacus and an adding machine can be helpful in calculations but have not replaced numbers; a refrigerator stores food, a financial bank stores money, and a blood bank stores blood, but these technologic storage devices have not led to the replacement of food, money, or blood by any other media. The computer can not perform a physical examination, nor can it take a good history. A well-organized computer program, suitably prepared in the types of form described earlier (Chapter 19, pages 337–339), might be helpful for obtaining certain "structured" aspects of a patient's history; a different type of computer procedure might be used for teaching medical students some of the intellectual strategies of history-taking;

but no inanimate observer of history-giving can ever cope with all the details of a patient's behavior and responses that must be perceived by the clinician directly.

A clinician fears that the computer may demolish the "art" of clinical medicine. The computer can only help remove some of the jargon, mysticism, intuitions, unverified judgments, and fallacious science that are now regarded as clinical "art". The computer cannot participate in the true art of medicine. It has none of the subtle sensory perception, intellectual imagination, and emotional sensitivity necessary for communicating with people and giving clinical care. It has neither the capacity to design a *complete* plan of clinical management nor the versatility to execute the plan.

A clinician fears that the computer may change the practice of medicine, as though medical practice has been unaltered by the technology of the printing press, the telephone, the airplane, the Roentgen ray, and the chemical laboratory. The clinician will assign to the computer any activities that he can teach it to do better than he can, or as well, just as he now often delegates roentgenograms to a radiologist, cytologic smears and tissues to a pathologist, and chemical and other tests to a laboratory technician. The clinician used to do blood counts, urinalyses, and microscopic inspection of white cells and urinary sediment himself; as soon as he learned to specify the performance of the procedures, however, he delegated them to a technician or to his office assistant. Similarly, the clinician will delegate to the computer the low-level intellectual task of storing and processing medical data, and a variety of other functions.

The clinician may not need a computer of his own. He may want only access to a computer in which he and his colleagues can jointly store, share, and analyze their data. From the computer's storage he can then later ascertain the characteristics of the patients he and his colleagues have seen in the past; how many patients there were; what treatments were used; and what happened afterward. He need not ask the computer to make a single clinical observation or a single clinical decision. All he may want the computer to do is store the data given to it, and, on command, to retrieve, sort, count, and print. But with this procedure, clinicians, for the first time in the long history of medicine, will be able to document their experience, to quantify their data, and to make their therapeutic decisions unimpaired by the fallible memory and limited vision of man.

If properly used, the computer will improve the practice of medicine by restoring attention to the *patient* in clinical science. The previous technology of the past century has pushed the patient out of the doctor's mind—replacing clinical evidence with the "scientific" data of disease or of human parts or fragments; replacing human symptoms and signs with the data of variables that had to be isolated and "controlled" because no mathematical or technologic models existed to deal with multiple, overlapping, simultaneously independent, discrete categories of information. The computer can help expand the human horizon of clinical medicine by enabling scientific attention to be given to the clinical and personal descriptions of sick people, instead of restricting "science" to the dehumanized dimensions of laboratory data. The new "rational technology" will resurrect the patient in the doctor's intellect because the clinician can now, at long last, "remember" all details of human information, and deal with them scientifically. The clinician can now contemplate all the patient's clinical evidence, not just the inferences; he can get information from other sources to complete gaps in his own immediate experience; he can manage the data with mathematical and quantitative agility; he can choose his treatment and give it not as scientist and healer, but as a scientific healer. After almost a century of clinical focus diverted to the laboratory, the clinican can once again observe the patient as a direct source of fundamental data in clinical science. To the source of what the clinician believes will give him science, he will surely give the attention and concern of his art.

What the clinician needs to fear today is not the computer, but his own absence from the efforts now being made to develop the application of computers in medicine, and his own lack of attention, as a research investigator, to basic clinical problems.

During the past few years, a new type of Ph.D. has entered the arena of medical research. The more conventional "medical" Ph.D. had been trained in some branch of biologic science—microbiology, anatomy, histology, biochemistry, and more recently, biophysics. The new Ph.D. who works in medicine is an "engineer"—trained to use the tools of statistics, computers, or some other branch of engineering science. In the contemporary rating system of scientific esteem in academic medicine, the new Ph.D. is often not regarded as a major scientific personage because he is "applied" rather than "basic", and an "engineer" rather than a "cellular biologist". Nevertheless, his contributions have been gratefully sought and accepted by the Ph.D.s, M.D.s, and clinicians who work in biomedical "basic science". The engineer has often been the designer of the apparatus—the gauges, pumps, ultracentrifuges, chromatographs, electron microscopes, radiation counters, multichanneled oscilloscopic polygraphs, spectrophotometers, and other technologic instruments—that make "basic science" possible. To get the data for the experiments of "basic science", an investigator must often depend on putting the tissues, cells, urine, or feces of an animal (or of a person) into a piece of "applied" equipment that was brilliantly conceived and produced by an "engineer".

The "engineer" has also begun to work on mechanical devices of clinical diagnosis and therapy—image intensifiers, internal cardiac pacemakers, external cardioverters, prosthetic limbs, and such surgical devices as vascular staples and artificial heart valves. More recently, via computer, the "engineer" has started to help investigate intellectual strategy in clinical diagnosis and therapy. To this rational clinical task, the statistician, electrical engineer, or computer scientist brings his own excellent intellect and knowledge, as well as his adroitness in operating statistical formulations and computers. He is willing and able to help.

But he is often asked not just to help. Because the clinician is either absent from the work or feels too insecure or ignorant about statistics and computers, and because the clinician often cannot express clearly what he wants to do and how he wants to do it, the "engineer" becomes, in essence, the director of the research, designing the investigation and deciding what questions to ask. The clinicians are happy about this arrangement because they think the "engineers" know more about "science", and will do a better job. The "engineers" accept the arrangement, because they want to make use of their talents and equipment. Both groups are happy, and the collaboration proceeds.

The flaw of this approach is that the "engineer" may be a connoisseur of statistics or computers, but not of clinical observation, and particularly not of clinical problems. He may be a connoisseur of numbers, but not of medical data; of stratagems and decisions, but not of clinical diagnosis and therapy. The "engineer" may not have been trained to observe like a clinician or, even if he has received an M.D. degree, to think like a clinician. He may not know the subtleties of human illness and of clinical experience that give a clinician his awareness of lanthanic patients, epidemiologic distributions, iatrotropic stimuli, spectrums of disease, therapeutic objectives, and therapognomonic clues that are the hallmark of clinical judgment. So the "engineer" designs intellectual clinical strategies that may be mathematically splendid, computationally effective, and statistically impressive, but clinically absurd.

To avoid using the "soft" and numerically unsatisfactory data of symptoms and signs, the "engineer" may write computer programs based primarily on demographic and laboratory data, thereby missing the point and the problems of clinical activities. He may, for purposes of insurance payments and other administrative necessities, arrange to calculate an "average length of patient hospital stay" that is farcical, depending on a preposterous concept of an "average" disease, and containing no provision for the many subtleties of illness, people, and treatment that determine the choice and duration of clinical therapy in or out of the hospital. In thinking diagnostically about symptoms and signs, the "engineer" may devise diagnostic strategies based on Bayes' theorem, a concept of inverse probability that is excellent when applied in appropriate situations but that cannot be appropriate for most clinical situations. Some of the many practical problems in using Bayes' theorem clinically have been cited elsewhere.[182] To apply the Bayesian concept in general clinical diagnosis requires assumptions about nature that are incompatible with realistic clinical activities. The types of data and the required "independence" of different variables in the Bayesian diagnostic calculations can be obtained only if clinicians ignore the epidemiologic realities of human ailments: many people have lanthanic or undiscovered disease, and many patients have multiple co-existing diseases.

The "engineer" may devise other diagnostic strategies based on types of diagnostic reasoning that astute contemporary clinicians have begun to abandon, because the clinicians are interested in precision, not probability. For example, no amount of statistics, probabilities, or hunches in clinical reasoning about jaundice can be as diagnostically precise as one revealing piece of tissue obtained through biopsy of the liver. Laënnec himself could interpret hemoptysis, chest pain, and rhonchi for us, but most modern diagnosticians would still pay more attention to the results of the roentgenogram and sputum tests. We might resurrect the celebrated Graves to deduce the cause of a patient's exophthalmos, heat intolerance, and weight loss without anorexia, but we would still like to know the results of the serum protein-bound iodine or radioactive iodine uptake before we definitely concluded that the patient had hyperthyroidism.

Seeking diagnostic accuracy, modern clinicians are often unconcerned with numerologic calculations of probability[183] that a particular disease exists in a selected patient. The main question in pathologic diagnosis is whether the disease is present or absent. If the diagnosis is made on the basis of eclectic intellectual criteria, then either the criteria are fulfilled or they are not. If the diagnosis is made on the basis of a certain item of para-clinical evidence—such as a biopsy, a roentgenogram, or a laboratory procedure—clincans will order the appropriate test, whenever feasible. Precise diagnosis has almost nothing to do with whether the probability of a disease's presence is 1/2 or 1/200 or 1/20,000. As long as the disease can possibly be present, clinicians will want to rule it out, when appropriate, by suitable tests. When satisfactory diagnostic proof exists, the disease exists, no matter what number is issued by the calculations of probability. If the disease can be neither specifically demonstrated nor ruled out, the clinician's decisions in managing the "undiagnosed" patient will depend on many features much more subtle than a simple calculation of diagnostic probabilities. The choice of a "working diagnosis" and initial therapy in such instances requires consideration of prognostic risks, therapeutic hazards, and many other clinical and personal circumstances often unrelated to the numerical statements of diagnostic likelihood.

Because the evidence to "rule in" or "rule out" specific diseases often comes from para-clinical tests, clincans will depend on the tests, rather than on clinical reasoning alone, in suitable situations. If such a test often provides a pathologic diagnosis more rapidly and accurately than the best of purely clinical diagnostic reasoning, how will the computer devoid of para-clinical data discover what the clinician already knows: that statistical probabilitites alone are not enough for precision in modern diagnostic science? If the result of the critical para-clinical test is to be obtained in advance and programmed into the computer, why bother using the computer? Why not just get the results of the test? Moreover, for those diagnoses whose precision depends not on para-clinical tests, but on intellectual clinical criteria, the computer can make no decisions unless standardized criteria are provided for it to use. For many diseases of modern medicine, however, no such criteria exist. In these situations, diagnosis by computer may be no more trustworthy than that provided by an elaborate, expensive ouija board.

Even in those situations where admirable progress has been made in developing the computer's observational performance of an adjunctive para-clinical test, such as electrocardiography,[182, 184, 185] the computer's basic problems with both patterns and criteria remain to be solved. The computer has not yet become able correctly to recognize the graphic pattern of an electrocardiographic tracing unless the inscribed baseline is perfectly straight. In those tracings that it can recognize, the computer provides mainly measurements rather than distinct diagnoses. It cannot interpret the data for critical diagnostic decisions because it does not have the criteria with which to do so; no such criteria exist. Clinicians all interpret electrocardiograms differently[186, 187] and have not yet established any fully validated or universally accepted standard criteria for general interpretation.

In one fundamental diagnostic problem of modern medicine, however, the computer's calculations of probability might be helpful. Although most of the current investigations of computers in diagnosis have been devoted to making a diagnostic decision from the assembled data, a much more important contemporary diagnostic problem is the choice of which data to assemble. This is a type of "on-line" problem, dealing with the strategy of the diagnostic work-up, rather than the selection of a diagnostic title. Which tests should be obtained, and in what order? When should we get a battery of tests simultaneously, and when sequentially? When can we dispose of a "battery" of tests and work with just a few? In which tests are the risks and costs greater than the significant information the tests may provide? How efficiently do clinicans organize the procedures of bedside examination and the timing of adjunctive tests? Are there some circumstances in which clinicians should obtain certain tests before examining the patient, or other circumstances in which a physical examination should precede the taking of an intensive history? Which routine diagnostic tests should be performed in the "work-up" of an asymptomatic patient, and what is their practical therapeutic value?

These are questions worthy of the clinican's intellect in using the computer's capacities. For the machine merely to produce a calculation of diagnostic names and probabilities gives the clinician relatively little effective help in his practical work. In such calculations, the computer may often yield only a tautologous re-iteration of a diagnostic statement already obtained from a para-clinical test. On the other hand, in the "on-line" problems of diagnostic strategy for choosing tests, the computer's calculations of probability can be valuable. Unfortunately, however, such calculations cannot be performed by any "simulation" techniques, and almost no appropriate data for the calculations are currently available. To do such calculations, clinicians will have to design a series of "flow-charts" that demonstrate the intellectual pathways of diagnostic reasoning, and will have to assemble satisfactory data from which to compute the various probabilities at each step in the pathways. Because history-taking, physical examination, and diagnostic tests are performed in a sequence, and because the data obtained at each point in this sequence may alter the subsequent procedures and probabilities, the components of the sequence must be indicated by a "flow-chart" or "logical tree", from which each consecutive possibility can then be studied and the data analyzed.

The design of such "flow-charts", and the collection of the appropriate data at each step for calculating sequential costs, risks, and diagnostic efficacy of the procedures, are a new challenge in basic clinical research today. The challenge cannot be managed with abstract theoretical models, or imaginative maneuvers in information theory. There must be specific data, obtained from specific observation of diagnostic results in general populations of patients, and analyzed with perceptive clinical thought. Bayesian probabilities, statistical maneuvers, and computational procedures can all be helpful in the final activities—but they provide neither data, concepts, nor sense for the fundamental work, and, if used alone, they cannot possibly provide satisfactory answers.

In dealing with prognosis, rather than diagnosis, the "engineer" may not be aware of the totally different intellectual and temporal distinctions between the two types of reasoning. Instead of recognizing that each pertinent clinical subgroup in the spectrum of a disease should be dealt with differently in estimating the outcome of illness,[27, 188] the "engineer" may arrange to predict prognosis by means of multivariate regression equations that are biologically inappropriate and clinically inscrutable.

The most frightening aspect of the current clinical activities with computers, however, is that neither the "engineer" nor the clinician may be able to discern when the activities are done badly. The computer scientist, although well aware of the maxim that "a computer cannot convert garbage into fruit salad", may not have the clinical judgment to know when he begins with garbage. The clinician, on the other hand, may not be able to distinguish the different fruits, or may be so awed by the gilded container in which the processed garbage appears that he neglects to scrutinize the contents.

No, the intellectual problems of clinical medicine are not problems in statistics, computers, or engineering; they are problems in clinical medicine. Clinical research may be too important to be left to clinicians alone, but it certainly cannot be done without them. Clinicians are the only scientists with enough background for understanding the clinical subtleties well enough to ask the right questions and to plan the best tactics in research designed to solve the problems. In technologic simile, the computer may be likened to a jet airplane, of which the "engineer" is pilot and navigator. He enjoys using the plane, he uses it well, and he wants to use it effectively, but he needs a clinician to tell him what trips to take, when to take them, where to stop, and how to avoid using the plane for journeys that are better accomplished by walking or by other means of travel, such as elevators, horses, bicycles, automobiles, or boats. The clinician need not learn to pilot the plane, but he needs to understand enough about navigation to be effective in making critical decisions about where and when to go; and the more he understands, the better he can work with the pilot.

Not many knowledgeable clinicians, however, are active today in research for developing and regulating the clinical use of computers. Clinicians in full-time practice either are too busy, or believe they are too ignorant, or have not been asked to participate. Clinicians in the full-time academic world, who have the time for research, are generally not interested, preferring to conduct laboratory investigations with the methods of biochemistry, electron microscopy, or microbiology. The academic clinical investigator often believes that the basic intellectual problems of clinical therapy are too "applied" to warrant fundamental research—and, besides, to work with computer "engineers", he might have to learn a methodology quite different from the one he has developed for doing "basic science".

At present, therefore, there are very few research clinicians who bring the wisdom of clinical judgment and an awareness of problems in clinical criteria, classification, and data to the "engineering" activities. The programs are being written frenziedly, the computers are running constantly, the pile of "print-outs" is mounting incessantly, and the results are being disseminated widely, but the product that may emerge is not clarity but chaos, not clinical comprehension but mathematical mysticism, not a shining marvel of human science but a gaudy pastiche of electronic art.

The clinican may believe he can afford to wait. A generation of embryonic clinicians is now learning set theory and Boolean algebra in elementary school. These clinicians of the future, as part of their undergraduate curriculum, will have learned many of the formal principles of logical thought. The future clinicians will be intellectually equipped to regard clinical reasoning as a deliberate, exciting exercise of the human mind, not as a nebulous act of intuition. They will find computers as easy to use as today's clinician finds the telephone, the typewriter, and the adding machine. When this new group of clinicians arrives on the medical scene, they should readily be able to solve many of the intellectual problems that challenge clinicians today.

But the problems of 20 years from now will be different from those of today. After another 20 years of development without careful clinical supervision, the accumulated abuses of an unregulated computer technology will be so immense and obfuscating that a young clinician may be unable to find his way through the confusion. Moreover, the medical student 20 years from now may have no suitable teachers to give him an appropriate background for understanding clinical problems. Mesmerized by the molecular goals of "basic science", many medical schools have now begun to change their curricula, emphasizing the study of cells more than symptoms, of chemistry more than community, and of microscopy more than man. Although this laboratory concept of medical science may belittle the scientific worthiness of patients' statements and problems, and may disparage the clinician's efforts to be a *clinical* scientist, the concept has become a dominant theme in medical education today. The clinical departments of many medical schools have steadily increased their attention to research in laboratory matters, while steadily decreasing their research in clinical problems, their instruction in clinical topics, and their maintenance of a faculty skillful in understanding and teaching *clinical* medicine. By the time today's young student reaches medical school, after having been intellectually prepared to solve basic problems in clinical science, the existing medical schools may no longer be concerned with those problems. The schools may have been converted from scholarly shrines for sick people to cenobitic citadels of cellular biology.

The clinician cannot effectively counteract this trend with sentimental protests about art, tradition, and humanism. These protests carry no intellectual power in an age of science. If clinical tradition is worth preserving in modern medical science, the tradition itself must be demonstrated to have scientific value.

The sublime paradox of the computer is that it gives clinicians the opportunity to restore scientific respectability to clinical art. For almost a century, the clinician has been dismissed as a scientist because his therapy was not recognized as an experimental procedure or because he could not quantify the experiments. Without precise diagnosis, potent therapy, and a rational technology for managing the complexities of clinical data, clinicians had to settle for a medical science based on the reductionist technology of non-human laboratory experiments. Just as "dehumanized" laboratory procedures have paradoxically brought the clinician diagnostic precision and therapeutic potency, "dehumanized" computers now paradoxically bring him a rational technology for analyzing his data. As a constant experimentalist in treating human illness, the clinician can now convert his activities into science. For the technology of computers to do more good than harm in this science, however, the work must be developed properly before the accreted abuse becomes impossible to regulate.

The clinicians who work with computers now will not need to study the computer intensively; the clinician's job will be to solve the basic rational clinical problems whose solution is a prerequisite for the computer to produce useful clinical results. The clinician will have to ask the questions, get the data, and plan appropriate methods for the analysis. The work cannot be accomplished merely as a travelog of conferences in which groups of computer experts meet to develop new speculative theories from old speculative theories. There will have to be data, not merely concepts; programs, not merely algorithms;* and practical demonstrations of workable techniques, not merely newer hypotheses about newer conjectures. The basis for the clinical algorithms will be the questions and plans of analysis designed by clinicians. And the basis for everything will be the data—provided by clinicians.

Can suitable clinicians be found for such work? If man, for nationalism or for science, can assemble an army of people and an armada of machines to launch, observe, and retrieve a single astronaut in space, it should not be too difficult to gather the investigative clinical scholars for studies of human illness that can help all mankind. Many clinicians now in full-time practice are intellectually well qualified for these activities and could be solicited for part-time (or full-time) research, if appropriate funds were made available. Many

* An *algorithm* is the word often applied in computer work to describe the particular strategy of problem solving on which the details of a computer program are based.

thoughtful young clinicians completing residency training and interested in an academic career, but unwilling to "grind enzymes" as a path to success, could easily be attracted to such clinical research if the appropriate positions and inducements were offered. Many academic clinical investigators who now waste their talents doing second-rate biochemical or immunologic research might want to study clinical problems if they believed that grants and academic advancement would be forthcoming.

Medical progress cannot afford to wait for a future generation of doctors to begin scientific research that affects a clinician's priceless intellectual possession—his reasoning—and his oldest tradition and main problem—the treatment of patients. The work of clinical regulation for computer technology and for the other technologies of medical diagnosis and treatment is too basic to risk any further delay. The time to begin is now.

*　　　　*　　　　*

There is still one more doubt, however—one more unresolved anxiety—that may beset the clinician: the nagging suspicion that he himself may become dehumanized in these acts of clinical science. If he begins to regard himself as the apparatus of the bedside and undergoes "standardization", if he begins to teach a machine to think like himself and if he learns, in the process, to think like a machine, how will he distinguish himself from the machine? How will he prevent his own conversion to automaton? What will keep him a human being, a person, a self?

These questions have been thoughtfully answered by J. Bronowski in his latest book, *The Identity of Man*.[189] As a biologic engine and as a cerebral calculator, says Bronowski, man is a machine, but man is always a self in that "his procedures for getting experience cannot all be formalized"; he "constantly grows and changes [with] ... new experiences" and he can "identify with the inner environment of others", being able to understand anger, tenderness, fear, curiosity, cruelty, fun, and every higher-order intellectual and emotional attribute that distinguishes man from machine or beast. As Bronowski puts it,

> Science must give honor to those whose work is superseded as well as to the newcomer. It must treat the truth of the past, and the way it was found, with dignity. It must respect the man's way of

> working more than what he finds. . . . Here is the point at which the values of science and self meet and complement one another; and it does not matter whether we call the tight complex of common values tolerance or respect or human dignity. In all of them, science seeks the dignity of the work, and we as men seek the dignity of man. . . .
>
> By identifying ourselves with the experience of others, we enlarge our knowledge of ourselves as human beings: we gain self-knowledge. . . . To be conscious is both to know and to imagine, and our humanity flows from this deep spring. When we imagine nature outside ourselves into the future, we create the mode of knowledge which is science. And when we imagine ourselves alive into the future, we create another mode: knowledge of the self. They are the inseparable halves of the identity of man.[190]

As humanist and artist, the clinician need not fear that medicine will be dehumanized by improved scientific methods for observing and analyzing the intact body, mind, existence, and clinical treatment of man. The traditional human values of clinical medicine may seem threatened today, but not by a technology or science that draws the clinician closer to the study of human beings. The threat comes from beliefs that give the label of "science" to a dissection of a patient's protoplasm but not to a description of his pain; from the concept that a "disease" is the derangement of a molecule or the dysfunction of a cell, but not the illness of a person; from devices that perceive man as a reduced fragment, but not as an intact whole; and from other false scientific dogmas, intolerant of the dignity of the past, that have distracted clinicians from their ancient domain: the care of the sick.

21. The Scientific Domain of the Investigative Clinician

When brief reports of scientific research are published in such journals as *Nature* and *Proceedings of the National Academy of Sciences,* each report is classified in a particular category of science. The list of categories includes many topics ancillary to clinical medicine: anatomy, biochemistry, cytology, genetics, histology, immunology, microbiology, pathology, pharmacology, and physiology. The categories, however, do not include clinical medicine itself, or any of its subdivisions, such as internal medicine, pediatrics, and surgery.

The categories designated as science are not confined to work that is "actively" experimental, since the list includes such primarily observational domains as astronomy, geology, and paleontology. The quality of science is not the main consideration in choosing categories, since acknowledgment is given to anthropology and sociology, which are generally considered to be less "scientific" than clinical medicine. The topics regarded as categories of science are not even required to contain observations of nature, since the list includes statistics, which is a purely methodologic discipline. Nevertheless, as an entity of its own, clinical medicine has no recognized status among the scientific domains into which modern scholarly investigation has been partitioned.

To outside editors, critics, and observers, clinical medicine apparently has no scientific identity and produces no research that warrants attention in the intellectual community of human science. Clinical medicine seems to be regarded as merely an "application" of concepts and technology in certain "basic sciences" on which the clinician's work presumably depends, and from which will come the "basic research" of clinical medicine. These two doctrines—that clinical medicine is merely an application of something else and that the something else can be called a "basic science"—have permeated the thought of doctors for almost a century. It is time the concepts were re-examined.

If "basic research" was difficult to define, "basic science" is impossible. What does the phrase "basic science" mean? Does it refer to the size of the particular object that is studied? If so, then physics, which deals with the smallest particles known to man, is the only and ultimate basic science. Does "basic science" refer to experimental work that has no hypothesis and no purpose? Surely not, for such decerebrate investigation cannot be regarded as either "basic" or "science". Does "basic science" refer to a challenge that man pursues for its own sake because it is there, without regard to any subsequent significance or practical value? If so, then mountain climbing is basic science. Does "basic science" refer to a certain collection of knowledge that is so fundamental, so all-encompassing, and so intellectually eminent that all other knowledge must flow from it? If so, then nothing is basic science, since no domain of human scholarship can fulfill this arrogant concept of "basic". Does "basic science" refer to knowledge, collected in one domain, that may be applied in another domain? If so, then everything is basic science, since every human activity depends on something else and is also applied in something else.

For any selected domain, the intellectual chain of "basic to" and "applied from" is always a circle, beginning with whatever domain is chosen, and eventually returning to that domain. One such circular conceptual chain is shown in Figure 38. Clinical medicine makes use of physiology, which contains many applications of biochemistry. Biochemistry depends on chemistry, which is an application of physics. Mathematics is basic to physics, but depends on philosophy. Semantics is basic to philosophy, linguistics to semantics, and human speech to linguistics. Human speech depends upon human development, which depends upon human health, which depends upon clinical medicine.

Every aspect of human knowledge is constantly, inevitably basic to something and applied from something else. There is no such thing as "basic science". The term is a misnomer, and the concept is a malformed mental mirage.

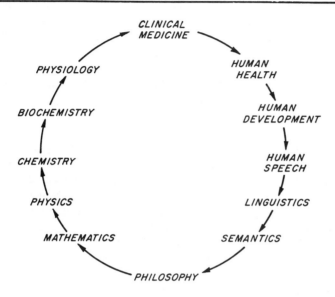

FIGURE 38

The chain of conceptual dependency in "basic" and "applied" science.

The realm of human biology pertinent to the work of a doctor of medicine contains ideas and technology from many non-clinical as well as clinical sources. As an arbitrary convention in the curriculum of many medical schools, the non-clinical instruction given to medical students is *pre*-clinical because it is given before the students begin bedside work. The non-clinical topics do not become "basic science" because of their temporal position in the current pedagogic sequence, however, and there is no omnipotent reason for maintaining the tradition of teaching them first. After a brief introduction to certain fundamentals of human structure and function, a medical student might well proceed directly to the study of sick people, and reserve the intense study of human parts until after, or while, he learns the behavior of the whole. To learn to sail a boat, a yachtsman is not required to know the molecular construction of canvas and wood, or the internal design of mechanisms for measuring wind velocity.

Instead of learning all the details of cytology, microbiology, and biochemistry before starting clinical work, a medical student might just as profitably study anthropology, sociology, and symbolic logic as his pre-clinical subjects. The knowledge to be learned in these subjects is often more basic and germane to the care of sick people than many of the clinically esoteric or irrelevant concepts of contemporary cytology, microbiology, and biochemistry. Many of these non-clinical concepts might be more meaningful and better taught if they were studied post-clinically, after the medical student has met man, and is ready to contemplate man's components.

Nor is clinical medicine just a domain of applied physiology, applied biochemistry, applied cellular biology, or applied anything. Clinical medicine is not a mere application of these subjects, any more than physiology is merely reduced clinical medicine, or biochemistry merely reduced physiology, or cellular biology merely a pragmatic application of chemistry and physics. This mistaken concept of applied extrapolation from some basic subject is responsible for many of the problems modern clinicians have in dealing with human beings. The clinician who has been taught physiology by observing a dog, biochemistry by observing a test tube, cytologic function by observing a cell, a pathology by observing a cadaver has not learned the art and science he needs for observing a sick person. When the observed patient does not behave like the materials of "basic science", the clinician may be unprepared for the distinctions between human reactions and those of animals or inanimate substances. He may have been taught no concepts, no explanations, and no intellectual methods to help reconcile the disparities, and to clarify the confusion.

The determining feature of a domain of nature is the particular entity that is observed. Each whole natural entity has distinctive patterns of behavior that establish the methods and goals of the scientific domain in which the entity is studied. The forest is different from the trees, the trees from the twigs, the twigs from the leaves, the leaves from the chlorophyll. Although the many different entities of nature are inter-related, each entity—from neutron to nation—constitutes a domain of its own. Each domain has a different basic particle or group of particles to be observed, each has different units of observation, each has different quantities of measurement for those units, each uses different methods, and each has different goals.

To regard clinical medicine as a mere application of what is learned from animals, test tubes, cells, and human cadavers is a fundamental misconception of a basic law of nature: a whole is *not* the mere sum of its parts. The instant that a scientist changes the unitary whole that he observes, it becomes a different entity, with different attributes and behavior that cannot be predicted from a knowledge of either the source or the parts.

We can take apart a clock and study the size of its wheels, the ratio of their gears, and the composition of their metal, but we would never discover, in this fragmented state of the clock, what it does only as a whole: indicate time. We can study the individual properties of two man-made satellites, but we cannot safely predict from their separate behavior how they will function when joined together in space. We can understand the composition of neuroglia, but must study separately what happens when they combine to form a brain; we can know every detail of structure of a dead human brain without understanding its function as a living mind.

The basic particle that is a unitary whole in the domain of physiology is a functional system of internal organs or cells; in biochemistry, a molecule; in philosophy, an idea; in semantics, a word. The basic particle that is a unitary whole in the domain of clinical medicine is a sick person; the basic units of observation are signs, symptoms, and personal attributes; the basic quantities of measurement are words and occasionally numbers; the basic methods are those of clinical examination, clinical reasoning, and clinical therapy; the basic goal is to prevent illness that has not yet occurred and, when illness already exists, "to cure occasionally, to relieve often, and to comfort always".[191]

To achieve this goal, a clinician will want to know about many things derived from other scholars who have studied disease and man. A clinician will want to know about the structure of man's parts and the way they function, alone and together, in health and in sickness; he will want to know about the names, causes, and mechanisms of disease; he will want to know about the inanimate and rational technologies that he can use to get and analyze data; he will want to know about the agents he can use in treatment; and he will want to know about the many ways in which man—as an individual particle and in groups—lives, creates, loves, and works. The clinician will borrow, apply, and sometimes add knowledge in all of the domains that deal with these separate aspects of disease and man. But none of these ancillary realms of natural knowledge is the clinician's basic domain; his own fundamental, unique domain—the realm of nature in which he observes, investigates, and constantly performs experiments—is the illness of man.

In studying the natural course of a patient's illness, a clinician—like an astronomer, geologist, or paleontologist—observes an experiment arranged by nature, not by man. In estimating prognosis for each of these natural experiments in human illness, a clinician's reasoning is exactly analogous to an astronomer's prediction of orbital pathway. By the act of therapy, the clinician imposes an active experiment upon the one he has passively observed, and tries to alter its anticipated natural outcome. In designing and appraising those therapeutic experiments, the clinician's reasoning is exactly analogous to that used in a chemist's or physicist's experimental attempts to alter nature.

If clinicians have not made their domain into a recognizable or better science, the problem arises from the clinicians' neglect of the basic entity of the domain, and from their depreciation of the scientific potential contained in clinical skills. Bewitched by the precision and standardization of laboratory technology, clinicians have abandoned or failed to improve precision and standardization in their own clinical observations and clinical reasoning. Clinicians have often rejected their own human sensory and cerebral capacities as inheren' defects, irremediable flaws, scientifically undesirable elements that must be avoided and removed by inanimate technology.

The fallacy of this belief is its exclusion of the human mind as an adjunct in the exploration of human complexity. The complexity of man is the very reason why many human attributes cannot be observed in animals, or reduced to dimensional measurement and automated observation in man. The total function of human beings extends beyond their gross or molecular structure, and cannot always be assessed by the terminology and techniques used for morphologic structure in man, or for function in lower animals. The behavior of man as a social, political, intellectual, or familial organism, and his clinical and psychic reactions in human illness, cannot all be measured in dimensional numbers or observed by inanimate devices. These functions can be discerned, defined, catalogued, and enumerated scientifically, however, if they are properly assessed by the only apparatus capable of the performance—by the sole instrument astute, versatile, perceptive, and adaptable enough to examine man as man—a human observer.

Despite the experimental investigative challenges offered clinicians by modern diagnosis, drugs, and surgery, the efforts of most clinical investigation and experimental medicine in human disease today are directed at etiology and pathogenesis of disease, not at prognosis and therapy of patients. For studying pathogenesis of disease, the methods of laboratory research are almost mandatory, since human morality prevents the general use of man as an animal in which to induce disease. For pathogenesis of degenerative or neoplastic diseases, however, laboratory research using man as the animal would be inadequate, even if permissible, since investigators do not yet know how to induce the human disease whose development they would like to study. The proper investigation of etiology of disease demands studies not merely of laboratory phenomena, but of large human populations. Even for the infectious diseases whose agents have been revealed by laboratory research, investigators still have little knowledge of the human or environmental features that predispose and mediate the infections in their hosts.

Whatever be the merit, site, and optimal material of research in etiology and pathogenesis of disease, the domain of prognosis and therapy for human illness surely belongs to the clinician. The domain is his to explore, since only he has the necessary clinical skills with which to question and to observe. The exploration of this domain has been increasingly neglected by many contemporary "clinical investigators" who use their clinical training only as background orientation for research in etiology or pathogenesis, performed with the methods of various laboratory domains in "basic science". Such investigators often regard the study of natural history in human illness and the taxonomic problems of clinical data as archaic, and they dismiss research in therapy as mere "drug testing"; they prefer the challenges of dissecting human function into molecular structures, and their search is for cause and mechanism, rather than care and management, in human disease. The very phrase "clinical investigation" has become increasingly transmogrified into a label for laboratory research, performed by a member of an academic clinical department, in which the material is not human and the direct orientation is not disease.

Laboratory investigation of this type is obviously desirable and necessary, but its intellectual stature is not inherently greater, and its performance is no more preferable, than clinical forms of clinical research. The clinical investigator must do many types of laboratory research to explain the clinical phenomena he observes and to apply the advances learned in the domains of "basic science", but he does a disservice to both clinical medicine and "basic science" if he abandons the precise identification of clinical phenomena and the clinical application of laboratory advances. Neither the clinical nor the non-clinical domains of science can function effectively if they become intolerant or suppressive of each other, or unconcerned with their inter-relationship. If not correlated with carefully delineated clinical and biologic phenomena, the advances of "basic science" are doomed to an isolated, meaningless existence.

The "basic scientist" often forgets the intellectual debts he owes the clinician for demonstrating what to explore. The current era of "molecular biology" in clinical research did not arise *de novo* from triumphs obtained in the laboratory alone; the triumph came from correlating precise laboratory observations with precise clinical observations. The era began with application of electrophoresis and other "molecular" techniques to study the hemoglobin of patients with sickle cell anemia.[192] A prerequisite to this research was the earlier observation, by hematologic clinicians, of the particular cluster of disease called *anemia,* and the clinicians' specific isolation and classification of the *sickle* entity. Had the laboratory techniques for assessment of hemoglobin molecules been applied merely to a general population of anemic patients, instead of to the specific group clinically identified as having sickle cell anemia, the "basic scientists" would have found nothing but diverse, insignificant variations. The primogenitive event that created the era of "molecular biology" in medicine would have been stillborn.

The clinical investigator has many important incentives for studying and applying laboratory techniques in the vagaries of disease and illness, but he forsakes his clinical training and function if he fails to correlate, to analyze, to regulate, and to teach the clinical significance of what he finds. The clinicians who treat patients, the clinicians who do clinical research or laboratory research, and the M.D.s and Ph.D.s who do purely laboratory research all need each other. They destroy their opportunities for mutual progress if laboratory workers scorn clinical activities as unscientific art, or if clinicians reject laboratory research as impractical abstraction. Every scientist owes full allegiance and respect to the whole that is his own domain, but he forgets, at his peril, that his domain is a mere part of the whole of natural science and human life.

The clinical academician has no guarantee that a knowledge of molecular structure will explain *all* the higher biologic and psychic functions that distinguish people from molecules or rats, and no assurance that all disease will vanish once the mechanisms and causes are known. Much of the laboratory research now being done in cancer and other chronic diseases has been ineffectual because the clinical entities under scrutiny have not yet been adequately observed, identified, and correlated. Conversely, the brilliant elucidation of molecular mechanism in sickle cell anemia has not yet brought practical prophylactic or remedial benefit to a single patient suffering from this disease. Until every human illness is abolished, clinicians will continue to face the basic challenges of prognosis and treatment, and will need separate scientific exploration of these challenges. For such work, the "investigative clinician" has a domain and a unitary entity different from that of his colleagues in laboratory research, and his scientific methods and purposes are therefore also different.

The scientific exploration of this clinical domain must come from apparatus that can supply human compassion as well as human cerebration, from activities that restore the patient to his rightful place as a source, as well as a beneficiary, of the data used for investigation. The clinician needs a renaissance of basic scientific research directed at himself and at patients. He needs to explore his basic methods for making exact clinical observations, for classifying them systematically, and for evaluating them with specific indexes, criteria, and analyses. The clinicians who undertake this investigation should have no scientific reluctance to call themselves clinicians. The work cannot be done by biochemists, electron microscopists, microbiologists, pharmacologists, physiologists, statisticians, or other investigators who lack clinical background or research interest in caring for sick people and in distinguishing the attributes of scientific variables unique to clinical and to human phenomena.

It is time that clinicians—whether working in an academic sanctuary or in the experiments of daily medical practice—stopped being scientifically ashamed of being clinicians, and stopped regarding science as either unobtainable in clinical work or as a threat to clinical "art". We need more basic research in clinical medicine today, not less; but first we need a more suitable definition of what is to be conceived and acknowledged as basic research in clinical medicine. For almost a century, the intellect of clinicians has been anesthetized by a dogmatic conceptual vapor that is as destructive to true clinical progress, and as fallacious, as the humors and miasmas of the past. The clinician has been taught to believe that "basic clinical science" includes all of biology except the clinical treatment of patients; that "basic clinical science" comes from manipulating a dog, fish, pigeon, or cell, but not from talking with a person; and that "basic clinical science" is a birthright granted in the laboratory and lost at the bedside or in the community.

The words "basic", "laboratory", and "science" are *not* synonymous in medical research. The importance of medical research does *not* depend on whether it is done in laboratory, ward, bed, armchair, library, or community. What is important in research is whether it is fundamental or trivial, good or bad. What makes it science is the effectiveness, not the type, of methods used by the investigator. What makes it fundamental is the type of goal it seeks, not the absence of a purpose; and how it is done, not where it is done. What makes it good is the way the investigator uses his artistic imagination and his intellectual discipline to choose problems, ask questions, design plans, execute procedures, analyze data, draw conclusions, and communicate results. These are the methods that produce "basic science"—whether the tools be stethoscope or spectrophotometer, conversation or chromatography, digital palpation or digital computer; and whether the material be men, books, rats, tissues, bugs, or brine.

The clinicians of the 17th, 18th, and 19th centuries, and many who worked much earlier, were superb observers and organizers of clinical data. They did this perhaps because they respected the scientific aspects of their craft, but also because it was all they knew how to do; there were almost no other types of data to be observed. The clinician of the 20th century must resurrect this respect for his primary skills. To form a powerful, coherent chain of therapeutic clinical science, he must bring strong links from the bedside to join the strength modern technology has given to the links provided from the laboratory.

The clinician has an ancient and honorable heritage, a tradition of enlightened thought and achievement, and a domain whose humanistic and scientific complexity can challenge the most demanding intellect or spirit, at levels of fundamental inquiry. He need not look for "basic science" elsewhere. He can make his own.

References*

1. MEDAWAR, P. B. Is the scientific paper fraudulent? Saturday Review **47**: 42–43 (Aug. 1), 1964. (*1*)
2. WOOD, H. F., SIMPSON, R., FEINSTEIN, A. R., TARANTA, A., AND STOLLERMAN, G. H. Rheumatic fever in children and adolescents: A long-term epidemiologic study of subsequent prophylaxis, streptococcal infections, and clinical sequelae. I. Description of the investigative techniques and of the population studied. Ann. Intern. Med. **60** (Supp. 5): 6–17 (Feb.), 1964. (*2, 257*)
3. BUTTERWORTH, J. S. AND REPPERT, E. H. Auscultatory acumen in the general population. J. Am. Med. Assn. **174**: 32–34 (Sept. 3), 1960. (*3, 324*)
4. FEINSTEIN, A. R. AND DiMASSA, R. The unheard diastolic murmur in acute rheumatic fever. New Eng. J. Med. **260**: 1331–1333 (June 25), 1959. (*3*)
5. AMERICAN HEART ASSOCIATION. Report of committee on standards and criteria for programs of care of the council on rheumatic fever: Jones criteria (modified) for guidance in diagnosis of rheumatic fever. Circulation **13**: 617–620 (Apr.) 1956. (*4, 83, 150, 183, 335*)
6. WITTS, L. J. Medical Surveys and Clinical Trials. 2nd Edition. Oxford University Press. London. 1964. An excellent bibliography on observer variability is contained on pages 43–49, at the end of the chapter, "Diagnosis in Group Research", by C. M. FLETCHER AND P. D. OLDHAM. (*4*)
7. FEINSTEIN, A. R., WOOD, H. F., SPAGNUOLO, M., TARANTA, A., JONAS, S. KLEINBERG, E., AND TURSKY, E. Rheumatic fever in children and adolescents: A long-term epidemiologic study of subsequent prophylaxis, streptococcal infections, and clinical sequelae. VII. Cardiac changes and sequelae. Ann. Intern. Med. **60** (Supp. 5): 87–123 (Feb.), 1964. (*6, 187, 255, 332, 347*)
8. FRIEDEN, J., SHAPIRO, J. H., AND FEINSTEIN, A. R. Radiologic evaluation of heart size in rheumatic heart disease. Studies in young patients. Arch. Intern. Med. **111**: 44–50 (Jan.), 1963. (*6*)
9. FEINSTEIN, A. R. AND SPAGNUOLO, M. The duration of activity in acute rheumatic fever. J. Am. Med. Assn. **175**: 1117–1119 (Apr. 1), 1961. (*6*)
10. FEINSTEIN, A. R., SPAGNUOLO, M., AND GILL, F. The rebound phenomenon in acute rheumatic fever. I. Incidence and significance. Yale J. Biol. Med. **33**: 259–278 (Feb.), 1961. (*6, 186*)

---

* Italic numbers in parentheses refer to pages in this book where the references are cited.

391

11. FEINSTEIN, A. R., KLEINBERG, E., AND SPAGNUOLO, M. The prognosis of acute rheumatic fever. Am. Heart J. **68**: 817–834 (Dec.), 1964. (*6, 150, 187, 211*)

12. FEINSTEIN, A. R., SPAGNUOLO, M., WOOD, H. F., TARANTA, A., TURSKY, E., AND KLEINBERG, E. Rheumatic fever in children and adolescents: A long-term epidemiologic study of subsequent prophylaxis, streptococcal infections, and clinical sequelae. VI. Clinical features of streptococcal infections and rheumatic recurrences. Ann. Intern. Med. **60** (Supp. 5): 68–86 (Feb.), 1964. (*6, 181, 186, 257*)

13. FEINSTEIN, A. R. AND STERN, E. K. Clinical effects of recurrent attacks of acute rheumatic fever: A prospective epidemiologic study of 105 episodes. J. Chron. Dis. **20**: 13–27 (Jan.), 1967. (*6, 186, 206–208*)

14. FEINSTEIN, A. R. Standards, stethoscopes, steroids and statistics. The problem of evaluating treatment in acute rheumatic fever. Pediatrics **27**: 819–828 (May), 1961. (*6, 332, 348*)

15. SPAGNUOLO, M. AND FEINSTEIN, A. R. The rebound phenomenon in acute rheumatic fever. II. Treatment and prevention. Yale J. Biol. Med. **33**: 279–298 (Feb.), 1961. (*6*)

16. FEINSTEIN, A. R., TAUBE, H., CAVALIERI, R., SCHULTZ, S. G., AND KRYLE, L. Physical activities and rheumatic heart disease in asymptomatic patients. J. Am. Med. Assn. **180**: 1028–1031 (June 23), 1962. (*6*)

17. FEINSTEIN, A. R. AND SPAGNUOLO, M. The clinical patterns of acute rheumatic fever: A reappraisal. Medicine **41**: 279–305 (Dec.), 1962. (*7, 8, 150, 185, 188, 211, 335*)

18. FEINSTEIN, A. R., ZAGALA, J. G., AND SPAGNUOLO, M. The pattern of symptoms, pre-treatment interval, and prognosis of acute rheumatic fever. Ann. Intern. Med. **57**: 563–571 (Oct.), 1962. (*7, 13, 186, 211*)

19. FEINSTEIN, A. R. AND SPAGNUOLO, M. Experimental reactivation of subsiding rheumatic fever. J. Clin. Invest. **40**: 1891–1899 (Oct.), 1961. (*7, 186*)

20. FEINSTEIN, A. R. AND SPAGNUOLO, M. Sore throats, streptococcal infections and prevention of rheumatic fever. J. Chron. Dis. **15**: 623–633 (June), 1962. (*8*)

21. FEINSTEIN, A. R. (Editorial). The basic elements of clinical science. J. Chron. Dis. **16**: 1125–1133 (Nov.), 1963. (*9*)

22. FEINSTEIN, A. R. Boolean algebra and clinical taxonomy. I. Analytic synthesis of the general spectrum of a human disease. New Eng. J. Med. **269**: 929–938 (Oct. 31), 1963. (*13, 170*)

23. MACDONALD, I. The individual basis of biologic variability in cancer. Surg., Gynec., & Obst. **106**: 227–229 (Feb.), 1958. (*13, 194*)

24. FEINSTEIN, A. R. Symptomatic patterns, biologic behavior, and prognosis in cancer of the lung. Practical application of Boolean algebra and clinical taxonomy. Ann. Intern. Med. **61**: 27–43 (July), 1964. (*13*)

25. FEINSTEIN, A. R. Symptoms as an index of biological behaviour and prognosis in human cancer. Nature **209**: 241–245 (Jan. 15), 1966. (*14, 116, 151, 153, 191, 194, 196, 197, 241*)

26. FEINSTEIN, A. R. Scientific methodology in clinical medicine. Ann. Intern. Med. **61**: 1964. I. Introduction, principles, and concepts, 564–579 (Sept.); II. Classification of human disease by clinical behavior, 757–781 (Oct.); III. The evaluation of therapeutic response, 944–965 (Nov.); IV. Acquisition of clinical data, 1162–1193 (Dec.). (*15*)

27. FEINSTEIN, A. R. AND KOSS, N. Prognosis by computer: Based on storage and retrieval of data for 5-year clinical course of 691 cases of lung cancer. J. Clin. Invest. **45**: 1007 (June), 1966. (Abstract). (*15, 375*)

28. Page 1193 in Ref. 26. (*16*)

29. BERNARD, C. Introduction à L'étude de la Médecine Expérimentale. 1st

Edition. J. B. Baillière et fils. Paris. 1865. A translation of this work, by H. C. GREENE, was reprinted, in paperback, as: An Introduction to the Study of Experimental Medicine. Collier Books. New York. 1961. Subsequent page references are all to this paperback edition (22).

30. LADIMER, I. AND NEWMAN, R. W. (Editors). Clinical Investigation in Medicine: Legal, Ethical and Moral Aspects. Law-Medicine Research Institute, Boston University. Boston. 1963. (23)

31. FREUND, P. A. Ethical problems in human experimentation. New Eng. J. Med. 273: 687–692 (Sept. 23), 1965. (23)

32. BEECHER, H. K. Ethics and clinical research. New Eng. J. Med. 274: 1354–1360 (June 16), 1966. (23)

33. INGLEFINGER, F. J., RELMAN, A. S., AND FINLAND, M. Controversy in Internal Medicine. W. B. Saunders Co. Philadelphia. 1966. (23, 116)

34. BATLEY, F. The dilemma of cancer statistics. Arch. Surg. 88: 163–166 (Feb.), 1964. (23)

35. WIENER, N. The concept of homeostasis in medicine. Trans. Stud. Coll. Physicians Philadelphia 20: 87–93 (Feb.), 1953. (Quotation reprinted on pages 156–157 of LUSH, B. [Editor]. Concepts of Medicine. Pergamon Press. London. 1961.) (24, 333)

36. FEINSTEIN, A. R., KOSS, N., AND AUSTIN, J. H. M. The changing emphasis of contemporary clinical research: I. An analysis of the submitted abstracts and selected programs at the annual "Atlantic City Meetings" during 1953–1965. Ann. Intern. Med. 66: 396–419 (Feb.), 1967. (32, 251, 292)

37. Page 101 in Ref. 29. (34)

38. PAYSON, H. E. AND BARCHAS, J. D. A time study of medical teaching rounds. New Eng. J. Med. 273: 1468–1471 (Dec. 30), 1965. (36)

39. Page 81 in Ref. 29. (39)

40. The Basic Works of Aristotle. Edited by R. MCKEON. Random House. New York. 1941. (41)

41. HEISENBERG, W. The Physical Principles of the Quantum Theory. University of Chicago Press. Chicago. 1930. (50)

42. Pages 108–111 in Ref. 29. (55)

43. MALAWISTA, S. E. On the action of colchicine. The melanocyte model. J. Exp. Med. 122: 361–384 (Aug. 1), 1965. (56)

44. Webster's New International Dictionary of the English Language. 2nd Edition. Unabridged. Edited by W. A. NEILSON. G. & C. Merriam Co. Springfield, Mass. 1935. (57, 70, 122, 134)

45. WITHERING, W. An Account of the Foxglove and Some of its Medical Uses. Swinney. Birmingham. 1785. (57)

46. KELVIN, W. T. (The closest formulation of Kelvin's actual quotation is: "When you cannot express it in numbers, your knowledge is of a meagre and unsatisfactory kind." Although this sentiment recurs in Kelvin's writing, no closer formulation could be found by T. S. KUHN, as reported in his chapter, "The Function of Measurement in Modern Physical Science", which appears on pages 31–63 of Quantification. Edited by H. WOOLF. Bobbs-Merrill Co. New York. 1961.) (61)

47. KNIGHT, F. Quoted on page 169 of Eleven Twenty-Six: A Decade of Social Science Research. Edited by L. WIRTH. Chicago. 1940. (62)

48. DARWIN, C. On the Origin of Species by Means of Natural Selection; or, The Preservation of Favoured Races in the Struggle for Life. 1st Edition. J. Murray. London. 1859. (66)

49. THOMPSON, D'A. W. On Growth and Form. Cambridge University Press. Cambridge. 1917. (66)

50. Szent-Györgi, A. Trans. First Conf. on Connective Tissue. Josiah Macy Jr. Foundation. New York. 1950. Page 32. *(66)*

51. Gregg, J. R. The Language of Taxonomy. Columbia University Press. New York. 1954. *(71)*

52. Simpson, G. G. Principles of Animal Taxonomy. Columbia University Press. New York. 1961. *(71)*

53. Beers, R. J. and Lockhart, W. R. Experimental methods in computer taxonomy. J. Gen. Microbiol. **28**: 633–640 (Sept.), 1962. *(71)*

54. Sokal, R. R. and Sneath, P. H. A. Principles of Numerical Taxonomy. W. H. Freeman & Co. San Francisco. 1963. *(71)*

55. Bronowski, J. The Common Sense of Science (Paperback). Vintage Books. New York. Date unstated. Page 47, Chapter 4. *(72)*

56. Faber, K. Nosography in Modern Internal Medicine. Paul B. Hoeber, Inc. New York. 1923. *(74)*

57. King, L. S. The Medical World of the Eighteenth Century. University of Chicago Press. Chicago. 1958. Chapter VII, Nosology. *(74)*

58. Page 2 in Ref. 56. *(75)*

59. Page 5 in Ref. 56. *(76)*

50. Page 9 in Ref. 56. *(76)*

51. Page 197 in Ref. 57. *(76)*

62. Page 198 in Ref. 57. *(76)*

63. Page 226 in Ref. 57. *(77)*

64. Ropes, M. W., Bennett, G. A., Cobb, S., Jacox, R., and Jessar, R. A. Proposed diagnostic criteria for rheumatoid arthritis. 1958 Revision. Bull. Rheum. Dis. **7**: 121–124 (Dec.), 1956. *(83, 335)*

65. Jones, T. D. The diagnosis of rheumatic fever. J. Am. Med. Assn. **126**: 481–484 (Oct. 21), 1944. *(83, 335)*

66. Ad Hoc Committee to Revise the Jones Criteria (Modified) of the Council on Rheumatic Fever and Congenital Heart Disease of the American Heart Association. Jones criteria (revised) for guidance in the diagnosis of rheumatic fever. Circulation **32**: 664–668 (Oct.), 1965. *(83, 335)*

67. Criteria Committee of the New York Heart Association. Diseases of the Heart and Blood Vessels. Nomenclature and Criteria for Diagnosis. 6th Edition. Little, Brown & Co. Boston. 1964. *(84, 98)*

68. Page ix in Ref. 67. *(84)*

69. Fletcher, C. M., Jones, N. L., Burrows, B. and Niden, A. H. American emphysema and British bronchitis. A standardized comparative study. Am. Rev. Resp. Dis. **90**: 1–13 (July), 1964. *(84)*

70. Burrows, B., Niden, A. H., Fletcher, C. M., and Jones, N. L. Clinical types of chronic obstructive lung disease in London and in Chicago. A study of one hundred patients. Am. Rev. Resp. Dis. **90**: 14–27 (July), 1964. *(84)*

71. Committee on Nomenclature and Classification of Disease of the College of American Pathologists. Systematized Nomenclature of Pathology. College of American Pathologists. Chicago. 1965. *(87)*

72. American Medical Association. Standard Nomenclature of Diseases and Operations. 5th Edition. Edited by E. T. Thompson and A. C. Hayden. Blakiston Division, McGraw-Hill Book Co. New York. 1961. *(87, 96)*

73. World Health Organization. Manual of the International Statistical Classification of Diseases, Injuries, and Causes of Death. Vols. I and II. Geneva. 1957. (A revision of this publication was issued in two volumes in 1962 by the U. S. Department of Health, Education, and Welfare under the title of "International Classification of Diseases, Adapted".) *(87, 96)*

74. BARNARD, W. G. Carcinoma of lung. Acta Un. Int. Cancr. **3:** 213–219, 1938. *(90)*
75. WILLIS, R. A. Pathology of Tumours. 3rd Edition. Butterworth & Co. London. 1960. *(90)*
76. KREYBERG, L. Histological lung cancer types. A morphological and biological correlation. Acta Path. Microbiol. Scand. Supp. **157:** 7–92, 1962. *(90)*
77. SHINTON, N. K. The histological classification of lower respiratory tract tumours. Brit. J. Cancer **17:** 213–221 (June), 1963. *(90)*
78. YESNER, R., GERSTL, B., AND AUERBACH, O. Application of the World Health Organization classification of lung carcinoma to biopsy material. Ann. Thor. Surg. **1:** 33–49 (Jan.), 1965. *(90)*
79. STOUT, A. P. Tumors of the Stomach. Atlas of Tumor Pathology. Section VI— Fascicle 21. Armed Forces Institute of Pathology. Washington, D. C. 1953. *(90)*
80. FRANTZ, V. K. Tumors of the Pancreas. Atlas of Tumor Pathology. Section VII—Fascicles 27 and 28. Armed Forces Institute of Pathology. Washington, D. C. 1959. *(90)*
81. SCHIMMEL, E. The hazards of hospitalization. Ann. Intern. Med. **60:** 100–110 (Jan.), 1964. *(93)*
82. COMMITTEE ON CARDIAC CLINICS OF THE NEW YORK HEART ASSOCIATION FOR THE PREVENTION AND RELIEF OF HEART DISEASE. Requirements for an ideal cardiac clinic and a system of nomenclature. Boston Med. & Surg. J. **189:** 762–768 (Nov. 15), 1923. *(94)*
83. GREENWOOD, M. The Medical Dictator, and Other Biographical Studies. Williams and Norgate, Ltd. London. 1936. Page 111. *(96)*
84. HODGINS, E. Listen: The patient. New Eng. J. Med. **274:** 657–661 (Mar. 24), 1966. *(97)*
85. AMERICAN THORACIC SOCIETY. Definitions and classification of noninfectious reactions of the lung. A statement of the Committee on Diagnostic Standards in Respiratory Diseases. Am. Rev. Resp. Dis. **93:** 965–981 (June), 1966. *(98)*
86. FEINSTEIN, A. R. Unpublished data.
87. McMANUS, J. F. A. The Fundamental Ideas of Medicine. Charles C Thomas. Springfield, Ill. 1963. Page 52. *(100)*
88. KING, L. S. (Editorial). On autopsies. J. Am. Med. Assn. **191:** 1078–1079 (Mar. 29), 1965. *(109)*
89. STARR, I. Potential values of the autopsy today. J. Am. Med. Assn. **160:** 1144– 1145 (Mar. 31), 1956. *(109, 112)*
90. SCHWARZ, G. S. Routine autopsy: Is it outmoded? Med. Opinion & Rev. (N. Y.) **1:** 12–15 (Feb.), 1966. *(109)*
91. LIEBOW, A. A. The autopsy room as a hall of learning. Am. J. Med. **21:** 485– 486 (Oct.), 1956. *(110)*
92. WILSON, R. R. In defense of the autopsy. J. Am. Med. Assn. **196:** 1011–1012 (June 13), 1966. *(110)*
93. McMANUS, J. F. A. The autopsy as research. J. Am. Med. Assn. **193:** 808–810 (Sept. 6), 1965. *(110)*
94. ANGRIST, A. Fitting the old-fashioned autopsy into the modern medical scene. Am. J. Clin. Path. **45:** 202–207 (Feb.), 1966. *(110)*
95. WILENS, S. L. My Friends the Doctors. Atheneum Press. New York. 1961. *(110)*
96. HEPPLESTON, A. G. The pathological anatomy of simple pneumokoniosis in coal workers. J. Path. Bact. **66:** 235–246 (July), 1953. *(112)*
97. SANTAYANA, G. The Life of Reason; or, The Phases of Human Progress. One volume edition revised by the author in collaboration with Daniel Cory. Scribner. New York. 1954. Page 82. *(116)*

98. Page 54 in Ref. 56. *(117–118)*
99. TROUSSEAU, A. Clinique Médicale de l'Hôtel-Dieu de Paris. J. B. Baillière et fils. Paris. 1861–1862. The citations here are from the translation, by J. R. CORMACK AND P. V. BAZIRE, of the 3rd revised and enlarged edition, published under the title of "Lectures on Clinical Medicine", Vol. I. Lindsay & Blakiston. Philadelphia. 1873. Page 35. *(121)*
100. Page 48 in Ref. 99. *(121)*
101. CHARCOT, J. M. De L'Expectation en Médecine. 1857. Quoted in: A New Dictionary of Quotations. Edited by H. L. MENCKEN. Alfred A. Knopf. New York. 1962. *(121)*
102. Page 454 in Ref. 99. *(121)*
103. ROGET, P. M. Roget's Thesaurus. 3rd Edition. Thomas Y. Crowell Co. New York. 1962. *(134)*
104. FOWLER, H. W. A Dictionary of Modern English Usage. 2nd Edition, revised by E. GOWERS. Oxford University Press. London. 1965. *(134)*
105. With the growing popularity of the "new math" in the curriculum of elementary schools, many good texts have been published on the subject. Some of my clinician colleagues, who were total novices in this field, have found the following two books particularly lucid and helpful:
    JOHNSON, D. A. AND GLENN, W. H. Sets, Sentences, and Operations. Webster Publishing Co. St. Louis. 1960.
    ROSENTHAL, E. Understanding the New Math. Hawthorn Books. New York. 1965.
    Of historical interest to readers who know the author for his non-mathematical writing is:
    CARROLL, LEWIS (C. L. DODGSON). Symbolic Logic and the Game of Logic. Reprinted in paperback by Dover Publications. New York. 1958.
    Readers who prefer a rigorous mathematical exposition can try one of the following:
    BIRKHOFF, G. AND MACLANE, S. A Brief Survey of Modern Algebra. 2nd Edition. The Macmillan Co. New York. 1953.
    ARNOLD, B. H. Logic and Boolean Algebra. Prentice-Hall, Inc. Englewood Cliffs, N. J. 1962.
    GOODSTEIN, R. L. Boolean Algebra (Paperback). Pergamon Press. Oxford. 1963.
    The original works by Boole and Venn are cited in the following two references.
106. BOOLE, G. An Investigation of the Laws of Thought. On Which Are Founded the Mathematical Theories of Logic and Probabilities. Original edition, 1854. Reprinted in paperback by Dover Publications. New York. 1951. *(161)*
107. VENN, J. Symbolic Logic. Macmillan and Co. London. 1894. (One of Venn's earlier works, The Logic of Chance, first published in 1866, was reprinted in 1962 by Chelsea Publishing Co., New York.) *(164, 189)*
108. STOLLERMAN, G. H., LEWIS, A. J., SCHULTZ, I., AND TARANTA, A. Relationship of immune response to Group A streptococci to the course of acute, chronic and recurrent rheumatic fever. Am. J. Med. **20**: 163–169 (Feb.), 1956. *(181)*
109. TARANTA, A., WOOD, H. F., FEINSTEIN, A. R., SIMPSON, R., AND KLEINBERG, E. Rheumatic fever in children and adolescents: A long-term epidemiologic study of subsequent prophylaxis, streptococcal infections, and clinical sequelae. IV. Relationship of the rheumatic fever recurrence rate per streptococcal infection to the titers of streptococcal antibodies. Ann. Intern. Med. **60** (Supp. 5): 47–57 (Feb.), 1964. *(181, 186)*
110. TARANTA, A., KLEINBERG, E., FEINSTEIN, A. R., WOOD, H. F., TURSKY, E., AND SIMPSON, R. Rheumatic fever in children and adolescents: A long-term

epidemiologic study of subsequent prophylaxis, streptococcal infections, and clinical sequelae. V. Relationship of the rheumatic fever recurrence rate per streptococcal infection to pre-existing clinical features of the patients. Ann. Intern. Med. **60** (Supp. 5): 58–67 (Feb.), 1964. (*181, 186*)

111. The data cited here were collected during the work reported in Ref. 25, but were not listed in that report. (*190*)

112. PROUDFIT, W. L., SHIREY, E. K., AND SONES, F. M. Selective cine coronary arteriography. Correlation with clinical findings in 1,000 patients. Circulation **33**: 901–910 (June), 1966. (*198, 256*)

113. ALFFRAM, P.-A. An epidemiologic study of cervical and trochanteric fractures of the femur in an urban population. Analysis of 1,664 cases with special reference to etiologic factors. Acta Orthop. Scand. Supp. **65**: 1–109, 1964. (*199, 200*)

114. EDWARDS, P. Fracture of the shaft of the tibia: 492 consecutive cases in adults; importance of soft tissue injury. Acta Orthop. Scand. Supp. **76**: 1–82, 1965. (*119, 201*)

115. MITCHELL, R. S., RYAN, S. F., PETTY, T. L., AND FILLEY, G. F. The significance of morphologic chronic hyperplastic bronchitis. Am. Rev. Resp. Dis. **93**: 720–729 (May), 1966. (*200, 202*)

116. WATANABE, S., MITCHELL, M., AND RENZETTI, A. D. Correlation of structure and function in chronic pulmonary emphysema. Am. Rev. Resp. Dis. **92**: 221–227 (Aug.), 1965. (*203*)

117. OSMER, J. C. AND COLE, B. K. The stethoscope and roentgenogram in acute pneumonia. Southern Med. J. **59**: 75–77 (Jan.), 1966. (*203*)

118. HALLEN, J. AND NORDEN, J. Liver cirrhosis unsuspected during life: A series of 79 cases. J. Chron. Dis. **17**: 951–958 (Oct.), 1964. (*203*)

119. LAWS, J. W., MOLLIN, D. L., AND COGHILL, N. F. Relation of radiological appearance to gastric function in simple atrophic gastritis. Lancet **1**: 510–512 (Mar. 5), 1966. (*203*)

120. ADLER, E. AND TAL, E. Relationship between physical disability and functional capacity in hemiplegic patients. Arch. Phys. Med. Rehab. **46**: 745–752 (Nov.), 1965. (*203*)

121. LAWRENCE, J. S., BREMNER, J. M., AND BIER, F. Osteo-arthrosis: Prevalence in the population and relationship between symptoms and X-ray changes. Ann. Rheum. Dis. **2**: 1–24 (Jan.), 1966. (*203*)

122. KLIBANOFF, E., FRIEDEN, J., SPAGNUOLO, M., AND FEINSTEIN, A. R. "Rheumatic activity". J. Am. Med. Assn. **195**: 895–900 (Mar. 14), 1966. (*203*)

123. WOOD, H. F., FEINSTEIN, A. R., TARANTA, A., EPSTEIN, J. A., AND SIMPSON, R. Rheumatic fever in children and adolescents: A long-term epidemiologic study of subsequent prophylaxis, streptococcal infections and clinical sequelae. III. Comparative effectiveness of three prophylaxis regimens in preventing streptococcal infections and rheumatic recurrences. Ann. Inter. Med. **60** (Supp. 5): 31–46 (Feb.), 1964. (*204*)

124. CONN, H. O., SMITH, H. W., AND BRODOFF, M. Observer variation in the endoscopic diagnosis of esophageal varices. A prospective investigation of the diagnostic validity of esophagoscopy. New Eng. J. Med. **272**: 830–834 (Apr. 22), 1965. (*204, 205*)

125. SPAGNUOLO, M., TARANTA, A., SNYDER, R., GERBARG, D. S., AND HOFFLER, J. J. Diagnosis from tape: A study of the auscultatory diagnosis of mitral regurgitation. Pages 146–151 in Proceedings, San Diego Symposium for Biomedical Engineering. La Jolla, Calif. 1963. (*204*)

126. RYTAND, D. A. Anticoagulants in coronary thrombosis with myocardial infarction. Arch. Intern. Med. **88**: 207–210 (Aug.), 1951. (*219*)

127. LOUIS, P. CH. A. Recherches sur les effets de la saignée dans quelques maladies inflammatoires, et sur l'action de l'émétique et des vésicatoires dans la pneumonie. Paris. 1835. An English translation by C. G. PUTNAM is the source of the references here: Researches on the Effects of Bloodletting in Some Inflammatory Diseases and on the Influence of Tartarized Antimony and Vesication in Pneumonitis. Hilliard, Gray & Co. Boston. 1836. *(220)*

128. Pages 123–142 in Ref. 83. *(220, 223)*

129. Pages 96–97 in Ref. 127. *(221)*

130. PAINE, M. Medical and Physiological Commentaries. Collins, Keese & Co. New York. 1840–1844. *(220)*

131. JACKSON, J. Preface and Appendix to Ref. 127. *(221)*

132. BOWDITCH, H. I. Brief Memories of Louis and Some of His Contemporaries in the Parisian School of Medicine of Forty Years Ago. Press of J. Wilson and Son. Boston. 1872. *(221)*

133. OSLER, W. Influence of Louis on American medicine. Bull. Johns Hopkins Hosp. **8**: 161–167 (Aug.–Sept.), 1897. *(221)*

134. MAINLAND, D. Elementary Medical Statistics. 2nd Edition. W. B. Saunders Co. Philadelphia. 1963. *(223)*

135. Page 42 in Ref. 56. *(223)*

136. Louis, P. CH. A. Anatomical, Pathological, and Therapeutic Researches on the Yellow Fever of Gibraltar of 1828. From observations taken by himself and M. Trousseau, as members of the French Commission at Gibraltar. Translated from the manuscript by G. C. SHATTUCK, JR. C. C. Little and J. Brown. Boston. 1839. *(223)*

137. Pages 52–57 in Ref. 99. *(223)*

138a. VIRCHOW, R. Quoted on page 76 of Ref. 87. *(223)*

138b. FRISCH, M. Homo Faber. Abelard-Schuman. New York. 1959. Page 165. *(224)*

139. ARMITAGE, P. Sequential Medical Trials. Blackwell. Oxford. 1960. *(240, 280)*

140. MAHER-LOUGHNAN, G. P., MACDONALD, N., MASON, A. A., AND FRY, L. Controlled trial of hypnosis in the symptomatic treatment of asthma. Brit. Med. J. (No. 5301): 371–375 (Aug. 11), 1962. *(225)*

141. WYLIE, C. M. AND WHITE, B. K. A measure of disability. Arch. Environ. Health **8**: 834–839 (June), 1964. *(225)*

142. FEINSTEIN, A. R. AND AREVALO, A. C. Manifestations and treatment of congestive heart failure in young patients with rheumatic heart disease. Pediatrics **33**: 661–671 (May), 1964. *(225)*

143. SHAPIRO, S., WEINBLATT, E., FRANK, C. W., SAGER, R. V., AND DENSEN, P. M. The H.I.P. study of incidence and prognosis of coronary heart disease: Methodology. J. Chron. Dis. **16**: 1281–1292 (Dec.), 1963. *(225)*

144. FRANK, C. W., WEINBLATT, E., SHAPIRO, S., SEIDEN, G. E., AND SAGER, R. V. The H.I.P. study of incidence and prognosis of coronary heart disease: Criteria for diagnosis. J. Chron. Dis. **16**: 1293–1312 (Dec.), 1963. *(225)*

145. GREEN, M. A. Criteria for discontinuation of therapy. Ann. Allergy **23**: 1–6 (Jan.), 1965. *(225)*

146. WORKING PARTY ON THE EVALUATION OF DIFFERENT METHODS OF THERAPY IN LEUKAEMIA. First report to the medical research council. Treatment of acute leukaemia in adults. Comparison of steroid therapy at high and low dosage in conjunction with 6-mercaptopurine. Brit. Med. J. (No. 5322): 7–14 (Jan. 5), 1963. *(225)*

147. KAUNG, D. T., WHITTINGTON, R. M., AND PATNO, M. E. Chemotherapy of chronic lymphocytic leukemia. Arch. Intern. Med. **114**: 521–524 (Oct.), 1964. *(225)*

148. WILSON, R. H., HARGIS, B. J., HORN, R. L., AND SHIELDS, D. O. A clinical and

laboratory method of determining the degree of pulmonary disability, with a proposed classification. Am. J. Med. **37**: 251–262 (Aug.), 1964. (*255*)

149. KORST, D. R., FRENKEL, E. P., AND NIXON, J. C. Multiple myeloma. Studies of mouse plasma cell tumor and human myeloma responsiveness to cyclophosphamide (cytoxan). Ann. Intern. Med. **60**: 217–230 (Feb.), 1964. (*cf.* Appendix, page 230). (*255*)

150. KLINE, N. J. Criteria for psychiatric improvement. Psychiat. Quart. **31**: 31–40, 1957. (*255*)

151. CALKINS, E., BLACK, R. L., CLARK, G. M., HOLLANDER, J. L., MAINLAND, D., MIKKELSEN, W. M., RAGAN, C., AND SHORT, C. L. Therapeutic evaluation in rheumatoid arthritis. Arth. Rheum. **3**: 101–111 (Apr.), 1960. (*255*)

152. LARSON, C. B. AND MCEWEN, C. (Co-chairmen). Conference on criteria for, and evaluation of, orthopedic measures in the management of deformities of rheumatoid arthritis. Arth. Rheum. **7**: 550–613 (Oct.), 1964. (*255*)

153. CROOKS, J., WAYNE, E. J., AND ROBB, R. A. A clinical method of assessing the results of therapy in thyrotoxicosis. Lancet **1**: 397–401 (Feb. 20), 1960. (*255*)

154. AMERICAN MEDICAL ASSOCIATION COMMITTEE ON MEDICAL RATING OF PHYSICAL IMPAIRMENT. A guide to the evaluation of permanent impairment: Extremities and back. J. Am. Med. Assn. **166**: 1–109 (Feb. 15), 1958. (*255*)

155. IBID. The visual system. **168**: 475–488 (Sept. 27), 1958. (*255*)

156. IBID. The cardiovascular system. **172**: 1049–1060 (Mar. 5), 1960. (*255*)

157. IBID. Ear, nose, throat, and related structures. **177**: 489–501 (Aug. 19), 1961. (*255*)

158. IBID. The central nervous system. **185**: 24–35 (July 6), 1963. (*255*)

159a. IBID. The digestive system. **188**: 159–172 (Apr. 13), 1964. (*255*)

159b. IBID. The endocrine system. **198**: 195–208 (Oct. 10), 1966. (*255*)

160. HILL, A. B. The clinical trial. Brit. Med. Bull. **7**: 278–282 (No. 4), 1951. (*262*)

161. PEARSON, K. The Grammar of Science. 1st Edition. 1892. Reprinted in paperback by Meridian Books. New York. 1957. Chapter IV, Cause and Effect—Probability. Chapter V, Contingency and Correlation—The Insufficiency of Causation. (*268*)

162. POPPER, K. R. The Logic of Scientific Discovery. Basic Books. New York. 1959. (*268*)

163. USPENSKY, J. V. AND HEASLET, M. A. Elementary Number Theory. 1st Edition. McGraw-Hill Book Co. New York. 1939. Page 20. (*293*)

164. This statement is not original, but I cannot now recall where I read or heard it, and a check of several potential sources has been unproductive. (*312*)

165. RYLE, J. A. The Natural History of Disease. Oxford University Press. London. 1936. (To cite Ryle only in this context of symptom description does an injustice to the breadth of his scope and work. This book should be read by all clinicians interested in knowing about human illness in life, rather than in the restricted setting of the hospital. His outlook was years ahead of his time, and clinicians of the future will use his far-sighted vision of the integration of community and hospital for major new advances in epidemiologic research and understanding.) (*318*)

166. MCKUSICK, V. A. Cardiovascular Sound in Health and Disease. The Williams & Wilkins Company. Baltimore. 1958. (*325*)

167. FABER, J. J. AND BURTON, A. C. Biophysics of heart sounds and its application to clinical auscultation. Can. Med. Assn. J. **91**: 120–128 (July 18), 1964. (*325*)

168. BRUNS, D. L. A general theory of the causes of murmurs in the cardiovascular system. Am. J. Med. **27**: 360–374 (Sept.), 1959. (*326*)

169. MCKEE, M. H. Heart sounds in normal children. Am. Heart J. **16**: 79–87 (July), 1938, (*332*)

170. Lessof, M. and Brigden, W. Systolic murmurs in healthy children and in children with rheumatic fever. Lancet 273: 673–674 (Oct. 5), 1957. (332)

171. O'Brien, W. M., Burch, T. A., and Bunim, J. J. An evaluation of the A.R.A. criteria for the diagnosis of rheumatoid arthritis. Arth. Rheum. 7: 745–746 (Dec.), 1964. (Abstract). (335)

172. Seegal, D. and Wertheim, A. R. On the failure to supervise students' performance of complete physical examinations. J. Am. Med. Assn. 180: 476–477 (May 12), 1962. (342)

173. Feinstein, A. R. The stethoscope: A source of diagnostic aid and conceptual errors in rheumatic heart disease. J. Chron. Dis. 11: 91–101 (Feb.), 1960. (348)

174. Peabody, F. W. The Care of the Patient. Harvard University Press. Cambridge. 1927. (348)

175. Quotation cited on page 12 of Ref. 166. (354)

176. Wiener, N. The Human Use of Human Beings; Cybernetics and Society. Houghton Mifflin. Boston. 1950. (359)

177. Platt, J. R. Strong inference. Science 146: 347–353 (Oct. 16), 1964. (359)

178. Szilard, L. Quoted in Ref. 177. (359)

179. Commoner, B. In defense of biology. Science 133: 1745–1748 (June 2), 1961. (359)

180. Dubos, R. Hippocrates in modern dress. Perspect. Biol. Med. 9: 275–288 (Winter), 1966. (359)

181. Meador, C. K. The art and science of nondisease. N. Eng. J. Med. 272: 92–95 (Jan. 14), 1965. (363)

182. Bruce, R. A. and Yarnall, S. R. Computer-aided diagnosis of cardiovascular disorders. J. Chron. Dis. 19: 473–484 (Apr.), 1966. (372, 374)

183. Ledley, R. S. and Lusted, L. B. Reasoning foundation of medical diagnosis: Symbolic logic, probability and value theory aid our understanding of how physicians reason. Science 130: 9–21 (July 3), 1959. (373)

184. Caceres, C. A. and Abraham, S. Computer use in health and medical research —Role for computers in heart disease control. Am. J. Pub. Health 53: 582–592 (April), 1963. (374)

185. Pipberger, H. V. and Stallmann, F. W. Computation of differential diagnosis in electrocardiography. Ann. N. Y. Acad. Sci. 115: 1115–1128, 1964. (374)

186. Acheson, R. Observer error and variation in the interpretations of electrocardiograms in an epidemiological study of coronary heart disease. Brit. J. Prev. Soc. Med. 14: 99–122 (July), 1960. (374)

187. Hurst, J. W. and Wenger, N. K. (Editors); Cabrera, E., Estes, E. H. and Hellerstein, H. K. (Authors). Electrocardiographic Interpretation. Blakiston Division, McGraw-Hill Book Co. New York. 1963. (374)

188. Sonquist, J. A. and Morgan, J. N. The Detection of Interaction Effects. A Report on a Computer Program for the Selection of Optimal Combinations of Explanatory Variables. Monograph No. 35. Survey Research Center, Institute for Social Research, The University of Michigan. Ann Arbor. 1964. (375)

189. Bronowski, J. The Identity of Man. Natural History Press. Garden City, N. Y. 1965. (379)

190. From pages 101, 105, and 80 of Ref. 189. (379)

191. No author is known for this aphorism, which is quoted on Trudeau's grave at Saranac, N. Y., and often cited as the goal of a clinician. According to many historians, the expression is originally French, (guérir quelquefois; soulager souvent; consoler toujours), and is at least 14 centuries old. (385)

192. Pauling, L., Itano, H. A., Singer, S. J., and Wells, I. C. Sickle cell anemia, a molecular disease. Science 110: 543–548 (Nov. 25), 1949. (388)

Index

Abnormality, criteria for, 329
  components of, 331, 332
Algorithms, definition, 378
American Federation for Clinical Research, 31, 251
American Society for Clinical Investigation, 31, 251
Anticoagulants, difficulty in appraising therapy, 23, 40, 70, 219, 343–344
"Applied science", antagonism to "basic science", 357–360
Aristotle, adaptation of methods to material, 41, 44
Art in clinical examination, 298–305
  distinction from science, 291–297
  history-taking, 299, 300
  long-term studies, 303
  materials and methods, 293–297
  medical journals, 292
  physical examination, concern for patient, 300–303
  rounds
    "abstract", 301
    conduct of, 303
    "grand", 300
    patient's expectations, 302, 303
    teaching, 302
    "veterinary", 302
Auenbrügger, Leopold Joseph, clinico-pathologic correlation and, 117
Auscultation
  apical systolic murmur, 5

"biopsy" of valvular and septal defects, 305
descriptive criteria, ingredients of, 5
diastolic murmur, 2
objective techniques, 3
problems of human versus inanimate performance, 323–327
unheard murmurs, 2

Bacon, Francis, multi-temporal correlations and, 223
"Basic science", 35, 37, 38
  antagonism to "applied science", 357–360
  attitudes in, 357–361
  changes in medical curricula, 376, 377
  clinical experience as background for statistics, 227
  "clinical investigation" and, 387
  clinical judgment and, 27
  clinical medicine and, 382–384
  conceptual chain of, 382
    illustration, 383
  definition, 382
  definition of experimenter, 22
  diversion of academic clinical skills to, 251
  inappropriate extrapolation and, 384
  intellectual debts to clinical medicine, 388
  limited intellectual horizons, 359

401